Acknowledgments

I want to express my heartfelt thanks to both Drs. Larry R. Faulkner and James H. Scully, Jr., for their encouragement, support, and faith in me. In addition, I am honored by the outstanding contributions to this edition by all of our authors; they are truly leaders in their field. Thank you.

D1541832

NMS *Psychiatry*

5th EDITION

Editor

Joshua T. Thornhill IV, MD

Professor of Clinical Neuropsychiatry and Behavioral Science
Assistant Dean for Clinical Curriculum
University of South Carolina School of Medicine
Department of Neuropsychiatry and Behavioral Science
Columbia, South Carolina

 Wolters Kluwer | Lippincott Williams & Wilkins
Health
Philadelphia · Baltimore · New York · London
Buenos Aires · Hong Kong · Sydney · Tokyo

Acquisitions Editor: Nancy Anastasi Duffy
Managing Editor: Kelly Horvath
Marketing Manager: Jennifer Kuklinski
Production Editor: Julie Montalbano
Designer: Holly Reid McLaughlin
Compositor: Circle Graphics, Inc.
Printer: Quebecor World, Inc.—Dubuque

Printed in the United States of America

Fourth Edition, 2001

Library of Congress Cataloging-in-Publication Data

Psychiatry / editor, Joshua T. Thornhill. — 5th ed.
   p. ; cm. — (NMS)
  Includes bibliographical references and index.
   ISBN-13: 978-0-7817-6514-5 (alk. paper) 1. Psychiatry—Outlines, syllabi, etc. 2. Psychiatry—Examinations, questions, etc. I. Thornhill, Joshua T. II. Series: National medical series for independent study.
   [DNLM: 1. Psychiatry—Examination Questions. 2. Mental Disorders—Examination Questions.   WM 18.2 P973 2008]
   RC457.2.P78 2008
   616.890076--dc22

                                                    2006031951

To purchase additional copies of this book, call our customer service department at **(800) 638-3030** or fax orders to **(301) 223-2320**. International customers should call **(301) 223-2300**.

Visit Lippincott Williams & Wilkins on the Internet: http://www.LWW.com. Lippincott Williams & Wilkins customer service representatives are available from 8:30 am to 6:00 pm, EST.

07 08 09 10 11
1 2 3 4 5 6 7 8 9 10

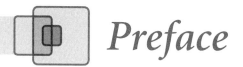

Preface

As we move forward into the twenty-first century, the scientific basis of psychiatry continues to expand. New medications have been developed for the treatment of individuals with schizophrenia, mood disorders, and severe anxiety disorders. Focused psychotherapeutic techniques have been proven as effective treatments. Because of the importance of evidence-based medical practice, we now have a number of scientifically based practice guidelines developed by the American Psychiatric Association. These guidelines, several of which are already in their second editions, have been used extensively in the preparation of this book.

In this fifth edition of *NMS Psychiatry,* each chapter as well as the drug appendix has been updated to include the latest medications and treatment protocols. Chapter 7 on substance-related disorders has been expanded to include "club drugs," and Chapter 10 on eating disorders has been given its own chapter to more clearly delineate these disorders from impulse disorders. In addition, we have continued to revise, update, and add new questions to each chapter and to the comprehensive examination to help students prepare for National Board of Medical Examiners (NBME) Subject examinations as well as the United States Medical Licensing Exam (USMLE) Step 2.

Finally, with this edition, we are fortunate to have added new contributors Drs. Campbell and Harper from the University of South Carolina School of Medicine and the Palmetto Health Alliance.

Joshua T. Thornhill IV, MD

Contributors

Robert J. Breen, MD
Associate Professor, HPI
Department of Neuropsychiatry and
    Behavioral Science
University of South Carolina
    School of Medicine
Medical Director
G. Werber Bryan Psychiatric Hospital
    and Earle E. Morris Alcohol and Drug
    Addiction Treatment Center
Columbia, South Carolina

Nioaka N. Campbell, MD
Assistant Professor of Clinical Neuropsychiatry
    and Behavioral Science
Department of Neuropsychiatry and
    Behavioral Science
University of South Carolina
    School of Medicine
General Psychiatry Residency Training Director
Palmetto Health Richland
Palmetto Health Alliance
Columbia, South Carolina

Richard L. Frierson, MD
Associate Professor of Clinical Neuropsychiatry
    and Behavioral Science
Director, Forensic Psychiatry Fellowship
Department of Neuropsychiatry and
    Behavioral Science
University of South Carolina
    School of Medicine
Columbia, South Carolina

Angela D. Harper, MD
Adult General Psychiatrist
Palmetto Health Alliance
Addictionologist
Department of Psychiatry
Richland Springs Hospital
Columbia, South Carolina

James H. Scully, Jr., MD
Medical Director
American Psychiatric Association
Arlington, Virginia
Clinical Professor of Neuropsychiatry and
    Behavioral Science
Department of Neuropsychiatry and
    Behavioral Science
University of South Carolina
    School of Medicine
Columbia, South Carolina
Clinical Professor of Psychiatry and
    Behavioral Sciences
Department of Psychiatry and Behavioral
    Sciences
George Washington University
    School of Medicine and Health Sciences
Washington, DC

Margaret A. Shugart, MD
Associate Professor
Department of Psychiatry and Behavioral
    Sciences
Emory University School of Medicine
Atlanta, Georgia

Joshua T. Thornhill IV, MD
Professor of Clinical Neuropsychiatry and
    Behavioral Science
Assistant Dean for Clinical Curriculum
Department of Neuropsychiatry and
    Behavioral Science
University of South Carolina
    School of Medicine
Columbia, South Carolina

NMS *Psychiatry*

Contents

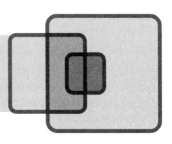

chapter 1

The Clinical Examination

JAMES H. SCULLY · JOSHUA T. THORNHILL IV

I OVERVIEW

A General psychiatric evaluation

1. The psychiatric evaluation differs from a routine medical examination in that it includes a **mental status examination** rather than a physical examination, although a physical examination may be included. The examiner asks the patient about **feelings and relationships,** not just historical facts. The psychiatric evaluation consists of:
   a. **Collecting data** from a careful history of the patient's problems
   b. **Conducting an examination**
   c. **Establishing a psychiatric diagnosis and developing a differential diagnosis** for further study
   d. **Constructing a treatment plan**

2. The primary method of obtaining data for a psychiatric evaluation is the face-to-face **interview.**
   a. **Sensitivity** is required because of the embarrassment many patients have about disclosing emotional problems. Special skills are necessary when taking psychiatric histories because many patients are embarrassed about disclosing their emotional problems. In general, people are less willing to discuss psychiatric symptoms than physical ones. Most patients are not psychotic, but many patients, especially those who are confused or disorganized, can be helped by the physician to give accurate details of their history.
   b. **Confidentiality** is important in all physician–patient interactions, especially when psychiatric issues are discussed. To maintain confidentiality, physicians should not discuss their patients in hallways or elevators. In teaching programs, case material must be presented, but it is important to maintain anonymity. Participants in any conference are bound by confidentiality.
   c. **Exceptions to the rule of confidentiality** are made when the need for safety is paramount such as in cases of child abuse or when threats are made to harm others.
   d. **Collateral sources,** such as record review and interviews of persons close to patients, may provide important additional information.

B Interview

1. **Verbal communication.** During the first few minutes of the interview, the physician should allow the patient to talk about any symptoms. The patient should feel comfortable enough to provide personal information.

2. **Nonverbal communication** such as facial expression and posture is equally important. It is also important to note how the story is told (e.g., tone of voice, feelings expressed).

C History of the present illness. Information should be obtained about the following:

1. **Onset, duration, or change of symptoms over time**

2. **Stressful events, especially losses,** including death of a loved one, job loss, or financial problems

3. **Patient perception of any change in her- or himself** or the perception of change in the patient by another individual (e.g., spouse, friend, supervisor at work)

4. **Previous psychiatric illness or treatment,** including medication, hospitalization, or other therapy, and responses to treatment (both positive and negative)

5. **Legal issues** with respect to the current illness (e.g., lawsuit, arrest, incarceration) or if the patient is a student, problems in school (e.g., truancy, suspension, expulsion)

6. **Secondary gain,** which is any benefit that the patient derives from the current problem (e.g., monetary compensation; relief from responsibilities at home, school, or work)

D Personal history

1. **Developmental milestones.** The physician should:
   a. Obtain information about the patient's **early development,** including details about the patient's mother's pregnancy and delivery. Information may be obtained from the patient, family members, or hospital records.
   b. Assess the patient's **temperament** as a child and determine any important family events (e.g., death, separation, divorce) that may have influenced the patient's temperament.
   c. Obtain information about the patient's **early experiences and relationships,** including school experiences (i.e., academic performance, delinquency), friends, family stability, early sexual experiences, and history of neglect or abuse. The patient's early relationships with parents, siblings, and friends can be important barometers of development.
   d. Assess important cultural and religious influences that affect the patient.

2. **Social history.** The physician should:
   a. Determine the breadth of the patient's **social life** (e.g., whether the patient is a loner, how difficult it is for the patient to establish friendships). The physician should assess both present and past levels of functioning in various social roles (e.g., marriage, parenting, work).
   b. Determine whether any **changes in personality** have been noted by the patient or by the patient's family or friends.
   c. Determine the patient's **marital status** or involvement in an intimate relationship, as well as the current level of **sexual functioning** and **sexual orientation.**
   d. Obtain the patient's **employment history,** including the number of jobs held and the reasons the jobs were terminated. Note any problems with alcoholism or antisocial behavior at work.
   e. Obtain the patient's **military service history** (if applicable), including the highest rank attained and a history of any disciplinary problems or combat experience.

3. **Family history.** The physician should:
   a. Ask the patient whether any **family members** have undergone **psychiatric hospitalization** or any other mental health treatment, attempted suicide, had problems with alcohol, or had other psychiatric problems. Families often deny significant psychiatric history.
   b. Determine **genetic risk factors** for mental disorders and **family attitudes** toward mental illness and treatment.
   c. Determine whether any family member is successfully using any **psychotropic medication** for the same illness. If so, there is a good chance that the medication will also help the patient.

4. **Previous psychiatric history**
   a. Note the **recurrence of an earlier problem** in the history of the current illness. List episodes of any **other psychiatric illness** chronologically.
   b. Note and record any **previous treatments in chronological order,** including the name and address of the therapist, length of treatment, medications and dosages, and outcome of treatment.

5. **Substance use and abuse**
   a. Ask screening questions about **alcohol and drug problems,** including whether family or friends have ever objected to the patient's drinking or drug use and whether the patient has ever thought that he or she has had a problem with alcohol or drugs, either legal or illegal. Also, consider the use of **tobacco.**
   b. Note any negative consequences of substance use, including tolerance, withdrawal, or effect on the present illness. The interviewer should be nonjudgmental but should ask specific questions about the consequences of alcohol or drug use, such as driving under the influence.

II PSYCHIATRIC EXAMINATION

The assessment of a patient with a psychiatric disorder should always include the psychiatric interview and the mental status examination. It may also include a physical examination, laboratory studies, and psychological tests.

A Psychiatric interview

1. **Physician–patient relationship**
   a. **Patients are often anxious** about a psychiatric evaluation. Although they may be self-referred, many patients are referred by another health care professional and may be ambivalent about the psychiatric examination. The physician should be courteous and respectful and should acknowledge the patient's feelings about being interviewed.
   b. The **environment** may affect the difficulty of the evaluation. The setting may range from a quiet, private office to a busy, noisy emergency department in a general hospital.
   c. Family members or others may provide important information. However, the physician should always obtain the **patient's permission to question family members.**
   d. Interruptions should be minimized, and **sufficient time should be allowed for completion of the interview.** Traditionally, the interview is 50 to 60 minutes long, but 20 minutes may be enough.
   e. The physician should sit at **eye level** with the patient.

2. **Mental status.** The **informal mental status examination** that includes an evaluation of the following patient characteristics begins immediately.
   a. Appearance
   b. Manner of relating
   c. Use of language
   d. Mood and affect
   e. Content of discussion (e.g., family problems, work issues)
   f. Perceptions
   g. Abstracting ability
   h. Judgment
   i. Insight

3. **Interview technique.** The examiner should:
   a. Lead the interview with the use of both open-ended and direct questions.
      (1) **Open-ended questions** allow patients to use their own words (e.g., "Tell me about your home life," "Tell me about your hospital stay").
      (2) **Direct questions** are used to elicit specific information (e.g., "Have you ever consulted a mental health professional before?" "Are you thinking about killing yourself?").
   b. Clearly communicate that he or she is listening.
      (1) **Attentive silence.** Nonverbal cues such as nodding and leaning forward demonstrate attention. The physician should establish eye contact and convey the message that he or she is interested in what the patient is saying.
      (2) **Facilitation.** Use of encouraging comments (e.g., "Tell me more about it") helps the patient focus while relating the history.
      (3) **Summarization.** By summarizing the patient's words, the physician lets the patient know that he or she is listening and allows the patient to correct any misunderstanding. The interviewer should summarize portions of the patient's story (e.g., "So, you have been increasingly sad for 3 weeks, during which time you have lost 7 pounds and have been waking up at 4:00 AM?").
      (4) **Clarification.** The role of clarifying statements is similar to summary statements but also includes connections that the patient may not recognize. A clarifying statement allows the interviewer to confirm the accuracy of the information and the patient to correct it if necessary. For example, the physician might say, "Your difficulty sleeping and your crying spells began in mid-September. Was this after your youngest child left for college?"

B Mental status examination   In contrast to the psychiatric history, which is a record of a patient's entire life, the mental status examination is an evaluation of a patient at one point in time. During the interview, the physician observes the following characteristics.

1. **Appearance.** The patient's overall appearance, dress, grooming, and any unusual features or gestures are noteworthy.

2. **Attitude.** How the patient relates to the interviewer (e.g., hostile, cooperative, evasive) may be important.

3. **Behavior and psychomotor activity.** Such features as gait, position, and overall level of activity may include unusual mannerisms, agitation, or psychomotor retardation. Manic patients may be unable to sit still, and schizophrenic patients may adopt bizarre postures or move stiffly and awkwardly.

4. **Speech**
   a. **Rate of speech** (e.g., rapid, slow, halting)
   b. **Amount of speech** (e.g., taciturn, lacking spontaneity, grandiose)
   c. **Tone of speech** (e.g., monotone, singsong, slurred)
   d. **Speech impairment** (e.g., dysarthria, stuttering, echolalia), accent, dialect, or any other obvious speech pattern
   e. **Aphasia** (a disorder of speech and language that is caused by neurologic illness). The patient may be either unable to speak normally or unable to comprehend speech properly. Aphasia that is caused by disorders of speech and language should be differentiated from aphasia that is caused by psychiatric illness.

5. **Mood and affect.** The emotional state that the patient experiences internally is known as **mood,** and the outward expression of the patient's internal emotional state is known as **affect.**
   a. **Mood in relationship to affect.** The interviewer notes whether the patient's mood and affect are the same. For example, a patient who has a depressed mood is likely to appear sad and quiet and to speak softly and slowly. However, some depressed patients have an agitated and anxious affect. On the other hand, a schizophrenic individual may act silly or unconcerned while discussing a sad event such as the death of a loved one. This inappropriate division between affective feeling and thought content led to the use of the term "schizophrenia," which means "split mind," not "split personality."
   b. **Depth and range of emotional expression**
      (1) **Labile affect** describes sudden shifts in emotional state. The patient may laugh one minute and cry the next without a clear stimulus.
      (2) **Flat affect** describes a shallow and blunted emotional state. Facial expression and voice lack spontaneity.

6. **Perception.** The presence of a perceptual problem is noted in the mental status examination or in the history. Perceptual abnormalities involve the sensory nervous system and include the following:
   a. **Hallucinations** are false perceptions of a sensory stimulus. Any sensory modality can be involved.
      (1) **Auditory hallucinations** are seen in psychosis. The hallucinations involve voices, not just sounds, that criticize, comment, or command.
      (2) **Visual hallucinations** are often seen with organic psychosis, especially toxic or drug-related states.
      (3) **Gustatory (taste) and olfactory (smell) hallucinations** should alert the physician to a disorder of the temporal lobe.
      (4) **Tactile hallucinations** are also seen in organic states such as alcohol withdrawal or cocaine and amphetamine abuse. **Formication** is the tactile hallucination of insects crawling over the skin.
      (5) **Kinesthetic hallucinations** include feeling movement when none occurs. The "out-of-body" experiences described in near-death situations may be kinesthetic hallucinations. People usually describe this phenomenon as floating above their body and looking down on the scene.
      (6) **Hypnagogic hallucinations** (brief hallucinations of any type that occur while falling asleep) or **hypnopompic hallucinations** (brief hallucinations of any type that occur while awakening) occur in normal individuals and are not considered serious or pathologic.
   b. **Illusions** are misinterpretations of an actual sensory stimulus. For example, a patient in the hospital may misperceive the movement of the bed curtain as a person and become frightened. Illusions occur in individuals with schizophrenia but are most common in delirium.

c. **Depersonalization and derealization** are alterations in an individual's perception of reality. With depersonalization, patients feel detached and view themselves as strange and unreal. Derealization involves a similar alteration in the patient's sense of reality of the outside world. Objects in the outside world may seem altered in size and shape, and people appear dead or mechanical.

7. **Thought process.** The pattern of a patient's speech allows the examiner to note the quality of the thought process, including its flow, logic, and associations. Abnormalities of the thinking process include the following:

   a. **Loose associations.** This abnormality involves the shifting of ideas from one to another with no logical connection, accompanied by a lack of awareness on the part of the patient that these ideas are not connected. The patient's thoughts are difficult for the examiner to follow.

   b. **Tangential thinking.** The patient wanders off the subject as new but related words are spoken. Usually it is possible to follow the patient's thoughts, but the patient often loses track of the interviewer's question.

   c. **Circumstantiality.** As with tangential thinking, the patient loses the point of what he or she is saying but stays within the general topic area. Irrelevant details cause digressions in conversation. These digressions are mild if the patient is merely anxious, but they can be severe if he or she is delirious and distractible.

   d. **Blocking.** This problem occurs when the thinking process stops altogether and the mind goes blank. It is found in individuals with acute anxiety and schizophrenia.

   e. **Perseveration.** This repetition of the same words or phrases occurs despite the interviewer's direction to stop.

   f. **Echolalia.** This problem is the direct repetition of the interviewer's words.

   g. **Flight of ideas.** This process, which is seen in mania, is characterized by rapid speech with quick changes of ideas that may be associated in some way, such as by the sound of the words. It may also involve loose associations.

8. **Content of thought.** Disturbances in thought content include:

   a. **Delusions** are fixed, false beliefs that are outside the patient's culture. For example, a belief that one's thoughts are being broadcast outside one's head is a delusion, but a belief in Santa Claus is not. Delusions may be paranoid (or persecutory), grandiose, nihilistic, somatic, or bizarre. **Delusions of reference** involve the belief that some person or object has special significance or power (e.g., a disc jockey is sending special commands to the patient).

      (1) Because delusions are fixed, false beliefs, they cannot be corrected by the physician. Contradiction of the patient's delusional belief may cause the patient to become angry and stop the interview.

      (2) The physician should not pretend to agree with the delusion but should take a neutral position and continue the examination.

   b. **Obsessions** are persistent, intrusive thoughts, ideas, or impulses. The patient realizes that the ideas do not make sense and are not being imposed from outside (i.e., delusion). An example is a man who is always fighting an impulse to run down the hall of an office building through a plate glass window at the end. He knows that this action is potentially life threatening, and he does not want to hurt himself, but he cannot stop thinking about it and feeling anxious. Other common obsessions include fears of contamination and unrealistic fears about physical health, as seen in hypochondriasis (see Chapter 8).

   c. Questions about **suicidal and homicidal thoughts** should be part of every mental status examination. It is important to exercise judgment and tact in discussing these issues. Assessment of **issues of safety** is one of the most important parts of the examination.

9. **Judgment.** By determining whether the patient understands the consequences of his actions, the clinician may assess the patient's social judgment. The physician may ask the patient a judgment question (e.g., "What would you do if you were stranded at Kennedy Airport with only $1.00 in your pocket?"). The examiner must recognize differences in cultural values when assessing judgment.

10. **Insight.** The physician should assess the patient's awareness of the problem, the cause of the problem, and what type of help is needed. Many people with serious mental illness such as bipolar disorder or schizophrenia lack insight and refuse necessary treatment.

11. **Cognition.** The mental status examination measures the ability of the brain to function. A formal mental status examination, a number of which are available, is necessary to adequately examine the patient's orientation, concentration, and memory. All mental status examinations are limited in scope compared with extensive neuropsychological tests, but the mini-mental state examination is a useful bedside clinical examination.

C **Physical examination** Assessment of the general medical or neurologic condition of the patient is sometimes necessary. An examination should be conducted if there is concern that an undiagnosed medical illness is contributing to or causing psychiatric symptoms. The examiner should note the following:

1. General appearance

2. Vital signs

3. Neurologic status, including motor, sensory function, gait, coordination, muscle tone, and any involuntary movements

4. Skin, with attention to scars from self-injury or tattoos

5. Any other area that has been noted in the history of present illness. Examination of the head, neck, heart, lungs, abdomen, and extremities may be indicated.

D **Clinical laboratory studies** The clinical laboratory is increasingly important in the diagnosis and treatment of psychiatric illness. The three functions of laboratory tests include screening for any underlying medical condition that might be causing the psychiatric symptoms, monitoring blood levels of psychotropic medications, and providing a baseline of biologic indicators as part of the diagnosis and treatment process. For example, obtaining an electrocardiogram (ECG) before giving tricyclic antidepressants (TCAs) may be appropriate.

1. **Screening tests for psychiatric illness caused by a general medical condition**
   a. **Nonselective studies**
      (1) Complete blood count (CBC)
      (2) Blood chemistry evaluation
         (a) Serum glucose level
         (b) Electrolyte levels, including calcium and phosphorus
         (c) Liver function tests, serum glutamic–oxaloacetic transaminase (SGOT), serum glutamate–pyruvate transaminase (SGPT), and bilirubin
         (d) Renal function tests, including blood urea nitrogen level and creatinine clearance
      (3) Urinalysis
      (4) Screening for syphilis
      (5) ECG
      (6) Thyroid function tests
      (7) Chest radiograph
      (8) Vitamin B_{12} and folate levels
   b. **Selective procedures** when clinically indicated (i.e., when results of routine laboratory studies are negative but a biological cause is suspected)
      (1) Arterial blood gas analysis
      (2) Blood alcohol level
      (3) Urine drug screen
      (4) Lumbar puncture and examination of the cerebrospinal fluid (CSF)
      (5) Special thyroid function tests
      (6) Heavy metal screen
      (7) Antinuclear antibodies
      (8) Serum and urine copper levels
      (9) Porphobilinogen and τ-aminolevulinic acid levels
      (10) Pregnancy test
      (11) Human immunodeficiency virus (HIV)
      (12) Monospot test for infectious mononucleosis

c. **Electroencephalography (EEG)**
   (1) The EEG is used to diagnose a variety of seizure disorders. The behavior associated with a temporal lobe seizure or partial complex seizure is sometimes difficult to distinguish from functional psychiatric disorders.
   (2) In delirium that is caused by metabolic problems, EEG results usually show high-voltage, slow-wave activity. These findings can be helpful in the differential diagnosis.

d. **Neuroendocrine tests**
   (1) **Dexamethasone suppression test.** Although the value of this test in diagnosing mental illness is limited, it can be used in a depressed patient to follow response to treatment. The patient is given 1 mg dexamethasone orally at 11:00 PM. Plasma cortisol levels are measured at 8:00 AM and 4:00 PM (rarely also at 11:00 PM). Dexamethasone ordinarily suppresses the patient's cortisol response. Plasma cortisol levels greater than 5 μg/dl are considered abnormal. Unfortunately, many conditions such as dehydration, alcohol abuse, hypertension, diabetes, and weight loss give a false-positive result. This test may help the patient accept diagnosis and treatment.
   (2) **Thyrotropin-releasing hormone (TRH) stimulation test.** Some depressed patients have a subclinical hypothyroid condition that causes depression. Other patients have lithium-induced hypothyroidism. The TRH stimulation test involves the intravenous injection of 500 μg TRH. TSH is measured after 15, 30, and 90 minutes. Normally, plasma TSH levels increase sharply to 10 to 20 μg/ml above the baseline level. An increase of less than 7 μg/ml is considered suppressed. This finding may correlate with the diagnosis of depression or subclinical hypothyroidism.

e. **Sleep studies: polysomnography.** Several medical problems associated with psychiatric symptoms such as sleep apnea, seizure disorders, headaches, sexual dysfunction, and insomnia can be evaluated by the sleep laboratory. Patients with major depression also have abnormal sleep patterns. The sleep laboratory uses the EEG, ECG, and electromyogram (EMG) in addition to the penile tumescence plethysmograph, oxygen saturation, and movement-measuring devices. In depression, findings include:
   (1) **Hyposomnia**
   (2) **Rapid eye movement (REM) latency,** which is a shortened time between the onset of sleep and the onset of the first REM period (< 65 minutes)
   (3) Greater proportion of REM sleep early in the night

2. **Plasma levels of psychotropic drugs.** The judgment of the clinician is the most important aspect of monitoring therapeutic efficiency of drugs. However, it is increasingly useful to monitor blood levels of certain psychotropic agents.
   a. **Lithium.** Because of the potential toxicity of lithium at blood levels close to therapeutic levels, monitoring lithium levels is mandatory. Plasma samples should be drawn 10 to 12 hours after the last dose.
      (1) Therapeutic levels range from 0.6 to 1.5 mg/L.
      (2) Toxicity usually occurs at levels greater than 2.0 mg/L but may occur at lower levels.
   b. **Carbamazepine.** A pretreatment CBC, reticulocyte count, and serum iron level should be performed. There is a small risk of agranulocytosis and aplastic anemia. During the first 3 months, weekly CBCs are indicated; thereafter, they can be performed monthly. Liver function tests are taken every 6 months.
   c. **Valproate.** Serum levels may be useful in following treatment; 45 to 50 mg/ml is considered therapeutic. Liver function tests are performed every 6 to 12 months.
   d. **Cyclic antidepressants.** Plasma levels of TCAs may be useful in adjusting dosages, assessing compliance, and minimizing toxic side effects.
      (1) **Nortriptyline and amitriptyline** have therapeutic windows (i.e., the therapeutic effect increases until an upper limit of the blood level is reached).
      (2) **Imipramine and desipramine** have a linear dose–response curve. Above certain levels, side effects outweigh therapeutic effects.
   e. **Neuroleptics.** Therapeutic levels for antipsychotic medications are not as well established as those for antidepressants. Blood levels may be used to evaluate compliance or nonabsorption.

    f. Clozapine. Use of this antipsychotic agent requires a weekly white blood count (WBC) and differential for the first 6 months followed by every other week for an additional 6 months and then once a month until it is discontinued because of potential toxicity.

3. Brain imaging for identifying biologic markers

    a. Computed tomography (CT). A CT scan can visualize lesions larger than 0.5 cm on cross-section. It also shows increased ventricle size associated with loss of brain cells. High ventricle:brain ratios (VBRs) are seen in patients with chronic schizophrenia and bipolar disorder.

    b. Magnetic resonance imaging (MRI). MRI scanning is based on measuring radiofrequencies emitted by nuclei when a strong magnetic field is applied. Detailed anatomy can be seen. MRI shows white matter lesions that are not seen by CT scan such as those that occur with demyelinating diseases (e.g., multiple sclerosis [MS]). With the exception of calcification, MRI generally provides superior detail compared with CT; as a result, it has generally replaced CT scanning as an imaging technique. It should be noted that the closed tube in which the patient is placed while an MRI scan is being performed often precipitates a claustrophobic response.

    c. Functional magnetic resonance imaging (fMRI). Computer enhancement with fMRI allows the detection of different levels of oxygenated blood. Increased brain activity causes increased blood flow; therefore, the functional activity of the brain can be measured indirectly. No radioisotopes are used. fMRI has been used to study organization of language in the brain, including problems such as dyslexia.

    d. Single-photon emission computed tomography (SPECT). Single-photon–emitting radio isotopes such as xenon 133 or iodine 123 are used. Xenon is inhaled, the isotopes are distributed to areas of the brain by blood flow, and brain activity is measured indirectly by photon detectors around the head.

    e. Positron emission tomography (PET). A PET scan shows specific areas of brain activity. Organic compounds such as glucose are labeled by short-lived, positron-emitting elements of oxygen, carbon, and nitrogen. A cyclotron is required to produce the labeled glucose, which limits widespread use of this technique. The prepared compound can be localized in the brain, showing biochemical activity of specific brain areas. For example, decreased activity in the frontal cortex is seen in patients with schizophrenia. PET scans do not show detailed anatomy or lesions smaller than 0.5 cm.

E Psychological tests These tests provide a standardized objective measure of certain patient characteristics, such as intelligence and personality.

1. Intelligence tests

    a. Most intelligence tests measure the **intelligence quotient (IQ),** which is arbitrarily defined as mental age divided by chronologic age multiplied by 100. An individual test score is compared with a standard or norm that is established by assigning the same tasks to a large group of people. These tests are influenced by culture and do not measure the entire intellectual capacity of the individual being tested. By definition, an average IQ is 100 (range, 90–110).

    b. The **Wechsler Adult Intelligence Scale (WAIS)** is the most widely used intelligence test for adults.

        (1) The WAIS has six verbal and five performance components, including information, comprehension, arithmetic, similarities, digit span, vocabulary, picture completion, block design, picture arrangement, object assembly, and digit symbol.

        (2) The WAIS generates a verbal IQ; a performance IQ; and a full-scale, or combined, IQ. A difference between the verbal and performance IQ scores of greater than 10 points suggests an organic brain syndrome.

2. Personality tests

    a. Minnesota Multiphasic Personality Inventory (MMPI). The MMPI consists of 550 yes-or-no questions. The results are given as scores in 10 scales: hypochondriasis, paranoia, masculinity–femininity, psychopathy, depression, hysteria, psychasthenia, schizophrenia, hypomania, and social introversion. The pattern of scores is interpreted by comparing the patient's score and subscores against standardized data. Although the test is objective, a trained psychologist should interpret the results.

b. **Rorschach test.** In this famous inkblot test, 10 standard ambiguous inkblots are shown to the patient in a predetermined order. The interviewer explores the patient's responses. This projective test shows the patient's thinking and association patterns.

c. **Thematic apperception test (TAT).** This test is also projective and consists of 30 pictures, not all of which are shown. The psychologist chooses a specific picture, depending on the psychological area to be examined. For example, one picture shows a seated young woman looking up at an older man. The patient is asked to create a story about the picture. This process indirectly reveals the patient's fantasies, fears, and conflicts. The test is not useful in developing a descriptive diagnosis.

d. **Sentence completion test.** This test is also used to elicit the patient's associations. It consists of a series of incomplete sentences that the patient is asked to complete (e.g., "I am afraid . . . ," "I feel guilty . . . ," "My mother is . . ."). The psychologist notes the themes and tone of the responses as well as any subject areas that the patient avoids.

e. **Draw-a-person test.** This test was originally used only with children, but it can also be used with adults. The patient is asked to draw a picture of a person. Then the patient is asked to draw a person of the sex opposite from the person in the first drawing. This test assumes that the drawing represents to some degree the patient's view of himself. The test can also be used to detect brain damage.

3. **Neuropsychological tests.** Specific aspects of brain function are tested by neuropsychological tests, which are usually given in a battery. Expertise is required to conduct these tests. Neuropsychological tests can detect subtle cognitive defects in patients who are not known to be demented and can assess strengths and weaknesses to aid in the rehabilitation of patients with brain damage.

a. **The Halstead-Reitan Neuropsychological Test Battery** includes:
   (1) The **trail-making test,** in which the patient is asked to connect alternating numbers and letters. This test assesses the patient's visuomotor perception.
   (2) The **rhythm test,** in which the patient is asked to identify pairs of rhythmic beats. It assesses auditory perception, attention, and concentration.
   (3) Other subtests that allow the neuropsychologist to evaluate a variety of brain functions such as perception, sensation, concept formation, visuomotor integration, and abstract thought.

b. The **Luria-Nebraska Neuropsychological Test Battery** and the **Bender-Gestalt Battery** are also used to diagnose brain damage.

III CLASSIFICATION OF MENTAL DISORDERS

[A] **Definitions** Although the term **"mental disorder"** does not have a precise definition, the *Diagnostic and Statistical Manual of Mental Disorders,* 4th edition (*DSM-IV*), defines it as a "significant clinical syndrome with behavioral and psychological symptoms, causing distress or impairment in functioning." Historically, mental disorders were dealt with separately from physical disorders. This practice perpetuates the belief of mind–body dualism.

1. **Causes of mental illness** can be:
   a. Biological
   b. Psychological
   c. Sociocultural–environmental

2. **Normal reactions to stressful events** such as the death of a loved one are not considered mental disorders.

3. **Socially unacceptable behavior** such as crime is not necessarily indicative of a mental disorder.

4. Few **diagnostic systems** consider mental disorders to involve both biological and psychological factors, but this split impairs the development of a comprehensive, integrated understanding of mental disorders.

[B] **Classification of mental disorders** The *DSM-IV* is based on empiric findings from literature reviews of data reanalysis and field trials. It uses a multiaxial assessment.

1. **Diagnostic axes**
   a. **Axis I: clinical syndromes.** These syndromes include organic mental disorders, schizophrenia, depression, substance abuse, and other conditions that may be a focus of clinical attention.
   b. **Axis II: personality disorders.** These disorders include prominent maladaptive personality features and defense mechanisms.
   c. **Axis III: general medical disorders.** These physical disorders are not necessarily causes of the psychiatric symptoms, but they are relevant to the treatment.

2. **Other domains for assessment**
   a. **Axis IV: psychosocial and environmental problems.** These problems include stresses that may affect the context in which the disorder developed. Generally, only psychosocial or environmental stresses that were present during the past year are listed. Stresses that occurred before the previous year are noted if they clearly contribute to the current disorder or treatment (i.e., history of trauma in a patient who is being treated for posttraumatic stress disorder [PTSD]). Common sources of stress include:
      (1) **Change in marital status** (e.g., engagement, marriage, separation)
      (2) **Parenting stress** (e.g., birth, illness of a child, or problem with a child)
      (3) **Interpersonal problems** (e.g., disagreement with friends, dispute with neighbors)
      (4) **Occupational problems** (e.g., trouble at school or work, unemployment, retirement)
      (5) **Change in living circumstances** (e.g., moving)
      (6) **Change in financial status,** especially loss
      (7) **Legal problems** (e.g., arrest, lawsuit, trial)
      (8) **Developmental milestones** (e.g., puberty, menopause)
      (9) **Physical illness or injury** (when related to the development of an Axis I disorder, it is listed in Axis III)
      (10) **Other stresses** (e.g., natural disaster, rape, unwanted pregnancy, death of a close friend)
   b. **Axis V: global assessment of functioning (GAF)** (Table 1–1). The physician rates the patient's level of psychological, social, and occupational functioning at the time of the evaluation. The GAF may also be used to rate the highest level of functioning for at least a few months during the past year.

IV PREVALENCE OF PSYCHIATRIC DISORDERS

The largest study of the prevalence of psychiatric disorders is the Epidemiologic Catchment Area (ECA) study (Table 1–2). Fifteen diagnostic categories from the *Diagnostic and Statistical Manual of Mental Disorders,* 3rd edition, revised (*DSM-III-R*), were studied in five sites. More than 20,000 people—a cross-section of the general population—were involved.

A In any one year, a mental disorder or substance abuse disorder affects 28.1% of the American population older than 18 years of age (> 52 million people). In comparison, nearly 50% of Americans have a respiratory illness, and more than 20% have a cardiovascular disease (Figure 1–1).

B Severe mental illness affects 2.8% of the American adult population, or approximately 5 million adults.

C Overall, the rates for men and women are approximately the same, but rates for men and women differ for specific disorders.

1. Men have higher rates of substance abuse and antisocial personality disorder.

2. Women have higher rates of depression, phobia, and dysthymic disorder.

D The **National Comorbidity Survey (NCS)** involved structured diagnostic interviews in more than 8,000 Americans.

1. Of respondents 15 to 54 years of age, 48% reported at least one mental disorder some time during their life. Thirty percent of these individuals reported at least one mental disorder in the previous year; 10% experienced major depression, 7.2% alcohol dependence, 2.8% drug dependence, 2.3% panic disorder, and 0.3% schizophrenia.

TABLE 1–1   The Global Assessment of Functioning (GAF) Scale

Consider psychological, social, and occupational functioning on a hypothetical continuum of mental health and illness. Do not include impairment in functioning caused by physical or environmental limitations.

Code (Note: Use intermediate codes when appropriate, e.g., 45, 68, 72.)

Code	
100	No symptoms; superior functioning in a wide range of activities; life's problems never seem to get out of hand; patient is sought out by others because of his many positive qualities
91	
90	Absent or minimal symptoms (e.g., mild anxiety before an examination); good functioning in all areas; interested and involved in a wide range of activities; socially effective; generally satisfied with life; no more
81	than everyday problems or concerns (e.g., an occasional argument with family members)
80	Symptoms are transient and predictable reactions to psychosocial stressors (e.g., difficulty concentrating after a family argument); no more than slight impairment in social, occupational, or school functioning (e.g.,
71	temporarily falling behind in school work)
70	Some mild symptoms (e.g., depressed mood, mild insomnia) or some difficulty in social, occupational, or school functioning (e.g., occasional truancy, theft within the household), but patient is generally functioning
61	ing well; has some meaningful interpersonal relationships
60	Moderate symptoms (e.g., flat affect, circumstantial speech, occasional panic attacks) or moderate difficulty in
51	social, occupational, or school functioning (e.g., no friends, unable to hold a job)
50	Serious symptoms (e.g., suicidal ideation, severe obsessional rituals, frequent shoplifting) or serious impair-
41	ment in social, occupational, or school functioning (e.g., no friends, unable to hold a job)
40	Some impairment in reality testing or communication (e.g., speech is sometimes illogical, obscure, or irrelevant) or major impairment in several areas, such as work or school, family relations, judgment, thinking, or mood (e.g., depressed man avoids friends, neglects family, and is unable to work; child frequently bullies
31	younger children, is defiant at home, and is failing at school)
30	Behavior is considerably influenced by delusions or hallucinations or patient has serious impairment in communication or judgment (e.g., sometimes incoherent, grossly inappropriate behavior, suicidal preoccupation) or is unable to function in almost all areas (e.g., stays in bed all day; has no job, home,
21	or friends)
20	Some danger of hurting self or others (e.g., suicide attempts without clear expectation of death, frequent violent behavior, manic excitement) or occasional failure to maintain minimal personal hygiene (e.g., smears
11	feces) or gross impairment in communication (e.g., largely incoherent or mute)
10	Persistent danger of severely hurting self or others (e.g., recurrent violence), persistent inability to maintain
1	personal hygiene, or serious suicidal attempt with clear expectation of death
0	Inadequate information

Adapted with permission from Endicott J, Spitzer RL, Fleiss, et al: The Global Assessment Scale: A procedure for measuring overall severity of psychiatric disturbance. *Arch Gen Psychiatry* 33:766–771, 1976; Shaffer D, Gould MS, Braic J, et al: Children's Global Assessment Scale (CGAS). *Arch Gen Psychiatry* 40:1228–1231, 1983; and Luborsky L: Clinicians' judgments of mental health. *Arch Gen Psychiatry* 7:407, 1962. Copyright 2008, American Medical Association. All rights reserved.

2. Fourteen percent of respondents reported three or more psychiatric disorders in their lifetime. This group reported 53.9% of all the lifetime disorders and 89.5% of the severe disorders in the past year.

3. Major depression was the most common disorder, with a lifetime incidence of 17.1%. It accounted for more "bed days"—people in bed and not at work—than any other disorder except for cardiovascular illness (National Institute of Mental Health [NIMH]). Alcohol dependence was associated with a lifetime history of 14.1%.

E Treatment

1. Only 42% of respondents with one or more disorders received any professional care. Only 26% received treatment in the mental health sector. Only one in 12 (8%) received treatment in substance abuse facilities.

2. Only 58.8% of respondents with three or more disorders (the most severely ill) received professional care. Of these patients, 41% received treatment in the mental health specialty sector and 14.8% received treatment in substance abuse facilities.

TABLE 1–2   Results of the Epidemiologic Catchment Area Study

Disorder	1 Month NUMBER IN MILLIONS (%)	1 Year NUMBER IN MILLIONS (%)
Any Mental Disorder Covered in Survey	28.9 (15.7)	51.7 (28.1)
Substance Abuse Disorders	7.0 (3.8)	17.5 (9.5)
Alcohol abuse or dependence	5.2 (2.8)	13.6 (7.4)
Drug abuse or dependence	2.4 (1.3)	5.7 (3.1)
Mood Disorders	9.6 (5.2)	17.5 (9.5)
Bipolar disorder	1.1 (0.6)	2.2 (1.2)
Major depression	3.3 (1.8)	9.2 (5.0)
Dysthymia	6.1 (3.3)	9.9 (5.4)
Schizophrenia	1.3 (0.7)	2.0 (1.1)
Anxiety Disorders	13.4 (7.3)	23.3 (12.6)
Phobia	11.6 (6.3)	20.1 (10.9)
Panic disorder	0.9 (0.5)	2.4 (1.3)
Obsessive-compulsive disorder	2.4 (1.3)	3.9 (2.1)
Somatization	0.2 (0.1)	0.4 (0.2)
Antisocial personality disorder	0.9 (0.5)	2.8 (1.5)
Severe Cognitive Impairment	3.1 (1.7)	5.0 (2.7)

V   EVALUATION AND MANAGEMENT OF PSYCHIATRIC EMERGENCIES

A **psychiatric emergency,** or **crisis,** is a stress-induced pathologic response that physically endangers the affected individual or others or significantly disrupts the functional equilibrium of the individual or the environment. The pathologic response may occur as an acute alteration in the individual's thoughts, mood, or behavior. The individual, the environment, or both may experience or react to the situation emergently.

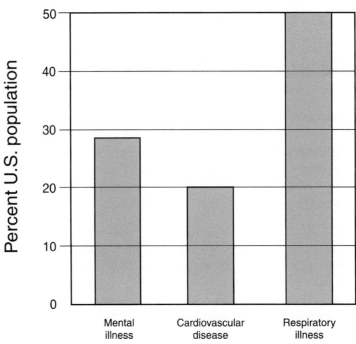

FIGURE 1–1   Percentage of U.S. population experiencing illness annually.

A Evolution of a crisis

1. **Stressors** from any source create a problem for an individual. In a crisis, the normal **coping mechanisms** of the individual are insufficient, and the individual is overwhelmed.

2. **Increased anxiety and disorganization** may follow the stressor and may further impair the individual's functional integrity and problem-solving capacity.

3. **Failure of adaptation** may cause an increasing sense of helplessness, accompanied by panic, depression, or both, and may result in further disorganization.

4. **Impulsive, maladaptive, and even desperate attempts by the individual to regain psychological equilibrium** are likely in this situation. The new equilibrium may help the individual cope and reduce dysphoria but may still be maladaptive because it limits the function of the individual or disrupts the environment required to maintain it. For example, an individual may use alcohol to lower anxiety and reduce the frequency of nightmares after a traumatic event. However, medical, social, and occupational complications may result from excessive alcohol use.

5. A **request for help** may occur at any time during this cycle, depending on the individual's response to the crisis and the social context. An individual with any psychiatric diagnosis or an individual with no preexisting disorder can have a psychiatric emergency. A diagnosis of a major mental disorder may be the result of an individual's maladaptive responses.

B Components of stress-induced responses   A dynamic interplay occurs among the stressor, the affected individual, and the social system that influences the individual's response. The severity of the psychopathologic response creates a psychiatric emergency out of a specific crisis.

1. **Stressors.** Although stressors depend on the interplay of individual and social factors, they are usually predominantly either internal or external.
   a. **Internal stress** occurs when individuals face a normal developmental task for which they are ill equipped or ill prepared. A normal environmental event may have great psychological meaning for a given person and may cause a disruptive increase in needs, a loss, or a conflict. Examples include an anxious adolescent who becomes disorganized when she leaves her family to attend college, and an aging, lonely woman who becomes suicidal after her cat dies.
   b. **External stress** results from a life event that is normally recognized as a significant source of stress such as the death of a family member, a divorce, or a serious illness.

2. **Nature of response.** Affected individuals determine whether a particular stress is major or minor and whether the response is adaptive or maladaptive. Healthy individuals may resolve a crisis in an adaptive, growth-promoting fashion.
   a. Healthy individuals may become so overwhelmed by stress that they have a pathologic adaptation. They are then more vulnerable to future stress.
   b. Individuals with significant disorders may decompensate with even minor environmental stress.

3. **Social system.** Individuals have varying needs for external support and structure and varying capacities to adapt to stress. Both the type of stress and the type of response affect the amount of environmental support that is available. Some individuals have many supportive resources that facilitate an adaptive resolution to a crisis.
   a. Some individuals have sources of support that are insufficient in the face of severe stress.
   b. Some individuals have sources of support that are easily overwhelmed or are even actively intolerant of their attempts to resolve the crisis. For these individuals, the external environment becomes another source of stress.

C Aims of evaluation   The practice guidelines for psychiatric evaluation of adults prepared by the American Psychiatric Association (APA) lists the goals of emergency evaluation.

1. To establish a provisional diagnosis responsible for the emergency, which may include other general medical conditions

2. To identify social, cultural, and environmental factors relevant to treatment decisions

3. To determine the level of cooperation the patient is willing and able to provide, any precautions that are needed to avoid harm to him- or herself or others, and whether involuntary treatment is needed

4. To develop a treatment plan, especially if hospitalization is needed

D Principles of evaluation

1. **Immediate assessment** of the condition and the dangerousness of the patient's behavior is essential. This assessment can be made on the basis of the following factors:

   a. **Patient behavior.** Loud, agitated, angry, and threatening behavior requires limit-setting and control before further evaluation can take place.

   b. **Arrival in the emergency department.** A patient who is brought in handcuffed or is otherwise restrained should be assessed cautiously despite calm or withdrawn behavior. The patient may be calm as a result of external control, and withdrawing this control prematurely may cause an escalation of the agitated behavior.

   c. **Reports on behavior.** Reports of dangerousness from family members and others must be investigated, even though the patient's history or behavior may be inconsistent.

2. **Thorough evaluation.** Secure surroundings that provide safety and comfort for both the evaluator and the patient should be available for a more extensive evaluation.

   a. **Steps that should be taken with all patients**

      (1) The **physical setting** should be quiet, open, and sparsely furnished. There should be a minimum of objects that may be used as weapons. Both the interviewer and the patient should have an unobstructed exit from the room. A call button to summon immediate help must be easily accessible to the interviewer.

      (2) **Trained assistants** who provide a show of force and can subdue an agitated patient should be readily available. It may be necessary to have help inside or just outside of the interview room.

      (3) **Mental status examination.** The physician should observe the patient's appearance, manner, and behavior during the evaluation.

   b. **Steps that may not be necessary with cooperative patients.** However, if indicated by the history or by an escalation of the patient's behavior, **these steps should be initiated before the evaluation can proceed safely.**

      (1) A **search for weapons** may be indicated by the history or the patient's behavior before further evaluation takes place.

      (2) **Verbal and nonverbal expressions of expectation regarding patients' self-control** and responsibility for their own behavior may be necessary. Patients may need to be reminded that external control is also available.

      (3) **Physical restraint** in the form of two- or four-point leather restraints is indicated if the patient cannot respond to verbal limit setting and reassurance. The need for safety for all people concerned supersedes the patient's requests, but the clinician should recognize the restrained patient's vulnerability and helplessness and treat the patient with respect and compassion.

         (a) If the patient arrives in restraints or handcuffs, adequate evaluation must take place before restraints are removed.

         (b) If an unrestrained patient cannot be controlled, he or she should be placed in leather restraints until the evaluation is completed. A patient should not be restrained in a supine position but should be on the side or with the head elevated to prevent aspiration if vomiting occurs. In addition, a patient in restraints requires constant monitoring.

3. **Identification of a crisis**

   a. **Overt.** A crisis may be immediately apparent from the patient's behavior or the circumstances surrounding arrival in the emergency department.

   b. **Covert.** A patient who is calm and superficially cooperative may still be potentially dangerous to him- or herself or to others. Empathic, detailed history taking with a high level of suspicion often shows the nature of the emergency. The following factors should raise the index of suspicion.

      (1) **Risk factors.** Certain historical data and mental status findings increase the probability of specific emergencies. Examples include a history of alcoholism or violence or findings of command hallucinations.

      (2) **Vague, evasive, or qualified answers** to questions in crucial areas such as suicide, homicide, and impulse control must be vigorously pursued. A patient's attempt to minimize

or ignore the consequences of observed or reported behavior should not be accepted without investigation. Discrepancies between the patient's history and the reports of others must be explored. The interviewer may need to meet individually with the other people to determine their true concerns.

    (3) **Feelings of discomfort on the part of the physician** should be examined. An intuitive, experienced physician who detects subtle discrepancies between patients' affect and their verbal content may identify a latent emergent situation.

4. **Symptoms and current illness**
   a. **Patient.** Interviewers can establish rapport by allowing patients to tell their own stories as much as possible. The examiner should obtain relevant information with the following questions:
      (1) What symptoms or problems led the patient to seek help?
      (2) Why is the patient seeking help now?
      (3) Why are these symptoms a problem at this particular time?
      (4) What are the patient's normal coping mechanisms in times of stress?
      (5) What is the patient's level of functioning in general?
      (6) How did the patient cope with similar stresses in the past?
      (7) How is the patient attempting to resolve the problem?
   b. **Others.** Family members, friends, employers, and coworkers may be able to answer many of these questions if the patient will not or cannot answer them accurately. Different individuals may accurately describe a particular aspect of the patient's situation or level of function, and the physician can use this information to compose an integrated picture of the patient.

5. **Patient history.** The level of detail provided in the history affects the accuracy of the picture of the patient. In a crisis, detailed history taking may not be feasible; however, the following areas should be explored.
   a. **Previous psychiatric illness.** The symptoms, circumstances, treatment, and response to treatment of previous illnesses should be outlined.
   b. **Dangerous behavior.** Previous episodes of self-destructive or assaultive behavior should be carefully explored because they have significant predictive value.
   c. **Medical history**
      (1) **Significant medical illness** may have a direct effect on the current crisis, may color the presentation, or may produce chronic vulnerability to stress.
      (2) **Drugs.** Prescribed medication, alcohol, and illicit drugs can profoundly affect thinking, feeling, and behavior. They may cause a crisis or significantly impair the patient's adaptive capacity.

6. **Physical examination.** A medical examination should be thorough, with particular attention paid to evidence of drug intoxication, withdrawal symptoms, and acute or chronic neurologic disease.

7. **Laboratory tests.** Laboratory studies should be guided by other findings and by the differential diagnosis. Blood and urine tests for toxic agents may be particularly helpful in an emergency situation.

E **Telephone calls**

1. **General issues.** People may call the emergency department for a variety of reasons, some of which may be covert or overt requests for help for any of the crises described. The physician can take limited action over the telephone, but some general principles should be followed.
   a. The patient's name, telephone number, and address should be obtained.
   b. The physician should attempt to establish an alliance with the patient without becoming too involved.
   c. The physician should encourage the patient to come to the emergency department as the next step in treatment.
   d. If the patient refuses to come in for evaluation, the physician's assessment of the patient's potential dangerousness dictates how persistently the physician and staff should encourage the patient to come to the clinic or hospital.

2. **Covert presentation.** The telephone request may be a subtle clue to a more serious problem. Use of the telephone may reflect the patient's conflict, discomfort, or embarrassment in seeking help.

If the patient reveals the underlying reasons for the call, he or she may feel less isolated and more receptive toward coming to the emergency department or referral to the appropriate resources. The physician should follow up the referral with both the patient and the agency or clinic to verify that contact is made.

3. **Overt presentation**
   a. **The cooperative patient.** A patient may describe a crisis overtly and may simply be requesting help to obtain treatment. In other cases, the patient's ambivalence may require the physician to make arrangements with family, friends, or the police to bring the patient to the hospital.
   b. **The uncooperative patient.** If the physician is concerned about imminent danger and the patient refuses to provide information, it may be necessary to trace the call and follow up any leads that the patient gives. Although it can be frustrating, the physician should attempt to build an alliance with the patient and should remind the patient of the limitations of telephone contact.

4. **Chronic callers.** Every emergency department has a contingent of chronic callers. Some of these people are lonely and need reassurance. Some are consciously or unconsciously expressing anger by repeatedly frustrating the staff.
   a. **Approach.** Whatever the motivation for the calls, the staff should attempt to place the caller in the appropriate treatment setting.
   b. **Plan.** Regardless of whether the callers go into treatment, a plan for handling them should be established. Identifying information (e.g., name, aliases, content) should be recorded. This process prevents new staff members from becoming tangled in a frustrating situation and minimizes the maladaptive gratification that these individuals receive from making calls.

VI SPECIFIC PSYCHIATRIC EMERGENCIES

A Suicide

1. **Clinical presentation**
   a. **Overt**
      (1) **Suicidal behavior.** Patients may ingest drugs or attempt suicide by slashing their wrists, taking an overdose, jumping out a window, or otherwise injuring themselves. Thus, patients often require medical or surgical intervention (e.g., gastric lavage, suturing) before a psychiatric assessment can be completed. Patients should be considered acutely suicidal until proven otherwise. Careful observation is needed to prevent another suicide attempt and to prevent the patient from leaving the emergency department.
      (2) **Suicidal ideation.** The patient may be obviously depressed, expressing concerns with little prompting and experiencing considerable pain and distress. The patient may ask for help in the control of suicidal impulses and for relief from depression.
   b. **Covert**
      (1) **Suicidal behavior.** Although patients may minimize or deny the implications of their behavior, they may have accidents that range from suspiciously to obviously suicidal. A patient who is unconscious of these self-destructive impulses may still be highly suicidal. A similar type of patient is one who appears homicidal or assaultive but whose behavior is primarily an attempt to provoke others such as the police to kill them.
      (2) **Suicidal ideation.** Patients may seek medical evaluation of a minor or severe somatic symptom. They may appear depressed or may disguise distress. Empathic questioning may prompt patients to reveal their feelings. Patients may show distress that is out of proportion to objective findings or may visit the emergency department many times over a short period. Although hoping to obtain help, patients may take the medication given for a somatic symptom in a suicide attempt.
   c. **Chronic suicidal ideation and behavior.** The patient repeatedly calls or visits the emergency department for suicidal ideation and attempts. Self-destructive behavior may be a means by which the patient attempts to manipulate the environment or relieve internal discomfort rather than an attempt to die. The patient evokes frustration and hostility in caregivers and is at great risk to be ignored or actively rejected. Because this type of patient is

also at great risk for suicide by design, miscalculation, or impulsiveness, careful evaluation is required.

2. **Risk factors**

   a. **Demographics**

      (1) The suicide rate in men is two to four times greater than that in women. However, women attempt suicide four times as often.

      (2) Whites and some Native American groups have much higher suicide rates than blacks and Hispanics. The suicide rate among African Americans is increasing, however.

      (3) Divorced, widowed, and separated individuals have higher suicide rates than married people.

      (4) White men older than 45 years have the highest suicide rate. There has been a significant increase in the suicide rate among adolescent boys in recent years. The elderly account for 10% of the American population and 25% of suicides.

      (5) Suicide rates do not differ significantly by economic status or occupation. Professional women, including physicians, have higher suicide rates than professional men.

   b. **Psychopathology.** Psychiatric illness is present in almost all people who commit suicide. Comorbidity (i.e., multiple psychiatric illnesses) is common.

      (1) **Mood disorder.** Major depression is the most common disorder and is present in approximately half of people who commit suicide.

      (2) **Substance abuse–related disorder.** Depression and substance-related disorders are present in two-thirds of all suicides. Alcohol is implicated in more than 25% of suicides. Other drugs such as marijuana and cocaine are seen in younger victims.

      (3) **Schizophrenia.** Approximately 5% of suicide victims have schizophrenia. About 10% of individuals with schizophrenia attempt suicide; 75% of these people are men. Individuals with schizophrenia have approximately the same risk for suicide as those with major depression.

      (4) **Delirium, dementia, and other cognitive disorders.** These disorders, as primary diagnoses, are found in 4% of people who commit suicide. Another psychiatric diagnosis is usually present as well.

      (5) **Panic disorder.** The diagnosis of panic disorder is statistically correlated with an increased incidence of suicide attempts. Most researchers believe that the presence of comorbid mental disorders such as depression and substance abuse–related disorder in patients with panic disorder is more important in predicting suicidal behavior than the diagnosis of panic disorder itself.

      (6) **Personality disorders.** Borderline and antisocial personality disorders occur in patients with suicidal behavior. Other psychiatric illnesses, especially substance abuse, are usually present as well.

   c. **Medical illness.** Poor health in the past 6 months increases the risk of suicide. Terminal illness accounts for fewer suicides than publicity suggests. Lack of postmortem examinations makes these risks unknown.

   d. **Genetics.** Most family studies involve mood disorders in which suicide is a factor, rather than suicide alone.

      (1) In one study of twins, suicides occurred only among monozygotic pairs, not among dizygotic pairs.

      (2) Family studies of an Amish community also show increased suicide rates in families with heavy genetic loading for unipolar, bipolar, and other mood disorders.

      (3) There appears to be a genetic risk of suicide that is independent of the risk of psychiatric illness.

      (4) Suicide risk is increased in families with psychiatric illness.

3. **Assessment of lethality (suicide risk)**

   a. **Episodic suicidal ideation and behavior.** Suicidal behavior may remit and relapse in response to patients' changing internal emotional and cognitive states and their environment. The patient, the environment, or both may require intervention to protect the patient.

   b. **Ambivalence of the suicidal patient.** The balance between the patient's wish to live and wish to die must be evaluated, including the factors that tip the balance one way or the other. Eight of 10 patients who eventually commit suicide give some warning of their intentions.

    c. Risk factors (predictors). In many cases, the patient's ambivalence and the episodic nature of suicidal behavior permit the behavior to be identified and prevented. The following predictors may aid the physician in determining which patients are at risk and to what extent.

      (1) Demographic indicators. Unemployed, divorced white men older than 45 years are at particularly high risk. Any of these factors, singly or in combination, should alert the physician to investigate the situation more fully.

      (2) Historical indicators. A recent loss, real or symbolic, or a change in the patient's status may precipitate a crisis, with the patient experiencing anxiety and depression.

        (a) Current illness. Patients who report hopelessness, helplessness, loneliness, and exhaustion are worrisome. An unexpected change in behavior such as giving away possessions or an unexpected change in attitude such as calmness or resignation in the midst of a distressing situation should be investigated. Overt or indirect talk of death should be followed up with specific questions about fantasies, wishes, plans, and means. In a patient who makes an unsuccessful suicide attempt, the following additional issues are important.

          (i) The patient's perception of the lethality of the attempt, expectations of rescue, and relief or disappointment at being alive are often more important than the objective dangerousness of the attempt, particularly in cases of apparent minimal danger.

          (ii) The extent to which the precipitating crisis is resolved or is being resolved may influence patients' wish to remain alive and their attitude toward the future.

        (b) History of suicide attempts. A history of previous attempts increases the risk of suicide, particularly if many attempts are made. The circumstances and lethality of the previous attempts should be determined. Forty percent of depressed patients who commit suicide have made a previous attempt.

        (c) Medical history. A history of chronic illness or an acute change in physical health increases the risk of suicide.

        (d) Family history. A family history of suicide is important both in terms of the patient's identification with the individual who died and the possibility of inheritance of an affective disorder. The patient may experience stress at the anniversary of the death or when he or she reaches the age of the person who died.

      (3) Diagnostic indicators. Depression, thought disorder, and impairment of impulse control, especially secondary to alcohol or drug abuse, are diagnostic indicators.

      (4) Mental status. The physician should assess the severity of depression, the presence of psychosis (especially command hallucinations), and any problems with impulse control. In addition, the physician should be aware of the patient's response to the interview (e.g., whether the patient feels understood; experiences some relief; and expresses more hopefulness or remains angry, pessimistic, and desperate).

      (5) Resources. The availability and support of family and friends are crucial. The physician should obtain their perceptions of the patient's lethality. They may need to be interviewed away from the patient to feel comfortable stating their concerns. In addition, in planning for treatment, the physician must be confident of their support and willingness to assume some responsibility for the patient. In particular, the physician must ascertain that there is no collusion with or covert encouragement of the patient's suicidal behavior.

   4. Countertransference reactions to suicidal patients. Countertransference refers to the physician's emotional reactions to the patient. These reactions may be unconscious or only dimly conscious. They may have a powerful effect on the physician's attitude toward the patient, approach to the patient, and even clinical judgment.

    a. Physician attitudes. Physicians have their own attitudes toward suicide and death, their own set of personal and clinical experiences, and conflicts about their own aggressive or self-destructive impulses. Unless physicians are aware of these reactions, they may minimize or distort patients' clinical data to accommodate their personal feelings or beliefs. Physicians may fear being overwhelmed if patients admit to suicidal ideation. Physicians may even fear that they will influence patients to commit suicide by talking about it.

b. Feelings of caregivers. The **patient's behavior** may produce **frustration, anger, and help-lessness in most caregivers.** A patient may evoke so much hostility that the physician may wish that the patient were dead. This reaction is serious because others in the patient's environment may feel similarly.

5. **Principles of emergency treatment**
   a. The patient must be **protected.**
   b. A **psychiatric consultation** must be sought if there is any question about the patient's lethality.
   c. **Treatment** must be considered. Treatment options include the following:
      (1) **Hospitalization.** Patients should be hospitalized if the lethality of their ideation or behavior is high. Lethality might be high because of the persistence of the patient's wish to die, the severity of concurrent psychopathology, or the absence of reliable sources of support in the patient's social environment.
         (a) Patients can be hospitalized **voluntarily** if they concur with the need for inpatient treatment.
         (b) Suicidal patients can also be hospitalized **involuntarily** if they refuse voluntary hospitalization. The length of time that patients can be held initially for treatment varies from state to state, but it is often in the range of 72 hours. Severely suicidal patients who resist treatment may require one-on-one observation to prevent escape or self-injury.
      (2) **Outpatient treatment.** Less restrictive treatment is indicated in patients who have some crisis resolution, mild concurrent psychopathology, environmental resources, and a therapeutic response to the interview. It usually involves a follow-up appointment within 48 hours and intensive crisis treatment thereafter. Somatic treatment can be initiated on an outpatient basis, but limited quantities of medication should be dispensed because of the potential for overdose.

B **Violence**

1. **Etiology.** Violent behavior is a result of the interplay between innate psychobiologic factors and the external environment.
   a. **Biologic factors**
      (1) **Neurotransmitters.** Serotonin metabolism appears to be involved in violent behavior in the same way that it is involved in suicidal behavior (i.e., lower levels of 5-hydroxy-indoleacetic acid [5-HIAA] are found in the CSF of offenders who kill with unusual cruelty than in the CSF of nonviolent offenders).
      (2) **Limbic system.** The role of partial complex seizures in violent patients is controversial. However, there appears to be no overall difference in the level of violent behavior in patients with psychomotor epilepsy compared with those without the condition.
      (3) **Endocrine abnormalities**
         (a) Because such a high percentage of violent acts are committed by men, there is speculation that androgens may be involved. However, no studies show this connection. With the exception of pedophilic behavior, antiandrogen treatment is not effective in decreasing violence.
         (b) **Premenstrual syndrome** is implicated in aggressive behavior in women and was once even used as a legal defense for violence. However, there is no scientific evidence of a causal link.
      (4) **Alcohol and drugs.** Alcohol decreases impulse control and inhibition and impairs judgment. There is a clear association between alcohol intoxication and violent behavior. Other drugs that have a similar effect on the brain and behavior include amphetamines, cocaine, phencyclidine (PCP), and sedative-hypnotic drugs. The aggressive and criminal behavior that is associated with obtaining these and other illegal drugs is also an indirect cause of violent behavior.
   b. **Psychosocial factors**
      (1) **Developmental factors.** A patient who was abused as a child is at increased risk of becoming an abusive adult. Witnessing abuse in childhood is also associated with increased violent behavior. Spousal abuse and family violence, even if not directed at the child, can influence the individual's later behavior.

(2) **Guns.** The number of deaths and injuries caused by firearms continues to increase. The risk of gun death among people 15 to 19 years of age increased 77% from 1985 to 1990. Guns are now the leading cause of death of adolescent males, replacing the automobile.

(3) **Environment**

(a) **Crowding** appears to be a factor in the increased potential for violence.

(b) **Weather** also has an effect on violence. Increased ambient temperature to the point of discomfort may produce increased aggression. However, aggressive behavior diminishes in very hot weather.

(4) **Socioeconomic factors.** Studies of race and violence have contradictory and controversial findings.

(a) Nonwhite populations experience higher rates of violence, as both victims and aggressors, than white populations.

(b) The best studies show that **severe poverty** and **marital disruption,** not race and economic inequality, are related to violence. The socioeconomic factors that disrupt the family structure also appear to increase the risk of aggression and violence in the children of affected families.

2. **Differential diagnosis.** Certain diagnoses are more likely to be associated with violence, although all patients may be potentially dangerous. Furthermore, accurate diagnosis permits the institution of specific treatment measures.

a. **Psychotic disorders**

(1) **Bipolar disorder: manic type.** Manic patients are often irritable and angry rather than amusing. They are pressured and hyperactive and may become aggressive if their grandiose, unrealistic plans are blocked. Their behavior may also be disorganized and unintentionally violent.

(2) **Schizophrenic disorders.** These psychotic disorders may be accompanied by considerable panic and agitation as well as deficient reality testing and impulse control. Schizophrenic individuals who refuse to take medication, who have a history of violence, and who have command hallucinations are particularly at risk for violence. More commonly, patients with paranoid schizophrenia exhibit violence. These individuals are hostile and fearful of attack, and they may act aggressively to defend themselves. Schizophrenic patients may experience command hallucinations that order them to hurt others.

(3) **Paranoid disorders.** Patients with paranoid disorders generally have stable, well-developed delusions but better reality testing and impulse control than patients with schizophrenia. However, their overly controlled and often denied hostility may erupt as murderous rage if the patient feels particularly threatened or experiences diminished impulse control.

b. **Nonpsychotic disorders**

(1) **Intermittent explosive disorder.** This disorder is more common in men than in women. These patients have discrete episodes of loss of control, and they commit serious assaults or destruction of property. Their behavior is grossly out of proportion to any precipitating psychological stressors. They may have genuine remorse about their actions afterward, but many of these patients enter prison or mental hospitals. A family history of violence is common.

(2) **PTSD.** Trauma victims who have also committed acts of violence (e.g., combat veterans) often fear a loss of control. Explosions of aggressive behavior may be unpredictable. These episodes may be associated with flashbacks and are triggered by something in the environment. Drug and alcohol use may complicate the situation, especially in patients with chronic feelings of rage and frustration.

(3) **Personality disorders. Substance abuse** increases the likelihood of acting out behavior in individuals with any type of personality disorder.

(a) Patients with **borderline personality disorder** have difficulty regulating their mood and behavior. Impulsive behavior, including violence, sexual promiscuity, suicidal gestures, and difficult and intense interpersonal relationships are seen.

(b) Patients with **antisocial personality disorder** exhibit outbursts of violence as well as pervasive antisocial behavior such as lying, stealing, and reckless actions that may endanger others.

(c) Patients with **paranoid personality disorder** are easily offended and are quick to react to any imagined or real insult. When two people with paranoid personality disorder are placed together, violence can easily result.

c. **Other disorders**

(1) **Substance abuse.** Alcohol intoxication is the most common cause of violent behavior in American culture. Other drugs that are associated with violence include sedative-hypnotics such as barbiturates and benzodiazepines as well as stimulants such as cocaine, amphetamines, and PCP. Glue sniffing and steroid use also increase violent behavior. Physicians should evaluate patients for dysarthria, nystagmus, unsteady gait, and tremors. Patients with PCP intoxication often exhibit confusion, disorientation, rage, and violent behavior.

(2) **Central nervous system (CNS) disorders.** Traumatic injuries to the brain, including birth injury, are associated with violent behavior. Postconcussion syndrome, which can be caused by apparently minor head injury, causes increased irritability and impulsive behavior. Any other organic mental disorder, including infection, degenerative processes, or ingestion of poison, can affect behavior.

(3) **Partial complex seizures.** Temporal lobe epilepsy is considered a cause of violence, although violence during a seizure is rare. Whether violent behavior is increased between seizures is a controversial issue. A patient who shows a repetitive pattern of poorly directed episodes of violence should undergo EEG with nasopharyngeal leads, regardless of whether other seizure activity is present.

(4) **Adult attention deficit (ADD) disorder.** Some patients continue to have symptoms of ADD after childhood. The symptoms include hyperactivity, poor concentration, low frustration tolerance, and poor impulse control. Treatment with methylphenidate may be effective.

3. **Assessment of dangerousness.** Although an accurate clinical diagnosis is important, it is only one element of an overall assessment of imminent and ongoing dangerousness. Future violent behavior is difficult to predict, but consideration of the following issues is helpful.

a. **Episodic violent behavior.** Because violent behavior is an infrequent event for most people, the difficulty of predicting future occurrences is increased. However, there is always a balance between an individual's internal state, including the degree of tension and the control over expression of aggression, and the environment. Certain combinations of internal and external factors may produce an assaultive crisis. An astute clinician can often identify when a patient is exceeding an acceptable expression of anger and frustration and approaching a loss of control and assaultiveness. Appropriate interventions at various points of this cycle may prevent the crisis or minimize the likelihood of serious injury.

b. **Internal control of violent impulses.** Factors that impair impulse control, either transiently or chronically, may be crucial in determining whether an individual merely fears a loss of control or actually acts on their impulses. In addition, violence is more likely to occur in certain contexts. The extent to which the current setting recreates a previous situation that resulted in a loss of control should be examined. Important factors are the patient's perception of external danger, whether real or imagined, and the need for self-protection.

c. **Risk factors**

(1) **Demographic indicators.** Boys and men who are 16 to 25 years of age are at particularly high risk for violent behavior. Because domestic violence is so prevalent, parents and spouses are at risk.

(2) **Historic indicators**

(a) A **recent major life change** may place an individual under increased stress and may lead to increased internal tension and frustration. The patient's feelings of internal pressure, frustration, anger, and potential explosiveness should be carefully explored.

(i) **Situations** (and individuals) **that influence the patient's feelings of tension** should be identified. The patient's attempts to cope with these feelings and the results achieved should be discussed.

(ii) The **patient's level of optimism or pessimism about preventing a violent action** should be assessed.

      (iii) The **patient's thoughts and fantasies about violence** are also important. Certain sadistic fantasies or violent ruminations may be directed toward a specific individual or group. Specific threats require investigation of the patient's relationship with and access to the threatened individual.

      (iv) **Specific plans and the availability of and familiarity with weapons** increase the danger.

      (v) The **patient's perception of what prevents him from carrying out the violent action** is also important.

      (vi) Current use of **drugs and alcohol** should be explored.

    (b) **History of violence**

      (i) A history of violent behavior is the most reliable predictor of future violence. This history includes fighting, assaults, arrests, and sanctioned violence (e.g., violent actions by soldiers and police).

      (ii) A history of impulsive or self-destructive behavior (e.g., accidents, arrests for speeding or reckless driving, self-mutilation) puts the individual at increased risk.

    (c) **Childhood history**

      (i) A history of neglect or abuse in childhood (witnessed or experienced) increases the likelihood of abuse and brutality directed toward the patient's children.

      (ii) A childhood history of cruelty to animals is also associated with continuing aggressiveness.

  (3) **Diagnostic factors.** The common diagnostic denominator is the degree to which the patient's thoughts are impaired in the contexts of hostility, irritability, and distorted perceptions of reality.

  (4) **Mental status.** Fluctuation in the patients' level of agitation throughout the interview should be noted. Patients' impulse control and judgment during the examination may contradict the content of their speech. Command hallucinations to hurt others are particularly worrisome, as are escalating delusional perceptions of external danger because these perceptions may be accompanied by frantic attempts at self-preservation. Sometimes delusional thinking places others in danger in the guise of protecting them. For example, a psychotic mother may believe that she must bathe her young daughter in scalding water to purify her. Any evidence of confusion or an organic mental disorder is significant because it suggests impairment of impulse control and judgment.

  (5) **Social system.** The thoughts of the patient's family and friends concerning the patient's potential for violence should be sought in separate interviews, especially if these individuals are potential victims. The family may provide reliable information about the patient's access to weapons. The clinician should assess whether a potential victim behaves in a challenging or provocative way toward the patient. If the patient appears calm, an interview with both the patient and the possible victim may be necessary to allow the physician to observe their behavior toward each other and to determine whether the crisis is resolved. The use of available community resources beyond those offered by family and friends (e.g., safe houses) should be assessed.

  (6) **Physician feelings.** Persistent feelings of fear or unease on the part of the physician may be important clues that further investigation and evaluation are necessary.

4. Countertransference reactions to violent patients

  a. **Physician reaction.** Angry, agitated, threatening patients are likely to frighten physicians. Physicians' lack of awareness of this fear, previous personal experiences with violence, and conflicts over their own aggressive impulses may affect their response to the patient.

    (1) **No reaction.** The physician may ignore or minimize the patient's concern with loss of control.

    (2) **Anger.** In response to their own fears, physicians may become angry and argue with patients. Physicians may challenge and humiliate patients, escalating already dangerous situations.

    (3) **Counterphobic reaction.** In response to unconscious fear and feelings of lack of control, the physician may act as though they, he, or she are in control of the situation.

(4) **Overly frightened reaction.** The physician may overestimate the patient's violent potential and feel unnecessarily anxious and self-protective.

b. **Consequences.** Intense, unacknowledged countertransference reactions can interfere with clinical judgment and treatment. Behavior may range from being overly concerned with control, or even punitive, to releasing the patient prematurely or permitting the patient to escape to avoid dealing with the patient. Either way, the patient may receive an inadequate evaluation and inappropriate treatment, and potential victims may remain in considerable danger.

5. **Principles of managing a violent patient**
   a. **Safety**
      (1) An adequate number of trained staff members must be available to restrain the patient physically if necessary.
      (2) Staff members should treat the patient firmly but compassionately.
   b. **Behavioral techniques**
      (1) It is important to act calmly.
      (2) The clinician and staff members should speak softly in a nonauthoritarian way.
      (3) Both the patient and the examiner should sit during the interview.
      (4) Staff members should check for the presence of weapons and confiscate any that are found.
      (5) There should be immediate access to an exit from the examining room.
      (6) Seclusion and restraint can be used to prevent imminent harm to others.
   c. **Psychopharmacologic approach**
      (1) **Neuroleptics** are the most commonly used medications in emergency situations. Haloperidol 5 to 10 mg may be given intramuscularly or orally every 30 minutes until agitation is controlled. The maximum dosage is 100 mg/day. Alternatively, ziprasidone 10 mg may be given intramuscularly every 2 hours. The maximum dosage is 40 mg/day. Neuroleptics should be avoided in patients who are experiencing alcohol or drug toxicity or withdrawal.
      (2) **Benzodiazepines** may be used with neuroleptics and in cases of withdrawal. Lorazepam 2 to 4 mg is given orally or parenterally every 4 to 6 hours. In some patients, benzodiazepines disinhibit violent behavior.
      (3) **Phenobarbital** in dosages of as much as 640 mg/day orally or amobarbital 200 to 500 mg intravenously (in 10% solution) is effective in managing aggressive behavior in patients with seizures. Side effects include decreased pulse rate and blood pressure.
      (4) **Other medications** that are useful in managing violent patients include the following agents:
         (a) **Lithium** is useful in treating bipolar illness but is not effective for treating other conditions.
         (b) **Carbamazepine** 600 mg/day is effective in decreasing aggressive behavior in some patients with schizophrenia and in those with partial complex seizures.
         (c) **Phenytoin** is effective in patients with episodic dyscontrol syndrome, although carbamazepine may be more effective.
         (d) **Propranolol** is effective in the treatment of patients with brain damage.
         (e) **Buspirone** helps control aggression in some elderly patients.
   d. **Responsibility to warn and protect others**
      (1) In American society, individuals are held responsible for their own actions, and information provided to a physician is considered confidential. However, as a result of the *Tarasoff* decision (*Tarasoff v. Regents of University of California,* 1976) and other legal cases involving attacks on third parties, clinicians are now expected to weigh the need for confidentiality against the need to protect others. In the *Tarasoff* case, the clinician was found liable for not warning the plaintiff that the patient had specifically threatened her.
      (2) If the patient makes a credible threat to harm a specific person, the clinician has a duty to warn that person. Good medical practice may also require involuntary treatment of the patient.

6. **Domestic violence: spousal abuse.** Violence in the home is pervasive, involving all socioeconomic classes. The most common pattern is battering of wives by husbands. Surveys indicate that one

of four women will be assaulted by a household partner in her lifetime. Sixty percent of female homicide victims are killed by someone they know.

a. **Clues.** The physician may consider the situation private family business and therefore avoid involvement. Because the situation may be chronic, with a certain equilibrium, both partners may resist intervention. In addition, the distinction between victim and perpetrator is not always clear. The following signs warrant further investigation.

  (1) **Unusual or unexplained trauma** suggests abuse, especially during pregnancy, which is often a time of particular stress.

  (2) **Vague somatic complaints** may reflect underlying psychological distress in either partner.

  (3) **Threats of violence** from either spouse should be investigated.

  (4) **Evaluation of any psychiatric symptoms,** especially chronic stress and depression, may result in disclosure of abuse at home.

  (5) **Overconcern of the patient's spouse or partner,** to the extent that the patient is not allowed to be alone or is rushed out of the emergency department, may disguise continuing abuse and a fear of exposure.

  (6) **Behavioral problems or psychiatric symptoms in children** may reflect chaos and violence in the home.

b. **Evaluation**

  (1) **Victim.** After establishing a supportive relationship with the patient, the physician should ask increasingly specific questions about violence, both past and current. The physician should not be deterred by evasive answers or initial denial but should recognize the vulnerable position of the victim (i.e., the patient may fear abandonment or retaliation if she is candid and may see no alternatives for herself). A discussion of resources and alternatives (e.g., safe houses) may be helpful early in the interview if the victim is fearful of cooperating.

  (2) **Abusive partner.** If present, the abusing partner should be evaluated with respect to dangerousness. If the abuser is not present, an assessment of the level of lethality of the situation should still be made. This assessment should include an evaluation of the partner's capacity for impulse control, the availability of weapons, the provocativeness of the victim, and the homicidal potential of both partners.

c. **Treatment.** The goal of treatment is to prevent further injury to either partner.

  (1) If there is any question about the lethality of the situation or the psychopathology of the partners, **psychiatric consultation** should be requested.

  (2) If lethality or the risk of future injury is high, the battered partner should not return home. Options include staying with friends or family, referral to a safe house, and hospitalization. If the victim refuses treatment, the physician should make her aware of resources and options but should not pressure her to accept help that she does not want unless she is returning to a life-threatening situation.

  (3) The physician should support the abused partner's decision not to return home, although the physician should not make the decision for the patient, except in the most serious of circumstances. Further treatment is often helpful to the patient during the process of separating from her partner and establishing an independent life. The patient may repeat the pattern of abuse by finding another abusive partner.

  (4) If the lethality of the current situation is low (i.e., the abusive partner wants help to prevent a recurrence), both partners can be referred for treatment, either as a couple or individually. Treatment should always be offered to the abusing spouse.

  (5) The **child welfare agency** should be notified because the children may also be experiencing physical or emotional abuse.

7. **Rape** is a crime of violence more than a crime of sexuality. It is the most common violent crime in the United States and also one of the most underreported. As many as 70% to 90% of rapes are unreported for a variety of reasons, one of which is continued victimization of affected women by police, courts, hospital staff, and even family and friends.

a. **Characteristics of the crime**

  (1) **Location.** Rape can occur anywhere from a deserted city street at night to a supermarket parking lot at midday to a woman's own home.

    (2) Violence. In all rapes, the woman's life is implicitly threatened. Explicit force is used 85% of the time, and victims are struck or choked 50% of the time. Five percent of women are severely beaten.

    (3) Victims. Although rape of men occurs, women are usually the victims. In addition, rape is the only violent crime, except perhaps spousal abuse, in which the victim's story is suspect unless she fights back. There is frequently an implication or even an accusation that the victim invited or encouraged the assault.

    (4) Assailants. The rapist is usually a man younger than 24 years of age. Most rapists have a police record, and many are sexually impotent before the rape.

b. Clinical presentation. The response of a victim to rape is similar to the response to stress in general and the response to other types of assault in particular. However, many issues intensify the conflicts and impair resolution. The following stages are usually observed, and an accurate diagnosis of the patient's stage of recovery can guide treatment.

    (1) Denial. The first stage involves shock and disbelief. The woman may describe a feeling of numbness that may last from a few minutes to several hours or days. The victim may appear shaken and drained but show little overt emotion. The absence of emotional reaction at this stage should not be mistaken for a lack of concern or lack of distress about the assault.

    (2) Emotional disorganization. The patient experiences denial, which alternates with periods of intense fear, anger, humiliation, and depression. These feelings may be associated with intrusive memories of the event, nightmares, phobias, hypervigilance, and anxiety. This stage may vary in intensity and may continue for months or years.

    (3) Resolution. The victim naturally attempts to resolve her disorganized state, which is distressing and disruptive to normal functioning.

        (a) Maladaptive resolution. The victim's attempts at resolution may be maladaptive and may cause chronic symptoms or new problems that are as bad as or worse than the initial event. The victim may make drastic changes in lifestyle that diffuse her anxiety about future attacks but are professionally and socially crippling. The victim may be unable to relate to others and often experiences a loss of sexual interest. In an attempt to reduce the level of anxiety and suppress intrusive memories and nightmares, the victim may abuse drugs or alcohol. Without active intervention, some victims may commit suicide.

        (b) Adaptive resolution. The victim, with or without treatment, gradually integrates the event. Intrusive recollections and feelings decrease as the victim returns to normal functioning in work and relationships. Similar situations or reminders of the attack may trigger transient reemergence of symptoms, but symptoms are usually less intense as time passes.

c. Evaluation and treatment. In cases of rape, it is difficult to separate evaluation and treatment. The physician, especially if male, must guard against repeating the humiliation by performing an intrusive interview and examination. It is helpful if the victim is treated and counseled by a female practitioner.

    (1) The **rape crisis team** or a psychiatric consultant should be called immediately to help assess the patient's current needs and support her during the examination.

    (2) The **patient's wishes and requests** should be respected. If the patient is alone and wants her family or friends contacted, she should be helped in contacting them. If she prefers not to contact anyone, this wish must be honored.

    (3) If the **patient is experiencing denial,** her distress should not be underestimated. When she feels safe, the patient may begin to express the feelings and disorganization associated with the next stage of recovery. If she continues to experience denial, the practitioner should explain that it is natural to have feelings and thoughts that may cause considerable distress and that talking about these thoughts will help her overcome them.

    (4) If the **patient is disorganized and upset,** she may feel considerable pressure to review the details of the event and to express her feelings. She may experience guilt, shame, responsibility, vulnerability, and helplessness.

    (5) If the patient arrives in the emergency department immediately after a rape, a **medical examination** should be performed after the patient is prepared. Obtaining details of the event is necessary to guide the physical examination. Specimens must be collected in case the patient wants to press charges. Discussion, treatment, and follow-up must take place because of the possibility of venereal disease or pregnancy.

(6) The **patient's resources** should be assessed. Meeting with family and friends separately (especially the victim's partner) may help them express their outrage and conflicting feelings away from the patient and, as a result, be more supportive.

(7) The **patient's decision** about returning home and obtaining subsequent treatment should be respected unless it is clearly unreasonable or dangerous. If the patient appears to be placing herself in jeopardy, physically or emotionally, it may be necessary to insist on further crisis intervention immediately.

(8) **Psychiatric follow-up** should be arranged. If the patient is resistant to treatment, periodic contact with a rape crisis center may be helpful.

BIBLIOGRAPHY

American Psychiatric Association: *Diagnostic and Statistical Manual of Mental Disorders,* 4th ed. Washington, DC, American Psychiatric Association, 1994.

American Psychiatric Association: *Practice Guidelines for Psychiatric Evaluation of Adults.* Washington, DC, American Psychiatric Association, 1995.

Gaw A: *Culture, Ethnicity and Mental Illness.* Washington, DC, American Psychiatric Press, 1993.

Hales RE, Yudofsky SC, Talbott JA: *Textbook of Psychiatry,* 2nd ed. Washington, DC, American Psychiatric Press, 1994.

Kessler R, McGonagle KA, Zhao S, et al: Lifetime and 12-month prevalence of DSM-III-R psychiatric disorders in the United States: Results from the National Comorbidity Survey. *Archives of General Psychiatry* 5:8–19, 1994.

Regier DA, Narrow WE, Rae DS, et al: The de facto US mental and addictive disorder service system: Epidemiologic catchment area prospective 1-year prevalence rates of disorders and services. *Arch Gen Psychiatry* 50:85–94, 1993.

Stoudemire A, Fogel BS: *Psychiatric Care of the Medical Patient.* New York, Oxford Press, 1993.

Winokur G, Clayton PJ: The *Medical Basis of Psychiatry,* 2nd ed. Philadelphia, WB Saunders, 1994.

Study Questions

Directions: *Each of the numbered questions is followed by answers. Select the ONE lettered answer that is BEST in each case.*

1. A 35-year-old lawyer has been evaluated in the emergency department for cardiac disease after an episode of palpitation and tightening of the chest. His medical condition is entirely normal, but he remains anxious. A psychiatric evaluation is considered. Special skills are required of the physician who conducts the examination for which of the following reasons?

- Ⓐ The patient may be embarrassed about disclosing emotional problems.
- Ⓑ The patient may threaten a lawsuit if psychiatric questions are asked.
- Ⓒ A male patient is generally unwilling to discuss psychological issues.
- Ⓓ The patient may still have cardiac disease that should be ruled out before a psychiatric evaluation is performed.
- Ⓔ The patient will deny any psychiatric problems if he thinks he has heart disease

2. A 38-year-old man is evaluated for psychiatric illness after being held hostage in a bank robbery in which he was a customer. He feels too upset to return to work, and he is on paid leave from his job. His request to remain on leave is an example of which of the following?

- Ⓐ Counterphobic reaction
- Ⓑ Malingering
- Ⓒ Perceptual distortion
- Ⓓ Psychotic distortion
- Ⓔ Secondary gain

3. During psychiatric evaluation of a 19-year-old college student who has attempted suicide by overdose, the examiner asks the question: "Did you take the pills before or after you talked to your boyfriend?" This is an example of which of the following kinds of interview techniques?

- Ⓐ Clarification
- Ⓑ Confrontation
- Ⓒ Facilitation
- Ⓓ Open-ended question
- Ⓔ Summarization

4. A 27-year-old man admits that he has persistent thoughts of curse words while attending church. Although he does not want to have the thoughts and is bothered by them, he cannot seem to stop them. He does not act on saying them aloud. Which of the following is the best description of this type of thinking?

- Ⓐ Delusional
- Ⓑ Derealization
- Ⓒ Obsessional
- Ⓓ Perseveration
- Ⓔ Referential

5. A young woman with schizophrenia is undergoing a psychiatric evaluation. The physician asks her why she has missed her last two appointments. The woman says that she does not want to be put in the hospital again and that the clinic reminds her of the hospital. Which of the following areas of the mental status examination best describes the problem?

- Ⓐ Association
- Ⓑ Cognition
- Ⓒ Delusion
- Ⓓ Insight
- Ⓔ Judgment

6. The dexamethasone suppression test is not used extensively in general psychiatric evaluations for which of the following reasons?

- (A) It is too expensive.
- (B) Its side effects include adrenal suppression.
- (C) It is contraindicated in pregnancy.
- (D) It has too many false-positive results.
- (E) It is associated with increased suicide.

7. A 40-year-old man with a history of chronic undifferentiated schizophrenia for more than 20 years is being evaluated. No medications have yet proved successful, and the man remains chronically psychotic. The best laboratory method to demonstrate decreased activity in his frontal cortex is which of the following?

- (A) Computed tomography (CT)
- (B) Magnetic resonance imaging (MRI)
- (C) Positron emission tomography (PET)
- (D) Rorschach test
- (E) Single-photon emission computed tomography (SPECT)

8. A 65-year-old woman is evaluated a few days after the death of her husband from a heart attack. She cries easily and says that she has difficulty sleeping, has trouble concentrating, and is not sure if life is worth living. Her condition is best described by which of the following?

- (A) Adjustment disorder
- (B) Major depression
- (C) Minor depression
- (D) Normal reaction to stress
- (E) Posttraumatic stress disorder (PTSD)

9. According to the National Comorbidity Survey (NCS), which involved diagnostic interviews of more than 8,000 Americans, the most common psychiatric disorder was which of the following?

- (A) Alcohol abuse
- (B) Depression
- (C) Generalized anxiety disorder
- (D) Panic disorder
- (E) Phobia

10. An 18-year-old college freshman is referred after midterm exams for crisis help because he wants to quit school and is anxious and depressed. Although his grades are As and Bs, he states he is "failing." In high school, he was a straight-A student, and he believes that he is a failure if he does not receive all As in college. The young man's symptoms are best described by which of the following mechanisms?

- (A) External stress-induced response
- (B) Impulsive disorganization
- (C) Internal stress-induced response
- (D) Maladaptive request for help
- (E) Underlying psychotic illness

11. A 25-year-old man is brought to the hospital by the police for emergency evaluation. He tried to assault the officer who was questioning him. He appears psychotic and confused. In evaluating his potential for violence, the physician should first assess which of the following?

- (A) Any history of hospitalization
- (B) Medication(s) the patient is using (if any)
- (C) Reports from relatives about the patient's recent behavior
- (D) Presence of command hallucinations
- (E) Any history of violence

12. A 19-year-old female college student is brought to the emergency department after a suicide attempt that involved self-ingestion of benzodiazepines and antidepressant medications. She states she no longer wishes to engage in any more self-destructive behavior. Initially, a physician should take which of the following management steps?

- [A] Perform a careful mental status examination
- [B] Perform gastric lavage
- [C] Hospitalize the patient—against her will if necessary
- [D] Obtain blood levels of the medications the patient took
- [E] Observe the patient carefully

13. You are a primary care physician treating a 59-year-old Puerto Rican lawyer for prostate cancer. He is divorced and living alone. In assessing his risk for suicide, which of the following demographic characteristics decreases his risk?

- [A] Age
- [B] Ethnicity
- [C] Marital status
- [D] Medical illness
- [E] Occupation

14. A 60-year-old woman is being treated for recurrent depression. She has attempted suicide twice in the past by overdose. After each attempt, she was hospitalized. Denying true suicide intent in the past, she admits that she uses suicidal gestures to control her family. The woman now expresses some suicidal thoughts. The physician's best course of action is which of the following?

- [A] Explore the patient's need to control others by threat.
- [B] Contact family members to assess stress at home.
- [C] Assess the level of the patient's ambivalence about suicide.
- [D] Assess the physician's own countertransference reaction.
- [E] Hospitalize the patient before further assessment.

15. Because the majority of violent acts are committed by men, testosterone has been considered a potential causative agent. Yet antiandrogen treatment has been shown to be effective in which one of the following disorders?

- [A] Alcohol dependence
- [B] Mania (bipolar I)
- [C] Pedophilia
- [D] Rape
- [E] Schizophrenia

16. A 29-year-old biker has been in an altercation with the police. A physician in the emergency department is suturing the man's laceration. Because the patient is angry and threatens to injure anyone who gets in his way, the physician becomes more controlling than is usual and sternly warns the patient to behave. Which of the following best describes the physician's behavior?

- [A] Authoritarian
- [B] Counterphobic
- [C] Limit setting
- [D] Overly frightened
- [E] Uninformed

17. A 20-year-old woman is brought to the emergency department after a rape. She states that her life was threatened with a knife by her assailant, but she appears unconcerned. She denies any feelings and states she just wants to be left alone. Which of the following best describes her mental state?

- [A] Delusional
- [B] Denial
- [C] Emotional disorganization
- [D] Malingering
- [E] Resolution

Directions: *Each set of matching questions in this section consists of a list of four to 26 lettered options (some of which may be in figures) followed by several numbered items. For each numbered item, select the ONE lettered option that is most closely associated with it. To avoid spending too much time on matching sets with large numbers of options, it is generally advisable to begin each set by reading the list of options. Then, for each item in the set, try to generate the correct answer and locate it in the option list, rather than evaluating each option individually. Each lettered option may be selected once, more than once, or not at all.*

QUESTIONS 18–20

Select the perceptual problem that most likely applies to each patient.

- A. Depersonalization
- B. Derealization
- C. Formication
- D. Illusion
- E. Olfactory hallucination

18. A 44-year-old chronic cocaine abuser is treated for self-inflicted skin excoriations; the patient feels that there are "bugs crawling all over me." He has scratched himself repeatedly in the past. He appears confused and admits to using cocaine that day.

19. A 29-year-old woman who is being treated for anxiety describes an episode at work in which everyone appeared to be mechanical and unfeeling. At times like this, she becomes frightened and thinks she is going insane. She has had this experience before, and it always passes after a few minutes.

20. A 60-year-old man in the coronary care unit becomes agitated because he believes the orderly mopping the floor is going to attack him with a club. The patient has been unstable medically, and his P_{O_2} is below normal.

QUESTIONS 21–24

Select the impairment in thought process that most likely applies to each patient.

- A. Blocking
- B. Circumstantiality
- C. Echolalia
- D. Flight of ideas
- E. Loose associations
- F. Perseveration
- G. Tangential thinking

21. A 50-year-old woman is asked during a psychiatric examination if she had ever been a patient in a psychiatric hospital. She responds, "That was the summer we were at the beach, it rained for 2 weeks. I was sad, but my sister Sarah did not help. She and I have never really gotten along."

22. A 22-year-old man is brought to the emergency department for evaluation. He appears confused but gives his name. When asked his occupation, he says, "Jesus was a carpenter. I am the right hand of God. I don't offend anyone."

23. A 30-year-old man who is being treated for bipolar illness has discontinued his medications for several months. He is brought to the clinic in an agitated state. When asked how he is feeling, he replies, "I am wonderful, the most wonderful in the universe. The universal gym is my invention, but Jim is just Dandy."

24. A 29-year-old woman with chronic schizophrenia rocks in her chair and does not seem to respond to an examiner's questions except to say, "No hope, no hope, no hope."

QUESTIONS 25–27

Select the Diagnostic and Statistical Manual of Mental Disorders (DSM) axis that is used to assess the situation described.

[A] Axis I
[B] Axis II
[C] Axis III
[D] Axis IV
[E] Axis V

25. A 32-year-old woman who has been treated for recurrent depression for 1 year has responded well to interpersonal psychotherapy and antidepressant medication. She tells her physician that her husband has just told her that he has been having an affair and wants a divorce.

26. A 58-year-old man is being treated for both recurrent depression and alcohol abuse. He has done well in treatment for both disorders, with an occasional slip in his drinking, and he has been sober for more than 1 year. He has just been told he has a liver mass that may be cancerous and is very upset.

27. A 24-year-old man suffers a severe head injury from a motor cycle accident. After awakening from a coma, he seems to be a different person, with poor social skills, gross and disgusting behavior, and foul language.

QUESTIONS 28–30

Select the diagnosis that most likely applies to the clinical situation.

[A] Antisocial personality disorder
[B] Bipolar disorder, manic type
[C] Intermittent explosive disorder
[D] Paranoid disorder
[E] Schizophrenia disorders

28. As the emergency department physician on call, you are asked to evaluate a 33-year-old man brought in by the police, who found him naked in the park. He attacked one of the policemen who questioned him. The man insists that he is the "emperor of the United States" and will "smite all who oppose him."

29. A 25-year-old unemployed construction worker is brought to the emergency department by the police. He denies intoxication but states several men in a bar challenged him "to prove himself." During the ensuing fight, the man broke both hands. The police report that extensive damage occurred. The man appears calm and somewhat content.

30. You are asked to evaluate a 29-year-old man arrested by the police for assaulting a drug dealer. The patient claims he is seeing visions of God, who talks to him. His mental status examination is otherwise normal. The man says that he is sorry he had to injure the drug dealer but knows that God will forgive him.

Answers and Explanations

1. The answer is A [*I A 2 a*]. Sensitivity is required in conducting a psychiatric evaluation because many people (not just men) find it difficult to discuss emotional issues. Malpractice suits may arise from failure to perform the appropriate examination when indicated. The examination should not be delayed until all other illnesses have been ruled out.

2. The answer is E [*I C 6*]. Secondary gain is any benefit that the patient derives from the current problem such as paid leave from work. The man may have an anxiety disorder such as posttraumatic stress disorder (PTSD), and he may not be faking or malingering. Perceptual and psychotic distortions have not been discussed. A counterphobic reaction would involve confronting the fear rather than avoiding it.

3. The answer is A [*II A 3 b (4)*]. Clarification statements may be similar to summary statements but also may include connections that the patient may not recognize (i.e., the relationship between the suicidal gesture and the phone call). The question, which is direct rather than open ended, does not need to be confrontational in tone.

4. The answer is C [*II B 8 b*]. The curse words are persistent and intrusive thoughts, which makes them obsessions. The patient is aware that the ideas make no sense, so the patient is not delusional. The ideas may be repetitive, but the patient does not perseverate in saying them.

5. The answer is D [*II C 10*]. The young woman shows a lack of insight into her illness, which can lead to a refusal of needed treatment. Although poor judgment may result, the problem is primarily caused by a lack of insight.

6. The answer is D [*II D 1 d (1)*]. The dexamethasone suppression test shows a lack of suppression of plasma cortisol levels not only in patients with depression but also in those with other conditions such as dehydration, alcohol abuse, and weight loss. This lack of specificity is the major reason why it is not widely used; it is not expensive, and it does not have any serious side effects.

7. The answer is C [*II D 3 e*]. Positron emission tomography (PET) shows specific areas of brain activity better than other scanning techniques. PET is more expensive than single-photon emission computed tomography (SPECT), which has limited its use. Computed tomography (CT) and magnetic resonance imaging (MRI) are used to visualize brain structure rather than function.

8. The answer is D [*III A 2*]. The death of a spouse is a highly stressful event, and strong responses do not constitute mental illness. There is a wide range of "normal" reaction to death of a spouse, and cultural influences may also be important.

9. The answer is B [*IV E 3*]. The National Comorbidity Survey (NCS) found that major depression was the most common psychiatric disorder, with a lifetime incidence of 17%. This condition accounts for more bed days than any other disorder except for cardiovascular illness.

10. The answer is C [*V B 1*]. The patient is facing a normal developmental task of college but is unable to deal with his own unrealistic expectations. Although it is appropriate to experience some anxiety when leaving home for college, this young man's usual coping skills are insufficient. Whether or not he has an underlying illness, his request for help is adaptive.

11. The answer is D [*V D 3 b (1)*]. In a patient with psychotic thinking who is being evaluated for dangerousness, violent command hallucinations are a significant acute risk factor for violence. Previous history of violence is also important, but it is not the first topic that needs to be assessed. No prescription medications are known to induce violence. Recent behavior may also be somewhat helpful in assessment but less so than command hallucinations. Past hospitalization history is not useful.

12. The answer is B [*VI A 1 a (1)*]. Initial treatment should involve removal of the ingested substances because whatever the patient's motives, the substances could be lethal. Obtaining blood levels and performing a mental status examination are secondary tasks. Whether the patient needs hospitalization or not is not yet apparent.

13. The answer is B [*VI A 2*]. Culture and ethnicity, which affect suicide rates, should be considered. Suicide rates are lower among Hispanics. Professional status does not significantly affect suicide rates. All of the other demographic characteristics of this patient (e.g., age, gender) increase the risk of suicide.

14. The answer is E [*VI A 3*]. The patient may be ambivalent about suicide; most people who kill themselves are. Because the patient has multiple risk factors for suicide, the safest course is to protect the patient while assessing her lethality.

15. The answer is C [*VI B 3*]. Some patients with pedophilia have responded to antiandrogens, which decrease sex drive and thus violent acts that involve sex. Rape is not usually considered a psychiatric disorder, and the other disorders listed that are associated with violence do not respond to antiandrogens.

16. The answer is B [*VI B 4 a (3)*]. Although the physician may think he is setting limits, he is responding as though there is no danger and he is in control. This unconscious, ill-advised reaction is primarily counterphobic.

17. The answer is B [*VI B 7 b (1)*]. In general, the first stage of response to the trauma of rape is similar to the reaction to overwhelming stress. Feelings of numbness may last for several hours or even days. The absence of emotional reaction should not be mistaken for a lack of concern or distress about the assault.

18. The answer is C [*II B 6 a (4)*]. Tactile hallucinations are seen in organic states such as cocaine abuse. Formication is the hallucination of insects crawling over the skin.

19. The answer is B [*II B 6 c*]. The patient describes derealization. Derealization involves an alteration in the sense of reality of the outside world. Objects may seem altered in size and shape, and people may appear dead or mechanical.

20. The answer is D [*II B 6 b*]. Patients in coronary care units are susceptible to delirious states. Illusions are common in delirium. The patient misperceived an actual sensory stimulus (i.e., the mop in the hands of the orderly) as a weapon.

21. The answer is B [*II B 7 c*]. The patient has not responded to the question but is in the general topic area. The irrelevant details represent digressions.

22. The answer is E [*II B 7 a*]. Loose associations are difficult to follow. There is no logical connection between patient statements, and the patient does not appear to be aware that the ideas are not connected.

23. The answer is D [*II B 7 g*]. This man, who is in a manic state, exhibits flight of ideas, which is seen in mania. In this case, this thought process involves rapid changes of ideas that are associated by the sound of the words.

24. The answer is F [*II B 7 e*]. The repetition of the same words or phrases despite the interviewer's direction to stop is perseveration.

25. The answer is D [*III B 2 a*]. Axis IV is the domain of psychosocial and environmental problems, including interpersonal problems and change in marital status. These stresses may affect another axis such as the one that represents the disorder for which the patient is being treated.

26. The answer is C [*III B 1 c*]. The knowledge that the liver mass may be cancerous is likely to influence the man's treatment for depression. However, the tumor may also be a consequence of the alcohol abuse.

27. **The answer is A** [*III B 1 a*]. Although this may appear to be a personality disorder (Axis II), the disorder is a newly acquired clinical syndrome caused by brain injury. Physical causes of mental disorders (formerly called organic brain disorders) are listed on Axis I.

28. **The answer is B** [*VI B 2 a (1)*]. This psychotic, hyperactive patient is manic. Public nakedness is nearly always pathognomonic for mania. When others attempt to control manic patients, they can be violent.

29. **The answer is C** [*VI B 2 b (1)*]. Intermittent explosive disorder, a nonpsychotic disorder, is associated with violent episodes. Alcohol may be involved, and the behavior is grossly out of proportion to any precipitating stressor.

30. **The answer is A** [*VI B 2 b (3) (b)*]. The patient appears to have been involved in criminal activity. Although his story is not consistent with psychotic illness, it is possible. The examiner looks for inconsistencies in the history and a clear secondary gain (i.e., avoiding legal consequences) to be had from feigning illness. If the patient had acted because of psychotic illness, one would expect a more disorganized mental status.

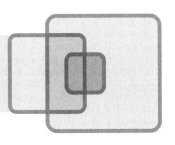

chapter 2

Personality Disorders

ROBERT BREEN

 INTRODUCTION

Each of us has a repertoire of coping devices or defenses that allows us to maintain an equilibrium between our internal drives and the world around us. This repertoire is **personality—the set of characteristics that defines the behavior, thoughts, and emotions of individuals.** The characteristics become ingrained and dictate people's lifestyles.

[A] Personality traits In general, personality traits are viewed as the result of cultural and societal influences as well as the child-rearing practices of the individual family. Recent studies in child development suggest that genetically determined temperamental factors may also be involved in personality development. Certain genetic characteristics may make the occurrence of a specific behavioral response more likely, thus leading to a specific personality style. When this stable pattern of response leads to problems, a personality disorder may exist. **A personality disorder is present when personality traits are inflexible and maladaptive, causing either significant impairment in social or occupational functioning or subjective distress.** Manifestations of a personality disorder are usually recognized by adolescence and continue into adulthood. However, symptoms may become less obvious in later years.

[B] Expression of symptoms Personality disorders are among the most common emotional disorders seen in psychiatric practice, particularly in the outpatient clinic. The patient's perception of the problem and the expression of symptoms, however, are different from those demonstrated in other psychiatric illnesses, making treatment difficult. Patients with personality disorders may complain of mood disturbances, particularly depression or anxiety. They may exhibit:

1. **Ego-syntonic symptoms,** in which patients do not recognize that anything is wrong with them that needs to be changed. They view existing disturbances as being the result of the world's being out of step with them.

2. **Ego-dystonic symptoms,** in which patients may be experiencing internally distressing symptoms that are self-induced but are still unable to alter their behavior.

[C] Clinical picture Symptoms of personality disorders generally affect other individuals and involve work, play, and all relationships.

1. **Individuals have trouble in their work settings.** They have often had many jobs and work below their capacities.

2. **Social relationships are disrupted or absent.** Individuals with personality disorders can be irritating and infuriating to those involved with them, and the reactions of these involved individuals are often more pronounced than the disorder itself.

3. **Patients may seek help as a result of a concurrent medical or surgical problem or because of a primary emotional distress.** In any case, these patients may elicit strong negative reactions in the physicians and other health care personnel who take care of them.

4. **In general, patients with personality disorders tolerate stress poorly** and seek help to alleviate the outside stress rather than to change their character. If stress is great, as it can be in those who are physically ill, patients may regress.

D Biology

1. **Genetics.** Twin and adoption studies show strong genetic components to **personality traits.** Less is known about **personality disorder.**

2. **Familial associations.** There is an increased risk of both Axis I and Axis II disorders in families of persons with personality disorders.

E Diagnosis

1. **Comorbid Axis I disorders are common.** The majority of persons with personality disorder also have one or more Axis I disorders. It is sometimes difficult to diagnose a specific personality disorder when a patient has a mix of traits. However, the ***Diagnostic and Statistical Manual of Mental Disorders,* 4th edition (*DSM-IV*), allows for the diagnosis of more than one personality disorder if a patient meets the diagnostic criteria for several disorders.** Diagnosis of a personality disorder should be made carefully in individuals who are reacting to a major environmental or social stress; for example, some young men develop maladaptive coping mechanisms in the military that they do not otherwise use.

2. **Axis I disorders make the assessment of personality disorder more difficult.** For example, a diagnosis of personality disorder should not be made in a person with schizophrenia unless the personality disorder *clearly* preceded the onset of schizophrenia.

3. Diagnosis of a personality disorder is only made after we can determine dysfunction in **at least one of the following four areas:**
   a. Cognition (perceiving or interpreting oneself, others, or events)
   b. Affect (range, intensity, lability, or appropriateness of emotional response)
   c. Interpersonal functioning
   d. Impulse control

II CLUSTERS OF PERSONALITY DISORDERS

Ten specific personality disorders are described in the *DSM-IV*. Because of the similarities in symptoms or traits, they are grouped into three clusters: cluster A is the odd or eccentric group; cluster B is the dramatic, emotional, and erratic group; and cluster C is the anxious and fearful group.

A Cluster A   The **odd or eccentric group** includes the **paranoid, schizoid, and schizotypal personality disorders.**

1. Affected individuals use the **defense mechanisms of projection and fantasy** and may have a tendency toward psychotic thinking.
   a. **Projection** involves attributing to another person the thoughts or feelings of one's own that are unacceptable (e.g., prejudice, excessive fault finding, paranoia).
   b. **Fantasy** is the creation of an imaginary life with which the patient deals with loneliness. A fantasy can be quite elaborate and extensive.
   c. **Paranoia** is a feeling of being persecuted or treated unfairly by others. Paranoid patients may feel that others are talking about or making fun of them.

2. Biologically, patients with cluster A personality disorders may have a **vulnerability to cognitive disorganization when stressed.**

3. **Schizotypal patients** have been found to have some of the same biologic markers seen in schizophrenic individuals, including low levels of monoamine oxidase (MAO) activity in platelets and disorders of smooth pursuit eye movements.
   a. It has been speculated that not everyone who has a genetic vulnerability to schizophrenia becomes psychotic, but some of these individuals may be diagnosed as having a schizotypal personality disorder.
   b. In families with a history of schizophrenia, the number of relatives with schizotypal personality disorder is also increased.

B Cluster B   The **dramatic, emotional, and erratic group** includes **histrionic, narcissistic, antisocial, and borderline personality disorders.**

1. Affected individuals tend to use certain **defense mechanisms such as dissociation, denial, splitting, and acting out.**
   a. **Dissociation** involves the "forgetting" of unpleasant feelings and associations. It is the unconscious splitting off of some mental processes and behavior from the normal or conscious awareness of the individual. When extreme, this can lead to multiple or disorganized personalities.
   b. **Denial** is closely associated with dissociation. In denial, patients refuse to acknowledge a thought, feeling, or wish but are unaware of doing so.
   c. **Splitting,** often seen in patients with borderline personalities, occurs when these individuals view other persons as "all good" or "all bad." Affected patients cannot experience an ambivalent relationship and cannot even be ambivalent in regard to their own self-image.
   d. **Acting out** involves the actual motor expression of a thought or feeling that is intolerable to a patient; this can involve both aggressive and sexual behavior. Patients with these types of personality disorders may be biologically vulnerable to stress (i.e., a tendency to low cortical arousal causes them to easily overstimulate) and a wide variation of autonomic and motor activities. Thus, a psychobiologic pattern may develop, which increases the potential for acting out that is not associated with any particular anxiety.

2. **Mood disorders** are common and may be the chief complaint.

3. **Somatization disorder** is associated with histrionic personality disorder.

C Cluster C   The **anxious and fearful group** includes **avoidant, dependent, and obsessive-compulsive** personalities.

1. Affected individuals use **defense mechanisms of isolation, passive aggression, and hypochondriasis.**
   a. **Isolation** occurs when an unacceptable feeling, act, or idea is separated from the associated emotion. Patients are orderly and controlled and can speak of events in their lives without feeling.
   b. **Passive aggression** occurs when resistance is indirect and often turned against the self. Thus, failing examinations, clownish conduct, and procrastinating are aspects of passive-aggressive behavior.
   c. **Hypochondriasis** is often present in patients with personality disorders, particularly in dependent, passive-aggressive patients. Biologically, these patients may have a tendency toward higher levels of cortical arousal and an increase in motor inhibition. Thus, stressful stimuli may lead to high anxiety or affective arousal.

2. Twin studies have demonstrated some **genetic factors** in the development of cluster C personality disorders. For example, obsessive-compulsive traits are more common in monozygotic twins than in dizygotic twins. **Patients with obsessive-compulsive disorder (OCD) are not at increased risk for obsessive-compulsive personality disorder and vice versa.**

III   SPECIFIC CLUSTER A PERSONALITY DISORDERS

These disorders—schizoid, paranoid, and schizotypal personality disorders—do not occur exclusively during the course of schizophrenia, which is a mood disorder with psychotic features, another psychotic disorder, or a pervasive developmental disorder. If criteria are met before the onset of schizophrenia, a premorbid condition exists (e.g., schizoid personality disorder [premorbid]).

A Schizoid personality disorder

1. **Definition.** This disorder is characterized by a pervasive pattern of detachment from social relationships and a restricted range of expression of emotions in interpersonal settings that begins by early adulthood.

2. **Symptoms.** Schizoid personality disorder is present in a variety of contexts, as indicated by **at least four** of the following:
   a. **No desire or enjoyment of close relationships,** including being part of a family
   b. **Choice of solitary activities** (almost always)
   c. **Little,** if any, **interest in having sexual experiences** with another person

      d. Enjoyment of few, if any, **activities**

      e. Lack of close friends or confidants other than first-degree relatives

      f. Apparent indifference to the praise or criticism of others

      g. Emotional coldness, detachment, or flattened affect

3. **Prevalence.** Because **patients** with schizoid personality disorder **rarely seek treatment,** the **prevalence** of this condition is unknown.

4. **Medical–surgical setting.** Illness brings these patients into close contact with caregivers, which is often seen as a threat to their equilibrium. Patients may intensify their aloofness and are likely to leave the hospital against medical advice if they are intruded on too much. Physicians should respect the patient's distance, should expect the development of trust to take a long time, and should not demand emotional reactions from the patient.

5. **Treatment.** Individuals with schizoid, paranoid, and schizotypal personality disorders do not usually seek treatment. If treatment is sought, physicians should be respectful but scrupulously honest in dealing with patients.

    a. Individual psychotherapy is usually the preferred approach.

    b. Group therapy can be more successful if patients can tolerate it.

B **Paranoid personality disorder**

1. **Definition (*DSM-IV*).** A pervasive and unwarranted suspicion and mistrust of people, hypersensitivity to others, and an inability to deal with feelings are characteristic. Individuals are neither psychotic nor schizophrenic. Although many paranoid individuals are careful observers and are often energetic and capable, they routinely misinterpret the actions of others as deliberately demeaning or threatening.

2. **Symptoms.** Paranoid personality disorder is indicated by **at least four** of the following:

    a. Suspicion, without sufficient basis, of exploitation or deceitfulness on the part of others

    b. Preoccupation with unjustified doubts about the loyalty or trustworthiness of friends or associates

    c. Reluctance to confide in others because of unwarranted fear that the information will be used maliciously against oneself

    d. Reading hidden, demeaning or threatening meanings into benign remarks or events

    e. Persistently bearing grudges (i.e., unforgiving of insult, injuries, or slights)

    f. Perception of attacks on character or reputation that are not apparent to others; **quick, angry reactions** or counterattacking

    g. Recurrent suspicions, without justification, regarding the fidelity of a spouse or sexual partner

3. **Prevalence.** The prevalence of paranoid personality disorder is believed to be 0.5% to 2.5% of the general population. People tend to group themselves in esoteric religions and pseudoscientific and quasipolitical groups. Groups of paranoid individuals who set themselves apart and see others as "the enemy" tend to provoke negative reactions from the outside, which reinforces their paranoid views.

4. **Medical–surgical setting**

    a. Patients. Illness tends to exacerbate the personality style of paranoid patients. Affected individuals tend to become more guarded, suspicious, and quarrelsome. In addition, they are frequently overly sensitive to slights and project their concerns onto others. They complain more often.

    b. Physicians. Clinicians should not expect to be trusted and should not impose closeness on these patients but should remain professional and even a little aloof. Although physicians should be courteous and honest and should respect the defenses of paranoid patients, they should be straightforward about all necessary diagnostic tests and procedures, laboratory results, and treatment regimens.

5. **Treatment.** Individuals with paranoid personality disorders, like those with schizoid personalities, rarely seek treatment. If treatment is sought, physicians should be respectful but scrupulously honest. For example, if a patient finds something amiss (e.g., lateness for an appointment), the therapist should admit fault and apologize immediately. The goal of treatment is to help patients understand that not all problems are caused by others.

    a. Individual therapy is usually the preferred approach.

       b. Occasionally, patients can tolerate **group therapy,** but great care must be taken in the selection of patients.

       c. Therapists need to avoid getting too close to patients too quickly. Some patients may become agitated and threatened, which causes a hostile defensiveness. **Limits** then must be set.

       d. **Antipsychotic medications** can be used in small doses for short periods of time to manage agitation. However, physicians should explain the side effects.

C Schizotypal personality disorder

  1. **Definition.** The central features of this disorder are pervasive patterns of "strange" or "odd" behavior, appearance, or thinking. These peculiarities are not so severe that they can be termed schizophrenic, and there is no history of psychotic episodes.

  2. **Symptoms.** A pervasive pattern of social and interpersonal deficits marked by acute discomfort with, and reduced capacity for, close relationships is indicative. Cognitive or perceptual distortions and eccentricities of behavior also occur. Schizotypal personality disorder is indicated by the presence of **at least five** of the following:

       a. **Ideas of reference** (excluding delusions of reference)

       b. **Odd beliefs or magical thinking** that influence behavior and are inconsistent with subcultural norms (e.g., belief in superstitions, clairvoyance, telepathy, or "sixth sense"; in children and adolescents, bizarre fantasies or preoccupations)

       c. **Unusual perceptual experiences,** including bodily illusions

       d. **Odd thinking and speech** (e.g., vague, circumstantial, metaphorical, overelaborate, or stereotyped)

       e. **Suspiciousness or paranoid ideation**

       f. **Inappropriate or constricted affect**

       g. **Behavior or appearance that is odd,** eccentric, or peculiar

       h. **Lack of close friends** or confidants other than first-degree relatives

       i. **Excessive social anxiety** that does not diminish with familiarity and tends to be associated with paranoid fears rather than negative judgments about oneself

  3. **Prevalence.** Several studies indicate that 3% of the population has this disorder.

  4. **Medical–surgical setting.** The problems posed by treating patients with schizotypal personality disorder and a medical or surgical illness are similar to those encountered with schizoid patients. Schizotypal individuals tend to put off caregivers. Illness threatens their isolation.

  5. **Treatment.** If treatment is sought, physicians should be honest in dealing with patients. The odd behavior of these patients can cause uneasiness in physicians, who must avoid all ridicule. Physicians should not expect to develop a warm relationship with patients and should respect the patients' need for psychological distance.

       a. Group therapy is associated with a greater chance of success than individual psychotherapy.

       b. However, only certain patients can tolerate group therapy.

IV   SPECIFIC CLUSTER B PERSONALITY DISORDERS

A Antisocial personality disorder

  1. **Definition.** Individuals have a **history of continuous and chronic antisocial behavior in which the rights of others are violated.**

       a. The **essential defect** is one of character structure in which affected individuals are seemingly **unable to control their impulses** and postpone immediate gratification.

       b. Affected individuals **lack sensitivity** to the feelings of others. They are egocentric, selfish, and excessively demanding; in addition, they are usually free of anxiety, remorse, and guilt.

       c. Violation of the law and customs of the local community is characteristic. The terms "sociopath" and "psychopath" have been applied to individuals with particularly deviant antisocial personalities.

       d. Personality disorders are considered lifelong conditions, and the signs of conduct disorder must be present in adolescence. The criteria for conduct disorder (i.e., a childhood pattern of antisocial and oppositional behavior) should be met.

    e. Persons who use illegal substances satisfy many of the criteria of antisocial personality disorder as a result of their pursuit of these substances. However, the diagnosis of antisocial personality disorder is not appropriate if the diagnostic criteria are all drug related and the patient shows some remorse about victimizing others.

  2. Symptoms. Factors indicative of antisocial personality disorder include:

    a. Current age of **18 years or older**

    b. Evidence of a **conduct disorder** (e.g., a childhood pattern of antisocial and oppositional behavior) with onset before age 15 years

    c. A pervasive **pattern of disregard for and violation of the rights of others** occurring since age 15 years, as indicated by at least three of the following:

      (1) Failure to conform to social norms with respect to lawful behaviors, as indicated by repeatedly performing acts that are grounds for arrest

      (2) Deceitfulness, as indicated by repeated lying, use of aliases, or conning others for personal profit or pleasure

      (3) Impulsivity or failure to plan ahead

      (4) Irritability and aggressiveness, as indicated by repeated physical fights or assaults

      (5) Reckless disregard for safety of oneself or others

      (6) Consistent irresponsibility, as indicated by repeated failure to sustain consistent work behavior or honor financial obligations

      (7) Lack of remorse, as indicated by being indifferent to or rationalizing having hurt, mistreated, or stolen from another person

    d. Antisocial behavior that does not occur exclusively during the course of schizophrenia or a manic episode

  3. Prevalence. In the United States, it is estimated that 3% of men have the disorder. The Epidemiologic Catchment Area (ECA) study suggests that lifetime prevalence for men may be over 7% and for women, 1%.

  4. Etiology. The etiology of antisocial personality disorder is unclear.

    a. There is often **a family history** of antisocial personality disorder in both men and women. Both **environmental and genetic factors** play a role. A sociopathic father is predictive of an antisocial personality regardless of whether the child is reared in the presence of the father. Family problems with alcoholism also increase the risk of antisocial behavior.

    b. Some antisocial behavior is precipitated by **brain damage secondary to closed-head trauma or encephalitis.** In these cases, the proper diagnosis is **personality change caused by a general medical condition.** The causative factors are generally believed to be biologic.

    c. Other studies indicate that **inconsistent and impulsive parenting** can be more damaging than the loss of a parent.

  5. Medical–surgical setting. The emergency department is a common site of interaction between physicians and patients with antisocial personality disorder. Impulsivity may lead to fights, suicide attempts, or other injuries. Substance abuse is a common complication.

    a. Patients may be superficially charming when under stress and not cause any particular problems initially. However, they tend to be manipulative if given a chance and resist following the rules of the hospital.

    b. Young patients have particular difficulty with the authority of physicians and tend to be noncompliant with treatment. In the hospital setting, they are generally disruptive, and when threatened, they are likely to leave the hospital against medical advice.

  6. Treatment

    a. Setting **firm behavioral limits** is crucial. In general, **inpatient settings** are the only places where behavior can be controlled. Outpatient treatment is rarely satisfactory because patients avoid treatment as soon as they experience any unpleasant effects.

    b. Group therapy is more helpful than individual therapy because the patient sees it as less authoritative. Inpatient groups can confront antisocial behavior because a group of antisocial personalities is made up of experts at recognizing this behavior. Group treatment may involve therapeutic communities as well.

    c. Medication to control aggression may be useful in patients with brain dysfunction. Beta-blockers, selective serotonin reuptake inhibitors (SSRIs), and bupropion have been used.

    d. Treatment of comorbid substance abuse is often necessary.

B Borderline personality disorder

1. **Definition**
   a. **Origin of term.** The term "borderline" originated with the concept that this disorder was on the border between neurosis and psychosis. The disorder has also been called borderline schizophrenia, pseudoneurotic schizophrenia, and ambulatory schizophrenia, but it is now thought to be distinct from schizophrenia.
   b. **Important features.** Essential features are **instability of self-image, interpersonal relationships, and mood.** An identity disturbance is usually present and is manifested by an uncertainty about sexual orientation, goals, types of friends, and self-image.

2. **Symptoms.** A pervasive pattern of instability of interpersonal relationships, self-image, affects, and control over impulses beginning by early adulthood is characteristic. Borderline personality disorder, which may be present in a variety of contexts, is indicated by **at least five** of the following:
   a. **Frantic efforts to avoid real or imagined abandonment**
   b. **Unstable and intense interpersonal relationships** characterized by alternating between extremes of idealization and devaluation
   c. **Identity disturbance;** that is, persistent and markedly disturbed, distorted, or unstable self-image or sense of self
   d. **Impulsivity** in at least two areas that are potentially self-damaging (e.g., spending, sex, substance abuse, reckless driving, binge eating)
   e. **Recurrent suicidal behavior,** gestures, or threats, or **self-mutilating behavior**
   f. Affective instability caused by a **marked reactivity of mood** (e.g., intense episodic dysphoria, irritability, or anxiety usually lasting a few hours and only rarely more than a few days)
   g. **Chronic feelings of emptiness**
   h. **Inappropriate, intense anger** or **lack of control of anger** (e.g., frequent displays of temper, constant anger, recurrent physical fights)
   i. **Transient, stress-related paranoid ideation** or severe dissociative symptoms

3. **Prevalence.** This disorder may be present in 1% to 2% of the population. The diagnosis is made twice as frequently in women. Of the individuals with this diagnosis, 90% also have one other psychiatric diagnosis, and 40% have two other diagnoses.

4. **Etiology.** Almost all theories related to the cause of the borderline personality have postulated problems in early development. **Severe abuse in childhood** (verbal, physical, and sexual) is a common finding. **Neurocognitive deficits** and **decreased serotonin** levels are also found.

5. **Medical–surgical setting.** When individuals with a borderline personality become ill, they exhibit an increase in stress and the potential for an exacerbation of symptoms related to the personality disorder.
   a. The illness can signify a threat to any emotional homeostasis that has developed.
   b. **Splitting** is used as a defense to divide others (see II B 1 c). The hospital staff may unconsciously take sides and, with the patient, view situations or people as "all good" or "all bad." This split often occurs between physicians and nurses. The intensity of the feelings provoked by patients may make medical treatment difficult.

6. **Treatment**
   a. **Psychological therapy.** This type of treatment may involve three approaches.
      (1) The **psychodynamic approach** aims to understand the underlying psychopathology. In general, standard long-term psychotherapy is difficult because patients tend to regress, and the reactions of therapists are intense.
      (2) **Treatment oriented toward supportive reality** is confrontational rather than interpretational. Therapists help patients recognize the feelings that are being provoked and their connection with behavior. Therapists set limits and provide structure. This approach is more appropriate in the general hospital setting.
      (3) **Dialectic behavioral therapy,** a form of cognitive therapy, has been developed to help individuals with borderline personality disorder gain better control of unstable emotions and impulsive actions. This form of therapy focuses on helping patients achieve some behavioral stability before beginning the sometimes volatile work of therapy for **trauma and abuse.**

    b. Pharmacologic treatment. This type of therapy is clinically important, and modest improvement in patient mood and behavior can be obtained with pharmacotherapy.

        (1) Modern **antidepressants** such as SSRIs have helped some patients control impulsivity and self-injury while improving their mood. The older MAO inhibitors (e.g., tranylcypromine) have been effective in improving mood but not in causing behavioral changes.

        (2) **Anticonvulsants** such as carbamazepine and valproate have helped decrease behavioral dyscontrol and stabilize mood.

        (3) Both typical and atypical **antipsychotic medications,** when given in low doses, have been shown to be effective in decreasing behavioral dyscontrol and reducing occasional psychotic symptoms.

        (4) **Benzodiazepines** are usually contraindicated for most patients because they may cause disinhibition, and drug abuse problems are common.

C **Narcissistic personality disorder**

    1. Definition. Individuals have a grandiose sense of their own importance but are also extremely sensitive to criticism. They have little ability to empathize with others, and they are more concerned about appearance than substance.

    2. Symptoms. Narcissistic patients have a pervasive pattern of grandiosity (in fantasy or behavior), need for admiration, and lack of empathy that begins in early adulthood and is present in a variety of contexts. Narcissistic personality disorder is indicated by **at least five** of the following:

      a. A grandiose sense of self-importance (e.g., **exaggeration of achievements and talents,** expectation for recognition as superior without commensurate achievements)

      b. Preoccupation with fantasies of unlimited success, power, brilliance, beauty, or ideal love

      c. Belief in being "special" and unique and can only be understood by, or should associate with, other special or high-status people (or institutions)

      d. Requirement for excessive admiration

      e. A **sense of entitlement** (i.e., unreasonable expectations of especially favorable treatment or automatic compliance with her views)

      f. Behavior that is **interpersonally exploitative** (i.e., takes advantage of others as a means to achieve her own ends)

      g. Lack of empathy (i.e., unwilling to recognize or identify with the feelings and needs of others)

      h. Jealousy or belief that others are envious (often)

      i. Arrogance; demonstration of haughty behavior or attitude

    3. Associated features

      a. Depression or a depressed mood is common.

      b. Painful preoccupation with appearance occurs.

      c. Features of other cluster B disorders are often present.

    4. Prevalence. The prevalence of narcissistic personality disorder is believed to be about 1% of the general population. Although the diagnosis has been made more often in recent years, this is likely to result from a greater interest in this disorder rather than to increased prevalence.

    5. Medical–surgical setting

      a. Patient reactions. Individuals react to illness as a threat to their sense of grandiosity and self-perfection. Intensification of characteristic behavior and either overidealization or devaluation of physicians is usually apparent. Patients expect special treatment.

      b. Physician or caregiver reactions. Patients tend to provoke negative reactions in caregivers. Feelings of both anger and boredom can be expected. Narcissistic personality traits are sometimes encountered in physicians, complicating work with difficult patients.

    6. Treatment

      a. Individual psychotherapy, with an attempt at understanding the pain suffered by patients, is the treatment of choice.

        (1) The therapist must deal with transitions from being overidealized to being devalued.

        (2) These transitions can be stormy, and they occur when the therapist has misunderstood the patient or has not been perfectly empathic. It is important that the physician not be defensive about mistakes.

   b. Group therapy in combination with individual therapy can be useful in helping patients obtain feedback about the effects they have on others.

D Histrionic personality disorder

1. **Definition.** Affected individuals are flamboyant, seek attention, and demonstrate an excessive emotionality. Their emotions are shallow and shift rapidly. Typically, they are attractive and seductive and, like narcissistic persons, overly concerned with their appearance. The disorder was formerly called "hysterical personality," but that term was discarded because of the many meanings of the word "hysterical."

2. **Symptoms.** A pervasive pattern of excessive emotionality and attention seeking that begins by early adulthood and is present in a variety of contexts is characteristic. Histrionic personality disorder is indicated by **at least five** of the following:
   a. Feeling of discomfort in situations in which the individual is not the **center of attention**
   b. Interaction with others that is often characterized as **inappropriately sexually seductive** or **provocative**
   c. **Insincere affect** (i.e., display of rapidly shifting and shallow expression of emotions)
   d. Consistent **use of physical appearance to draw attention** to oneself
   e. **Speech that is excessively impressionistic** and lacking in detail
   f. **Self-dramatization,** with a theatrical and exaggerated expression of emotion
   g. **Suggestibility** (i.e., easily influenced by others or circumstances)
   h. **Exaggeration of importance** of relationships and acquaintances

3. **Associated features.** As with all of the cluster B disorders, mood and somatization disorders, especially depression, are common.

4. **Prevalence.** The prevalence of histrionic personality disorder is estimated to be about 2% to 3% of the general population. The condition is diagnosed in women much more often than in men. Men who exhibit similar behavior patterns are often diagnosed as narcissistic.

5. **Medical–surgical setting**
   a. Physicians may find patients charming and fascinating, especially when they are of the opposite sex.
   b. Patients often think of illness as a threat to their physical attractiveness. They may view illness as a punishment for their thoughts or feelings, and men may see it as a threat of mutilation.
   c. Male patients may behave in an inappropriate sexual manner with female nurses and physicians; the sexual behavior may be a cover for deeper concerns about dependency. These patients learn that they can be taken care of by being sexually attractive, and this behavior is accentuated under the stress of illness. Physicians should approach patients as professionals and remind them that the roles are set. At the same time, it is important to remain noncritical.

6. **Treatment**
   a. **Psychotherapy,** either individual or group, is generally the treatment of choice. In general, therapists help patients become aware of the real feelings underneath the histrionic behavior.
   b. **Antidepressant medications,** especially MAO inhibitors and SSRIs, have been useful in treating mood disorders associated with this personality type.

V SPECIFIC CLUSTER C PERSONALITY DISORDERS

A Avoidant personality disorder

1. **Definition.** Although individuals with avoidant personality disorder are timid and shy, they do wish to have friends, unlike schizoid patients. Because they are so uncomfortable and afraid of rejection or criticism, they avoid social contact. In addition, they are self-critical and have low self-esteem. If affected individuals are given strong guarantees of uncritical acceptance, however, they will make friends and participate in social gatherings.

2. **Symptoms.** A pervasive pattern of social inhibition, feelings of inadequacy, and hypersensitivity to negative evaluation that began by early adulthood is indicative. Avoidant personality disorder, which is present in a variety of contexts, is indicated by at least four of the following:
   a. **Avoidance of occupational activities that involve significant interpersonal contact** because of fears of criticism, disapproval, or rejection

b. **Unwillingness to become involved with people** unless certain of being liked
c. **Restraint in intimate relationships** because of the fear of being shamed or ridiculed
d. **Preoccupation with worry about being criticized or rejected** in social situations
e. **Inhibition in new interpersonal situations** because of feelings of inadequacy
f. **Belief that they are socially inept, personally unappealing, or inferior** to others
g. **Unusual reluctance to take personal risks** or engage in any new activities because they may prove embarrassing

3. **Associated features.** Social phobias and agoraphobia may be present, but they are also separate disorders that need to be ruled out.

4. **Prevalence.** The prevalence of avoidant personality disorder is believed to about 0.5% to 1% of the general population. Little is known about sex ratios or familial patterns.

5. **Medical–surgical setting.** Unlike schizoid patients, avoidant patients may do well in the hospital, where they are undemanding and generally cooperative. Illness can allow them to be taken care of and establish relationships with the staff. However, avoidant patients are sensitive to criticism and may misinterpret equivocal statements as being derogatory or ridiculing and withdraw emotionally.

6. **Treatment**
a. **Psychotherapy,** either individual or group, can be useful. Patients respond to genuine caring and support.
b. **Assertiveness training** may provide new social skills.

B **Dependent personality disorder**

1. **Definition.** These passive individuals allow others to direct their lives because they are unable to do so themselves. Other people such as spouses or parents make all the major life decisions, including where to live and what type of employment to obtain.
a. The **needs of dependent individuals are placed secondary to those of the people on whom they depend** to avoid any possibility of having to be self-reliant. Dependent persons lack self-confidence and see themselves as helpless or stupid.
b. Some authorities believe that the presence of this disorder depends to a large extent on **cultural roles** (i.e., some groups of people are "expected" to assume dependent roles on the basis of certain criteria such as gender or ethnic background).

2. **Symptoms.** A pervasive and excessive need to be taken care of, which leads to submissiveness, clinging behavior, and fear of separation is characteristic. This behavior begins by early adulthood and is present in a variety of contexts, as indicated by **at least five** of the following:
a. **Inability to make everyday decisions** without an excessive amount of advice and reassurance from others
b. **Need for others to assume responsibility** for most major areas of their life
c. **Difficulty expressing disagreement** with others because of fear of loss of support or approval (realistic fears of retribution should not be included here)
d. **Difficulty initiating projects** or doing things on their own (as a result of a lack of self-confidence in judgment or abilities rather than a lack of motivation or energy)
e. **Goes to excessive lengths to obtain nurturance and support** from others, to the point of volunteering to do things that are unpleasant
f. **Feelings of discomfort or helplessness when alone** because of exaggerated fears of being unable to care for oneself
g. **Urgent seeking of another relationship** as a source of care and support when a close relationship ends
h. **Unrealistic preoccupation with fears** of being left to take care of oneself

3. **Associated features.** Children who have had a chronic physical illness or who have had separation anxiety may be at risk for this disorder in adulthood. Depression is common.

4. **Prevalence.** The prevalence is unknown, but passive-dependent traits are common. The diagnosis is more frequent in women and the youngest children in a family.

5. **Medical–surgical setting**
a. Being sick usually means being taken care of, and one might expect that dependent individuals would be good patients. However, **illness may provoke intolerable feelings of fear of abandon-**

ment and helplessness in these patients. There is a pull to regress to an earlier state of dependency, which may frighten patients because of its intensity. Feelings of dependency increase. Generally, dependent individuals become demanding and complaining when they are sick.

b. **Physicians need to set limits.** It is important for physicians, nurses, and other staff to meet with these patients to plan what kind of care is going to be given. For instance, it should be clear to patients how often the nurse will come by to check on them. If this is not done early, the negative reactions that these patients provoke can lead to punitive behavior on the part of the caregivers.

6. Treatment
   a. **Psychotherapy** can be very useful in the treatment of dependent patients. The focus is on the current behavior and its consequences. Therapists should be careful when there is a challenge to a pathologic but dependent relationship. Patients may leave therapy rather than give up such a relationship.
   b. Behavioral therapies, including **assertiveness training,** can be helpful.

C Obsessive-compulsive personality disorder

1. **Definition.** Affected individuals are perfectionistic, inflexible, and unable to express warm, tender feelings. They are preoccupied with trivial details and rules and do not appreciate changes in routine. **Obsessive-compulsive disorder (OCD)** is an Axis I anxiety disorder that involves irresistible obsessions and compulsions and should be distinguished from obsessive-compulsive personality disorder. Individuals with OCD may not have the personality disorder, and individuals with the personality disorder may not have the anxiety disorder.

2. **Symptoms.** Individuals with obsessive-compulsive personality disorder display a pervasive pattern of preoccupation with orderliness, perfectionism, and environmental and interpersonal control, at the expense of flexibility, openness, and efficiency. This behavior begins by early adulthood and is present in a variety of contexts, as indicated by at least four of the following:
   a. **Preoccupation with details, rules, lists, order, organization, or schedules** to the extent that the major point of the activity is lost
   b. **Perfectionism that interferes with task completion** (e.g., inability to complete a project because one's own overly strict standards are not met)
   c. **Excessive devotion to work and productivity** to the exclusion of leisure activities and friendships (not accounted for by obvious economic necessity)
   d. **Overconscientiousness, scrupulousness, and inflexibility about matters of morality, ethics, or values** (not accounted for by cultural or religious identification)
   e. **Inability to discard worn-out or worthless objects** even when they have no sentimental value
   f. **Reluctance to delegate tasks or to work with others** unless they submit to exactly their way of doing things
   g. Adoption of a **miserly spending style toward both oneself and others** (money is viewed as something to be hoarded for future catastrophes)
   h. **Rigidity and stubbornness**

3. **Associated features.** People with this disorder have few friends. They are difficult to live with and tend to drive people away. They may do very well in jobs that require detail and precision with little personal interaction. Hypochondriasis may develop later in life.

4. **Prevalence.** This disorder is more common in men and is believed to about 1% of the general population.

5. **Medical–surgical setting**
   a. Illness may be **perceived by compulsive individuals as a threat to their control** over impulses. Generally, stress increases compulsive behavior with an intensification of self-restraint and obstinacy.
      (1) Patients become more inflexible than before, which may lead to complaints about the sloppiness of the hospital and imprecision of the care being given.
      (2) When these patients are critical of failure to meet their standards, physicians should avoid defensive, authoritarian rebuttal. There is a fear of losing control of a situation on the part of these patients, and this may lead to a struggle for control with their physicians.

      b. Control should be shared with patients in as many ways as possible. Patients should be allowed to participate actively in the decisions and details of their actual medical care. This may include charting medication times, carefully calculating caloric intake, and monitoring fluid intake and output.

    6. Treatment. In general, individuals with compulsive personalities recognize that they have problems, unlike those with the other personality disorders. These patients know that they suffer from their inability to be flexible, and they realize that they do not permit themselves to have good feelings.

      a. Individual psychotherapy can be helpful, but treatment is difficult because these patients use the defense of isolation of affect. **Group therapy may be more useful.**

      b. Therapy should **focus on current feelings and situations,** and excessive time should not be spent on examining the psychological etiology of the condition. Struggles for control should be avoided. Depression, when present, should be treated.

VI   PERSONALITY DISORDERS NOT OTHERWISE SPECIFIED (NOS)

Patients may not always present with all the criteria for a specific personality disorder but still have clinically significant distress or impairment. In other situations, patients may present with symptoms of more than one personality disorder in a cluster. The NOS designation would then be appropriate if criteria were not met for any one disorder. This category also can be used when clinicians decide that a specific personality disorder not included in *DSM-IV* is appropriate.

A For example, **passive-aggressive personality disorder** was included in *DSM-III-R* but not *in DSM-IV* because studies indicated the diagnosis was too situation specific and described a cluster of symptoms more than a personality disorder.

B **Depressive personality disorder** has also been considered.

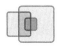 *Study Questions*

Directions: *Each of the numbered items in this section is followed by possible answers. Select the ONE numbered answer that is BEST in each case.*

1. A 28-year-old law student is admitted to the hospital for gallbladder problems. He is stubborn, rigid, and expects staff to adhere to his exact ways of doing things. He refuses to stop working on school papers. He reports that his girlfriend has threatened to leave him unless he changes his inflexible ways and throws out some of a large collection of useless junk. Which diagnosis appears more appropriate?

- [A] Antisocial
- [B] Avoidant
- [C] Histrionic
- [D] Obsessive-compulsive
- [E] Schizotypal

2. You expect the patient in Question 1 may act out in which of the following fashions when under stress in the hospital?

- [A] Strange behavior may put off caregivers
- [B] Sees hospitalization as a threat to his control
- [C] Can be charming but in a manipulative fashion; resists rules
- [D] Uses splitting, possibly dividing the staff, who might take sides
- [E] Likely to be cooperative and do well with the attention

3. You might recommend which of the following interventions to the staff regarding the patient in Question 1?

- [A] Set firm limits; consider an antidepressant.
- [B] Set firm limits on patient and staff roles; remain noncritical.
- [C] Odd behavior may make staff uneasy, but avoid ridicule.
- [D] Similar patients generally do well, but avoid criticism.
- [E] Share control with the patient in as many ways as possible.

4. Twin and adoption studies demonstrate which of the following characteristics?

- [A] Genetic factors do not affect personality disorder.
- [B] Axis I comorbidity is common.
- [C] Personality is too complex to measure biologically.
- [D] Cluster C disorders are inherited.
- [E] Personality traits have a strong genetic component.

5. When individuals with personality disorders are unable to see their role in the disturbances in their lives, the symptoms that develop are considered

- [A] Characterlogical
- [B] Ego dystonic
- [C] Ego syntonic
- [D] Internal
- [E] Self induced

6. You are called to the emergency room (ER) to see a 24-year-old woman who is waiting for stitches for a wrist laceration. She has been seen in the ER seven times previously for self-inflicted wrist lacerations. She reports rapid mood swings, impulsivity, a chronic feeling of emptiness, and periods in which she feels paranoid when under stress. Which diagnosis appears most appropriate?

- [A] Antisocial
- [B] Borderline
- [C] Obsessive-compulsive

    D. Paranoid

    E. Schizoid

7. You expect that this patient in Questions 6 may act out in which fashion when under stress in the hospital?

    A. Strange behavior may put off caregivers

    B. Can be charming but in a manipulative fashion

    C. Likely to be charming and fascinating; threatened attractiveness

    D. Uses splitting, possibly dividing the staff, who might take sides

    E. Likely to be cooperative and do well with the attention

8. For the patient in Question 6, you might recommend which of the following interventions to the staff?

    A. Be straightforward, explain everything, expect distrust.

    B. Odd behavior may make staff uneasy, but avoid ridicule.

    C. Set firm limits and consider an antidepressant.

    D. Similar patients generally do well, but avoid criticism.

    E. Share control with the patient in as many ways as possible.

9. A 35-year-old man presents requesting psychotherapy for problems with reacting angrily to his coworkers. The patient reports persistent fear that he will lose his job "due to a system that has it out for me." He reports distrust of others and a "look out for number one" philosophy. Which diagnosis appears most appropriate?

    A. Antisocial

    B. Avoidant

    C. Narcissistic

    D. Obsessive-compulsive

    E. Paranoid

10. You might recommend which form of treatment for this patient in Question 9?

    A. Start a MAO inhibitor antidepressant to reduce impulsivity.

    B. Refer him straight to group therapy.

    C. Start an antipsychotic and plan to explain treatment for side effects only if they occur.

    D. Cautiously begin individual psychotherapy.

    E. Tell the patient there is no hope for treatment and you will not take his money.

11. Persons who experience others as either "all good" or "all bad" and cannot experience an ambivalent relationship are exhibiting which of the following mechanisms?

    A. Denial

    B. Identification

    C. Projection

    D. Regression

    E. Splitting

12. The defense mechanism whereby an individual attributes to another individual thoughts or feelings of their own that are unacceptable is called:

    A. Dissociation

    B. Fantasy

    C. Isolation

    D. Projection

    E. Splitting

13. Which of the following medications has been useful in decreasing self-injury in patients with borderline personality disorder?

    A. Alprazolam

    B. Diazepam

    C. Diphenhydramine

⌐D⌐ Fluoxetine
⌐E⌐ Methylphenidate

14. Patients with which of the following personality disorders are most likely to handle the stress of hospitalization relatively well?

⌐A⌐ Antisocial
⌐B⌐ Avoidant
⌐C⌐ Borderline
⌐D⌐ Dependent
⌐E⌐ Schizotypal

15. A 35-year-old single man is admitted to the hospital for deep vein thrombosis. He has been inappropriately provocative and seductive toward the female staff. Dramatic and suggestible, he appears obsessed with his attractiveness. He exaggerates his familiarity with some staff members and displays shallow, shifting emotions. Which diagnosis appears most appropriate?

⌐A⌐ Antisocial
⌐B⌐ Avoidant
⌐C⌐ Histrionic
⌐D⌐ Obsessive-compulsive
⌐E⌐ Paranoid

16. You expect this patient in Question 15 may act out in which fashion when under stress in the hospital?

⌐A⌐ Aloof; may want to leave against medical advice
⌐B⌐ Will likely be charming and fascinating; his sense of attractiveness may be threatened by illness
⌐C⌐ Very guarded, suspicious, and quarrelsome
⌐D⌐ Will use splitting, possibly dividing the staff, who might take sides
⌐E⌐ Will see hospitalization as a threat to his control

17. For the patient in Question 15, you might recommend which of the following interventions to the staff?

⌐A⌐ Be straightforward, explain everything, and expect distrust.
⌐B⌐ Set firm limits and consider an antidepressant.
⌐C⌐ Similar patients generally do well, but avoid criticism.
⌐D⌐ Share control with the patient in as many ways as possible.
⌐E⌐ Set firm limits on patient and staff roles; remain noncritical.

18. A 19-year-old man with a 7-year history of legal charges is admitted for treatment of phlebitis secondary to intravenous drug abuse. On the ward, he was initially quite charming to the staff but became irritable and aggressive when denied requests for more pain medication. He is demanding to be discharged. When changing his bed, staff found syringes and needles he had taken from the drug cart when a nurse was tending to another patient. When the nurse was reprimanded by her supervisor, the patient showed no remorse for the consequences of his action. Which diagnosis appears most appropriate?

⌐A⌐ Antisocial
⌐B⌐ Narcissistic
⌐C⌐ Paranoid
⌐D⌐ Schizoid
⌐E⌐ Schizotypal

19. You expect this patient in Question 18 may act out in which of the following fashions when under stress in the hospital?

⌐A⌐ Aloof; may want to leave against medical advice
⌐B⌐ Strange behavior may put off caregivers
⌐C⌐ Will likely be charming and fascinating; his sense of attractiveness may be threatened by illness
⌐D⌐ Might suffer feelings of abandonment and helplessness
⌐E⌐ Can be charming but in a manipulative fashion; resists rules

20. You might recommend which of the following interventions to the staff for the patient in Question 18?

    A Set firm limits and consider an antidepressant.
    B Odd behavior may make staff uneasy, but avoid ridicule.
    C Set firm limits; anticipate a demand for discharge against medical advice.
    D Be straightforward, explain everything, and expect distrust.
    E Share control with patient in as many ways as possible.

21. You would recommend which of the following courses of treatment for this patient in Question 18 after discharge?

    A Treatment with benzodiazepines to reduce anxiety
    B Individual therapy focusing on building a strong patient–therapist relationship
    C Tell the patient there is no hope for treatment and you will not take his money
    D Group therapy with a particular therapist and patients
    E Volunteer work in a pain clinic to help develop more empathy

Directions: *Each set of matching questions in this section consists of a list of four to 26 lettered options (some of which may be in figures) followed by several numbered items. For each numbered item, select the ONE lettered option that is most closely associated with it. To avoid spending too much time on matching sets with large numbers of options, it is generally advisable to begin each set by reading the list of options. Then, for each item in the set, try to generate the correct answer and locate it in the option list, rather than evaluating each option individually. Each lettered option may be selected once, more than once, or not at all.*

QUESTIONS 22–29

For each patient description, select the appropriate personality disorder.

    A Antisocial
    B Avoidant
    C Dependent
    D Histrionic
    E Obsessive-compulsive
    F Paranoid
    G Schizotypal

22. Patients tend to group themselves in esoteric religious and pseudoscientific groups

23. Patients exhibit clairvoyance and telepathy.

24. Patients display behavior similar to that precipitated by brain damage.

25. Patients persistently bear grudges and are unforgiving of insults.

26. Patients believe that they are socially inept, personally unappealing, or inferior to others.

27. Patients are easily influenced by other people or by circumstances.

28. Patients have difficulty expressing disagreement with others because of fear of loss of support or approval.

29. Patients fear losing control.

QUESTIONS 30–34

For each characteristic listed, select the appropriate personality disorder.

- [A] Antisocial
- [B] Borderline
- [C] Narcissistic
- [D] Paranoid
- [E] Schizoid

30. Patients take offense quickly and question the loyalty of others.

31. Patients have a defective capacity to form social relationships.

32. Patients fail to plan ahead and are impulsive (e.g., may move without a job).

33. Patients form relationships that lack empathy; they idealize or devalue others.

34. Patients exude a sense of entitlement with the expectation of special favors but without assuming reciprocal responsibilities.

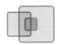 *Answers and Explanations*

1. The answer is D [*V C 2*]. Some diagnostic criteria for obsessive-compulsive personality disorder include preoccupation with details, perfectionism interfering with task completion, excessive devotion to work, scrupulousness, inability to discard collected belongings, reluctance to delegate, miserly spending style, rigidity, and stubbornness.

2. The answer is B [*V C 5*]. In the medical–surgical setting, persons with obsessive-compulsive personality disorder may become even more inflexible because the illness is perceived as a threat to their need for control.

3. The answer is E [*V C 5*]. In the medical treatment of persons with obsessive-compulsive personality disorder, sharing control with the patient may obviate the perceived threat to their need for control.

4. The answer is E [*I D*]. Twin studies have shown a strong genetic component to personality traits, but it has been difficult to demonstrate the same influence regarding personality disorders in cluster C (i.e., avoidant, dependent, and obsessive-compulsive personalities). Comorbidity has not been the focus of twin studies.

5. The answer is C [*I B*]. Patients with personality disorders perceive their problem and express their symptoms differently from patients with other psychiatric illnesses. Patients with personality disorders often believe that the disturbance in their lives is caused by the outside world, rather than internally, the symptoms of which are called ego syntonic. Symptoms of a personality disorder are caused by the characterlogical style of the patient. Symptoms include feelings of anxiety, depression, and anger, but these symptoms do not meet the criteria for a specific Axis I disorder.

6. The answer is B [*IV B 2*]. Some diagnostic criteria for borderline personality disorder include impulsivity, recurrent suicidal or self-mutilating behavior, rapid mood swings, chronic feelings of emptiness, and possible paranoia when under stress.

7. The answer is D [*IV B 5 b*]. In the medical–surgical setting, persons with borderline personality disorder may use splitting as a defensive mechanism, sometimes resulting in dividing the staff, who might take sides.

8. The answer is C [*V B 5*]. In the treatment of patients with borderline personality disorder, setting firm limits and providing structure can be therapeutic. Antidepressants can help some patients control impulsivity and self-injury while supporting mood.

9. The answer is E [*III B 2*]. Some diagnostic criteria for paranoid personality disorder include suspicion of being exploited or deceived, doubts about the loyalty of others, reluctance to confide in others, perceiving threats or attacks in benign remarks and actions, and angry reactions to perceived threats.

10. The answer is D [*III B 5*]. Patients with paranoid personality disorder may respond to treatment, but psychotherapy is preferred to pharmacotherapy. Low doses of antipsychotic medication can help at times, but side effects could be perceived as a threat. Individual psychotherapy is a better choice than referral straight to group therapy.

11. The answer is E [*II B 1*]. These patients "split" the good and bad aspects of a normal relationship because they cannot tolerate the emotions of ambivalence. The same person may be "all good" at one moment only to become "all bad" at another time. Caregivers sometimes begin to act toward the patient and each other in these stereotypical ways.

12. The answer is D [*II A 1 a*]. Projection is the defense mechanism whereby an individual attributes to another individual thoughts or feelings of their own that are unacceptable. Fantasy is the creation of an imaginary life. Regression is a retreat to earlier defenses. Splitting is attributing only all good or all bad qualities to an individual. Identification is the unconscious patterning of aspects of another individual's personality.

13. The answer is D [*IV B 6 b (2)*]. Modern drugs such as fluoxetine and other serotonergic antidepressants have shown some efficacy in reducing behavioral impulsivity and self-injury in borderline patients. Benzodiazepines such as alprazolam and diazepam should be avoided because they may cause disinhibition or be abused. Antihistamines such as diphenhydramine are sometimes used for sedation but do not effect self-injury. Stimulants are contraindicated unless the patient has another condition for which stimulants would be appropriate.

14. The answer is B [*V A 5*]. Patients with avoidant personality disorder are undemanding and generally cooperative. A medical illness allows them to be taken care of, which may help their psychiatric disorder. Patients with schizotypal, dependent, antisocial, and paranoid personality disorders all tend to have more problematic interactions with staff while hospitalized.

15. The answer is C [*IV C 2*]. Some diagnostic criteria for histrionic personality disorder include a need to be the center of attention, inappropriate seductive or provocative behavior, obsession with physical attractiveness, dramatic behavior and impressionistic speech, suggestibility, and exaggeration of the importance of relationships.

16. The answer is B [*IV D 5 a and b*]. In the medical–surgical setting, persons with histrionic personality disorder may give the impression of being charming and fascinating. The patient's dependence on their sense of attractiveness may be threatened by illness.

17. The answer is E [*IV D 5 c*]. In the treatment of persons with histrionic personality disorder, setting firm limits on patient and staff roles is critical. At the same time, staff should try to remain noncritical of behavior symptomatic of the disorder.

18. The answer is A [*IV A 2*]. Some diagnostic criteria for antisocial personality disorder include evidence of conduct disorder with onset before age 15 years, a pattern of disregard for or violation of the rights of others, irritable and aggressive behavior, deceitfulness, recklessness, and lack of remorse.

19. The answer is E [*IV A 5 a and b*]. In the medical–surgical setting, persons with antisocial personality disorder may give the impression of being quite charming but in a manipulative fashion. They may resist hospital rules and be noncompliant, and when challenged, they may leave treatment against medical advice.

20. The answer is C [*IV A 5 c*]. In the treatment of persons with antisocial personality disorder, setting firm limits is important but often triggers a demand to leave treatment against medical advice.

21. The answer is D [*IV A 5 c*]. Antisocial personality disorder can respond to treatment. Group psychotherapy can be effective, but an experienced therapist and particular group of patients are needed. Controlled substances may be abused by some persons with antisocial personality disorder.

22–29. The answers are: 22-F [*III B 3*], **23-G** [*III C 2*], **24-A** [*II A 4 b*], **25-F** [*III B 2*], **26-B** [*V A 2*], **27-D** [*IV D 2*], **28-C** [*V B 2*], **29-E** [*V C 2*]. Patients with the cluster A disorders, paranoid and schizotypal personality disorders, are odd and eccentric. Paranoid persons tend to form into eccentric groups and hold grudges. Schizotypal people have odd thinking such as clairvoyance.

Patients with the cluster B group of disorders, which includes histrionic and antisocial personality disorders, are dramatic and erratic. Histrionic patients are highly suggestible. Sometimes compulsive, antisocial behavior can be precipitated by brain damage.

Patients with the cluster C group of personality disorders display anxious and fearful features. Avoidant people fear that no one will like them because they are not "good enough." Dependent persons will do anything to keep from being left alone, and obsessive patients are fearful of losing control.

30–34. **The answers are:** 30-D [*III B 2 b*], 31-E [*III A 1 a*], 32-A [*IV A 2 c*], 33-B [*IV B 2*], 34-C [*IV C 2 c, d*]. Patients with paranoid personality disorder are suspicious about the motives of others and have a basic deficit in trusting others, so they easily take offense and question whether others are loyal.

Although all personality disorders cause problems relating to interpersonal relationships, people with a schizoid personality lack the capacity to form such relationships.

Irresponsibility and the inability to consider the consequences of impulsive actions are the features of patients with antisocial personality disorder. Whereas all personality disorders tend to cause problems in the workplace, antisocial people have particular difficulty being reliable.

A hallmark of individuals with borderline personality disorder is a pattern of unstable and intense interpersonal relationships. Splitting, in which people are experienced as "all good" or "all bad," can be seen in other disorders but is most often seen in those with borderline personality disorder.

People with narcissistic personality disorder expect to be treated specially without actually having achieved merit. They feel entitled and tend to exploit others. Although they need and seek admiration from others, they lack the ability to identify with others' feelings.

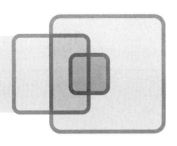

chapter 3

Psychotic Disorders

ROBERT BREEN

I INTRODUCTION

A Schizophrenia is a disorder characterized by derangement of thought processes, affect, and behavior. The disorder involves expression of positive and negative symptoms.

1. **Positive symptoms** are those that are added to the presentation such as delusions, hallucinations, catatonia, and agitation.
2. **Negative symptoms** are patient characteristics that appear missing from the presentation. This may involve affective flattening, apathy, social withdrawal, anhedonia, and poverty of thought and content of speech.

B Established biologic markers or pathognomonic clinical features that define schizophrenia do not exist.

1. The *Diagnostic and Statistical Manual of Mental Disorders,* 4th edition (*DSM-IV*), has been edited so that elements from previous diagnostic systems and from studies of the frequency of symptoms in different populations form the current diagnostic criteria for schizophrenia.
   a. The **diagnostic criteria** of the *DSM-IV* represent a departure from trends established by the *DSM-III* and the *DSM-III-R* in that they are **less specific concerning symptoms** of schizophrenia and oriented more toward the course of the disorder (Tables 3–1 and 3–2). Current criteria for the diagnosis of schizophrenia require that some symptoms be present for at least 6 months with significant disturbance for at least 1 month of that time. The actual course varies widely among individuals.
   b. The newer criteria are **more inclusive.**
2. The **International Pilot Study of Schizophrenia,** a World Health Organization study, attempted to discover reliable methods of diagnosing schizophrenia across different cultures and national boundaries.
   a. Using psychiatric interviews and the Present State Examination (PSE), researchers noted the **most common symptoms** (Table 3–3). However, these frequently occurring symptoms are also common in other conditions such as organic mental disorders and mood disorders.
   b. This diagnostic approach is of limited use with individual patients because it does not propose minimal or threshold criteria for the diagnosis in individual cases. Rather, it has been a basis for other diagnostic systems such as the *DSM-III-R* and, to a lesser extent, the *DSM-IV.*

C Even in research studies of schizophrenia, when rigorous diagnostic criteria are applied, the prognosis is highly variable.

II EPIDEMIOLOGY

It is difficult to draw precise conclusions concerning the epidemiology of schizophrenia. Studies have often conflicted because of difficulty in defining diagnostic criteria, difficulty in sampling methods for such a disabling psychotic illness, and differences in expression and prognosis across different cultures.

TABLE 3–1 *DSM-IV* Diagnostic Criteria for Schizophrenia

A. Two of the following for most of 1 month:
  1. Delusions
  2. Hallucinations
  3. Disorganized speech
  4. Grossly disorganized or catatonic behavior
  5. Negative symptoms
  (Note: Only one of these is required if delusions are bizarre or if hallucinations consist of a voice keeping up a running commentary on the person's behavior or thoughts or if there are two or more voices conversing with each other.)
B. Marked social or occupational dysfunction.
C. Duration of at least 6 months of persistent symptoms such as attenuated forms of group A symptoms (above) or negative symptoms. At least 1 month of this must include a group A symptom.
D. Symptoms of schizoaffective and mood disorder are ruled out.
E. Substance abuse and medical conditions are ruled out as etiological.

A **Incidence, prevalence, and cost**

1. **Incidence.** Reported values range between 0.11 and 0.70 per 1,000. The most recent studies indicate that the incidence of schizophrenia may have declined during the past 10 to 20 years. Problems with sampling and changes in diagnostic criteria may account for the decreased incidence.

2. **Prevalence.** As with the incidence of schizophrenia, developing countries generally have lower prevalence rates of schizophrenia, which reflects lower incidence rates and better prognostic

---

TABLE 3–2 Schizophrenia Subtypes

In all of the following subtypes of schizophrenia, the diagnostic criteria for schizophrenia must be met first, particularly criterion A symptoms:

Paranoid Type
A. Preoccupation with one or more delusions or frequent auditory hallucinations
B. Does not have prominent disorganized speech, disorganized behavior, flat or inappropriate affect, or catatonic behavior.

Disorganized Type
A. All of the following are prominent:
  1. Disorganized speech
  2. Disorganized behavior
  3. Flat or inappropriate affect
B. Does not meet criteria for catatonic type

Catatonic Type
The clinical picture is dominated by at least two of the following:
A. Motoric immobility as evidenced by catalepsy or stupor
B. Excessive motor activity (apparently purposeless and not influenced by external stimuli)
C. Extreme negativism or mutism
D. Peculiarities of voluntary movement such as posturing, stereotyped movements, prominent mannerisms, or prominent grimacing
E. Echolalia or echopraxia

Undifferentiated Type
Symptoms of schizophrenia criteria A are present, but the criteria are not met for paranoid, catatonic, or disorganized types.

Residual Type
A. Criterion A for schizophrenia is no longer met and criteria for other subtypes of schizophrenia are not met.
B. Evidence of the disturbance (evidenced by negative symptoms or two or more criterion A symptoms) is present in an attenuated form.

TABLE 3–3 **Symptoms of Schizophrenia**

Most Frequently Found Symptoms*	Highest Reliability of Symptoms	Lowest Reliability of Symptoms
Lack of insight	Suicidal ideation	Negativism
Auditory hallucinations	Elated thoughts	Perseveration
Verbal hallucinations	Ideas of reference	Stereotyped behavior
Ideas of reference	Delusions of grandeur	(e.g., lip smacking, chewing)
Suspiciousness	Hearing thoughts aloud	
Flatness of affect	Derealization	
Voices speaking to the patient	Lack of concentration	
Delusional mood	Hopelessness	
Delusions of persecution	Delusions of persecution and reference	
Inadequate description of problems		
Thought alienation		
Thoughts spoken aloud		

*In descending order.

expectations than in the industrialized world (e.g., schizophrenic patients in developing countries tend to recover from their illness at a higher rate than do schizophrenic patients in industrialized nations).

   a. **Point prevalence** (i.e., the number of cases at one moment in time) has been widely estimated to range between 0.6 and 8.3.

   b. **Lifetime prevalence** in the United States was estimated to be 1.3% in the Epidemiologic Catchment Area (ECA) study.

3. **Cost.** In the United States, the most recent cost estimate for has risen to $65 billion annually.

B **Gender**   In the Western world, schizophrenia occurs in men and women at approximately equal rates; however, men tend to develop the disease earlier than do women. In developing countries, men appear to suffer from schizophrenia at a rate that may be several times that of women. Perhaps because of the difference in age of onset, whereas men with schizophrenia tend never to have been married, affected women tend to be divorced or separated.

C **Role of socioeconomic status**   The prevalence and incidence of schizophrenia as well as disease course correlate with socioeconomic status.

1. **In the United States,** the highest rates are found in the **lower socioeconomic classes,** suggesting that either socioeconomic factors produce or precipitate schizophrenia or that schizophrenic patients tend to drift downward in socioeconomic status (i.e., **drift hypothesis**). According to the ECA studies, the risk of schizophrenia in people in the lowest socioeconomic quartile was eight times higher than in individuals in the highest quartile.

2. During the **Depression of the 1930s,** the outcome of schizophrenia in the United States and Great Britain was worse than either before or after that period of time.

3. **In India,** the highest rates occur in the upper castes, suggesting that social stress on a class of people, rather than drift, may be a major factor in precipitating schizophrenia.

4. **In cities with populations of more than 100,000,** the incidence increases in proportion to the size of the city, although this relationship does not hold true in rural areas and smaller cities.

D **Premorbid personality**   Although certain personality features seem to antedate the development of schizophrenia in about 25% of cases, research has not demonstrated specific personality features that reliably predict the development of schizophrenia. A study of home movies suggests that preschizophrenic children show greater negative affect than normal siblings, and female preschizophrenic children consistently show less joy in their facial expressions.

III ETIOLOGY

Just as Eugen Bleuler felt the need to refer to the "group of schizophrenias," we must think in terms of the "etiologies" of schizophrenia. The etiology of schizophrenia is complex and yet undetermined. No one set of theories can account for the complicated onset and far-ranging symptoms of schizophrenia. Schizophrenia transmission in families does not fit any known pattern of pure genetic transmission, and current theories suggest a pattern that may be activated through as yet unknown biologic, social, and psychological factors. Proposed etiologies include the following:

A Genetic theories   Genetic factors clearly play a role, but the actual manner of genetic transmission of schizophrenia is complicated. Recent evidence that schizotypal personality disorder is more common in relatives of persons with schizophrenia has bolstered genetic theories. (This association is also valid for adopted relatives.)

1. **Familial transmission.** Some studies show high rates of mental illness in relatives of patients with schizophrenia (not necessarily schizophrenia). Alternatively, positive traits such as creativity are found in some cases. The risk of disease in first-degree relatives of individuals with the illness is 3% to 7%. However, recent studies that involve narrower diagnostic criteria than those used previously suggest that the risk may be lower than once indicated.
   a. **Twins**
      (1) A simple single gene transmission of schizophrenia is no longer plausible. Findings indicate that monozygotic twins have a 53% risk of developing schizophrenia, despite having identical genotypes.
      (2) According to one study, whereas monozygotic twins raised together have a concordance rate of 91%, monozygotic twins raised apart have a concordance rate of 78%. Other studies of twins reveal a concordance rate of 40% to 50% for monozygotic twins and about 10% to 14% for dizygotic twins.
   b. **Parents.** If both parents are schizophrenic, a child's risk of developing schizophrenia ranges between 15% and 55%. Single gene transmission with variable penetrance is suggested by findings of increased risk in families with more than one schizophrenic member. The risk is 17% in persons with one sibling and one parent with schizophrenia and 47% in those with two parents with schizophrenia.

2. **Other genetic associations. Polygenic transmission** more easily accounts for some of the discord in genetic studies; it is consistent with the differences in severity of the disease and the variable rates of pathology in some families. To prove a polygenic basis of transmission will likely take more progress in efforts to map the entire human genome.
   a. Reports of a gene location on **chromosome 5** are associated with some patterns of familial transmission, but later studies have failed to replicate this finding.
   b. **Defects in smooth pursuit eye movements** have also been associated with some familial patterns of transmission. Although the association cannot explain all of the smooth pursuit ocular motor dysfunction in schizophrenia, it may prove useful in future studies of the genetic transmission of schizophrenia.

B Developmental theories   Rigorous research studies in the latter half of the twentieth century have suggested that developmental factors play a major role in the etiology of schizophrenia.

1. **Fetal exposure to risk factors**
   a. **Season of birth** appears to be correlated with the risk of developing schizophrenia. In both the Northern and Southern hemispheres, the risk for developing schizophrenia is greatest for individuals born in the late winter and early spring. **Prenatal exposure to a virus** such as influenza is implicated.
   b. **Prenatal malnutrition** has also been suggested. There was an increase in the risk of developing schizophrenia for persons born after the Dutch hardship winter (1945–1946) during World War II, when food was scarce in the Netherlands. Low birth weight is also associated with an increased risk of developing schizophrenia.

2. **Obstetric complications. Fetal hypoxia** is known to cause such neurologic conditions as cerebral palsy and mental retardation. Up to a ninefold increase in risk of schizophrenia is associated

with preeclampsia. However, schizophrenia is much less common than obstetric complications, so fetal hypoxia is not the sole etiologic factor.

C **Psychological theories**

1. **Psychological testing** is clearly abnormal in persons with schizophrenia and also in some of their relatives without expression of the disease. Biological differences more readily explain such testing abnormalities. Psychological testing shows:
    a. **Lack of creativity and imagination** on the Thematic Apperception Test and the Rorschach test in persons with schizophrenia. Test results indicate preservation of verbal intelligence but not performance intelligence quotient (IQ) on the Wechsler Adult Intelligence Scale (WAIS).
    b. **Attention deficits,** which are common on testing in both persons with schizophrenia and some of their relatives
    c. **Loss of executive function,** which makes it difficult for persons with schizophrenia to make choices and decisions about simple things such as what to wear and when to eat. Clinical loss of executive function may be a factor in the development of negative symptoms.

2. At one time, theories involving **family interaction** were a credible etiologic basis for schizophrenia, but the rapidly increasing mass of biologic data concerning the development of schizophrenia has negated these hypotheses.
    a. The theory that the illness was caused by mistakes in mothering by a so-called **"schizophrenigenic mother"** has been discredited.
    b. **Double-bind communications** are no longer thought to play an etiologic role in schizophrenia. Double-bind communication has the following characteristics:
        (1) An **intense relationship** between those involved
        (2) Two messages expressed on different levels that **conflict with or deny each other**
        (3) A child who is forbidden from commenting on or clarifying messages, which results in frequent "no-win" situations in which the child cannot avoid conflict no matter the response. The psychological distress created by such a situation was once thought to result in psychosis.
    c. **"Expressed emotions,"** with a high level of affect with criticism and overinvolvement, were once thought to cause schizophrenia. More recent research indicates that this style of communication does occur in some families but that it is more closely likely to cause an exacerbation of schizophrenia, not the first episode. Family education projects that attempt to change this style and make it more noncritical have had positive effects on outcome.

3. **Cultural causes** of schizophrenia have been investigated to explain differences in incidence between industrialized and rural areas. However, economic factors that affect access to nutrition, sanitation, and health care are more likely to account for any cultural differences.

D **Biologic mechanisms** Modern scientific study has attempted to explain schizophrenia through chemical or biological mechanisms. No one abnormality appears to account for the spectrum of symptoms in schizophrenia. Most likely, abnormal cell development or cell damage in multiple regions of the brain mediated by multiple chemical messenger systems cause the disease.

1. **Neurotransmitter system abnormalities**
    a. **Dopamine.** One of the oldest theories of the etiology of schizophrenia is that dopamine and dopaminergic neurons are the primary systems involved in the pathophysiology of schizophrenia.
        (1) Dopamine receptors, particularly D-2 receptors, are found in abnormal numbers in the brains of persons with schizophrenia. D-2 receptor blockade is the sine qua non of the antipsychotic effects of typical neuroleptics.
        (2) Positron emission tomography (PET) scans indicate increased activity of dopaminergic neurons in the limbic system, which is strongly correlated with hallucinations and other positive symptoms of schizophrenia.
        (3) PET scans also indicate decreased activity of dopaminergic neurons in the frontal lobes and prefrontal cortex, which is correlated with the negative symptoms of schizophrenia.
    b. **Serotonin.** Investigation into serotoninergic systems has been one of the most active areas of schizophrenia research and drug development over the past 2 decades.

        (1) Early investigation of some psychotomimetic compounds showed high levels of activity in serotoninergic systems of the brain.

        (2) Serotoninergic neurons are known to project from the midbrain into the prefrontal cortex and frontal lobes and a variety of other brain regions that may inhibit the function of dopaminergic neurons.

        (3) Abnormal levels of serotonin and its metabolite 5-hydroxyindoleacetic acid have been found in the cerebrospinal fluid (CSF) of persons with schizophrenia (and also in those who have committed suicide).

    c. Glutamate. An exciting new area of research into the biological dysfunction of schizophrenia is centered on the neurotransmitter glutamate.

        (1) Glutamate levels are reduced in the CSF of persons with schizophrenia. In addition, glutamate receptor antagonists such as phencyclidine can cause schizophrenia-like psychotic symptoms in normal research subjects.

        (2) In vivo testing using magnetic resonance imaging (MRI) spectroscopy and postmortem pathologic studies have both demonstrated signs of decreased glutamate activity in the pyramidal neurons of the prefrontal cortex.

        (3) Glutaminergic neurons interact with both serotonergic and dopaminergic systems.

    d. γ-Aminobutyric acid (GABA). Scientists also believe that GABA, a fast-acting neurotransmitter in the brain that plays a critical role in the expression of anxiety disorders, plays an inhibitory role with dopaminergic neurons. In this way, GABA may be responsible for terminating or controlling the activity within dopamine systems.

        (1) Low levels of GABA are found early in the course of schizophrenia.

        (2) Benzodiazepines, which work in part as GABA agonists, can relieve some symptoms of schizophrenia in some patients.

        (3) Baclofen, a GABA receptor antagonist, can exacerbate schizophrenia.

2. Structural abnormalities. More than 100 years of scientific research have revealed a wide range of structural abnormalities in the brains of persons with schizophrenia. Unfortunately, such studies have tended to be small, sometimes lacking rigorous controls.

    a. Enlargement of the lateral ventricles is the most consistent finding. With loss of brain mass through developmental failure or neuron death, the CSF would expand to fill the space. Up to now, it has been impossible to identify any one brain region as the primary site of neuron loss.

    b. Decreased size of the thalamus has been reported in several studies. The thalamus is an important area in the complex interconnection of various brain regions, and a dysfunctional thalamus may disrupt function of wide-ranging areas of the brain.

    c. Abnormalities in the size of the hippocampus is another frequent finding. Scores of studies have identified a smaller than usual hippocampus in schizophrenia. What is unclear is when cell loss occurs: in utero, in childhood, or upon development of symptoms.

    d. Abnormalities in the cell architecture in the **prefrontal cortex** have been reported. This condition may impair the effective transmission of neuronal impulses from the limbic system as well as from higher order association areas in the parietal and temporal regions.

3. Functional abnormalities. The development of **PET and MRI spectroscopy** allows viewing of the functioning brains of persons with schizophrenia with little risk of harm to the subjects.

    a. An **increase in activity in the limbic system** is closely correlated with the **positive symptoms** of schizophrenia. Administration of either **typical** or **atypical neuroleptics** can reverse this overactivity.

    b. A decrease in activity in the frontal lobes of persons with schizophrenia is closely correlated with the **negative symptoms** of schizophrenia. Administration of **atypical neuroleptics** can sometimes reverse this hypoactive state.

4. Other abnormalities

    a. Recent studies have found **abnormal levels of phospholipids** in some cell membranes of schizophrenia patients. Abnormal cell membrane function would disable normal neurotransmitter function.

    b. G proteins, another cell membrane constituent, may play a role in schizophrenia. G proteins have a key function: they relay messages from neurotransmitter receptors in the membrane to second messenger systems within the neuron. Activation of these second messenger systems can influence multiple intracellular processes, including genetic transcription within the nucleus.

IV CHARACTERISTIC FEATURES

Clinical expression of schizophrenia varies according to diagnostic criteria used to define the population and, to some extent, the etiologic models of the clinician or researcher. In general, features of schizophrenia reported by patients (e.g., hallucinations) tend to be more reliable than those observed by clinicians (e.g., poverty of thought content). Symptoms usually include disruptions in areas of psychological and social functioning. However, even in cases of severe disruption, some areas of functioning may be preserved (e.g., a hospitalized patient with chronic schizophrenia who exhibits bizarre behavior and severe disruptions of speech and thinking may retain the skills of a concert pianist). Symptoms of schizophrenia may change and become less severe over the course of the illness.

A **Form of thought** refers to the structure of thought as experienced by patients and displayed through verbal communication. Disturbances in the form of thought are defined as **formal thought disorder,** which may manifest in the following ways:

1. **Loosening of associations** is observed in speech when connections among the patient's ideas are absent or obscure. Listeners may feel as if understanding of the patient's thought had been suddenly lost. (In contrast, in the tangentiality and flight of ideas typical of mania and anxiety disorders, patients may express coherent ideas but lose the point of a string of ideas.) Examples of loosening of associations are listed below.

   a. **Word use may be highly idiosyncratic and individualized.** Words may be created (**neologism**) or selected by patients using their own internal logic and special symbolism.

   b. **Abnormal concept formation is a perceptual defect** in which patients are unable to exclude irrelevant or competing ideas from their consciousness; their thinking becomes overinclusive. Extraneous items and details that have specific meaning to patients are incorporated into the patients' communication but are difficult for listeners to follow.

   c. **Logic in schizophrenia may follow a primitive pattern** (in the piagetian sense). Illogical reasoning, exclusion of important information from the reasoning process, and frank distortion of logical connections occur in schizophrenic patients. Patients assume the existence of causal connections when others perceive no such connections. Patients may treat symbols as if they were actual objects or may inappropriately substitute them for other logical elements.

   d. **Concreteness may substitute for abstraction.** In general, patients with early-onset schizophrenia may experience greater deterioration of abstraction ability than patients with late-onset disease, as measured by psychological tests. Simultaneous preoccupation with symbols and abstractions, as well as the loss of the ability to process these, are features commonly seen among schizophrenic patients.

      (1) The ability to form abstract ideas may be severely impaired.

      (2) The ability to discern abstractions within ideas may become limited, and concrete interpretations of abstract ideas may become predominant.

      (3) The ability to understand metaphors and similes may be lost.

   e. **Language structural problems** are seen in individuals with schizophrenia, but many of these problems are rare. However, unusual, stilted language is common. Examples include:

      (1) **Neologisms**

      (2) **Verbigeration** (the persistent repetition of words or phrases)

      (3) **Echolalia** (a repetition of the words or phrases of the examiner, which is seen in severely disorganized psychotic states)

      (4) **Mutism** (a functional inhibition of speech and vocalization, which is seen in a variety of nonpsychotic and psychotic illnesses)

      (5) **"Word salad"** (a complete lack of language, which is seen in patients with psychosis and several very specific central nervous system [CNS] lesions)

2. **Poverty of content and speech** is seen in several of the schizophrenic spectrum disorders. Speech may be complex, concrete, or limited in overall productivity, but it generally lacks specific information content.

3. **Thought blocking** is an internal interruption in patients' speech and flow of thought. It may appear that a hallucination may interrupt patients, although they may not be able to identify the interruption.

B **Content of thought** refers to the most characteristic feature of schizophrenia, **delusions,** which are defined as fixed, false beliefs. Delusions cannot be changed by reasoning and are inconsistent with the beliefs of the patients' cultural group. However, they may have a culturally based content (e.g., Americans who believe that they are the targets of influence by the Central Intelligence Agency). In some cases, delusions may be so individualistic that no cultural connections can be made. Delusions may be relatively circumscribed or may pervade all aspects of patients' life and thinking. In some cases, delusions may appear relatively trivial to patients, but more commonly, they become an organizing force in patients' lives. Delusions may be simple in their organization or highly complex and systematized. Sexual, religious, and philosophical content of delusions are common.

1. **Delusions of persecution** are beliefs that others are trying to harm, spy on, influence, or humiliate patients or interfere with their affairs. Persecutory delusions are frequently pervasive and actively incorporate features of patients' lives.

2. **Delusions of reference** are beliefs that random events in the environment have special meaning and are directed specifically at patients (e.g., talking by strangers, television, or radio about patients; random events such as accidents that have been designed to harm or influence patients). **Ideas of reference** differ from delusions of reference in intensity rather than form.

3. **Delusions of influence** are beliefs that patients' thoughts and actions are controlled by outside forces. In extreme cases, patients feel as if they were robots without thoughts and actions of their own. Patients may believe that body parts, frequently the genitals, are manipulated by unseen forces. Likewise, patients may feel as if their thoughts have been removed and replaced by alien thoughts.

4. **Thought broadcasting** involves thoughts leaving a patient's head and going directly to objects in the environment. Patients may experience this as a physical sensation. For those who have not experienced this phenomenon, thought broadcasting is difficult to understand.

5. **Grandiose delusions** are more common in patients with mania than in those with schizophrenia. However, schizophrenic patients may feel as though they are central figures in the complex delusional systems in the environment. Patients' feelings of having special knowledge, special relationships with important figures, or of posing a threat to conspiracies may all be considered grandiose. These grandiose delusions are differentiated from the expansive and positive grandiose delusions that are typical of mania.

6. **Somatic delusions** in schizophrenic patients typically include feelings that the body has been manipulated or altered by outside forces. These somatic delusions must be differentiated from the somatic delusions of other disorders (e.g., having cancer or a decaying body), which are typical of major depression with melancholic features. Patients with somatic delusions may feel that:
   a. An electronic device has been placed in their body.
   b. Their body is under the control of others.
   c. Portions of their body are not their own.

C **Perceptual disorders** include a variety of distortions of sensory experiences and their interpretation. **Recent data suggest that a fundamental perceptual defect in schizophrenia is the inability to habituate and suppress extraneous environmental stimuli or internal thought processes.** However, it must be emphasized that **no perceptual disturbance is pathognomonic of schizophrenia.** Perceptual distortions may occur in healthy people as well as in patients with mood disorders or organic mental syndromes.

1. **Hallucinations** are sensory experiences that occur without corresponding environmental stimuli.
   a. **Auditory hallucinations** range from unformed buzzing sounds to complex voices holding conversations. The most characteristic auditory hallucinations of schizophrenia include hearing voices speaking about a patient in the third person, hearing voices making derogatory comments about the patient, and hearing one voice telling the patient to commit some action.
      (1) The voices may be muffled or distinct, familiar or unfamiliar, single or multiple, and of either gender. Patients may hear their own voice spoken aloud.

(2) Command hallucinations are a special form of auditory hallucination in which voices tell a patient to commit some action. In some patients, these hallucinations are so persistent that they become difficult to resist. Patients who hear command hallucinations telling them to harm themselves or others must be considered dangerous.

    b. **Visual hallucinations** are also experienced by schizophrenic patients, although they are more common in other disorders, particularly organic mental disorders. These hallucinations may be simple, but they are most characteristic of schizophrenia when they are complex and related to a patient's delusional system (e.g., a visit from aliens).

    c. **Other hallucinations may be tactile, gustatory, olfactory** (frequently an unpleasant and indescribable odor), or **somatic.** Similar to visual hallucinations, these hallucinatory experiences also occur in individuals with other disorders (e.g., olfactory hallucinations in complex partial seizures). In schizophrenic patients, they are frequently connected to delusional systems.

2. **Illusions** are misperceptions or misidentifications of identifiable environmental events or objects that may occur in any sensory modality. Illusions are common in a variety of disorders and occur in normal individuals as well. In schizophrenic patients, illusions may be variants of a normal experience given a delusional explanation.

    a. **"Déjà vu"** feelings are those in which unfamiliar situations feel strangely familiar. These illusions also occur as a normal phenomenon and in several forms of epilepsy.

    b. **"Jamais vu"** feelings are defined as those in which familiar situations feel novel and unfamiliar. These illusions also occur in epilepsy.

    c. **Hypersensitivity** to light, sound, or smell is common in schizophrenia and other disorders such as migraine headaches.

    d. **Distorted perceptions of time** also occur in a variety of conditions such as dissociative states and anxiety.

    e. **Misperceptions of movement, perspective, and size,** which are typical of organic conditions and anxiety, also occur in schizophrenia.

    f. **Changes in body perception** of one's own body or the body of others also occur.

D **Affect** is defined as the observable manifestations of mood and emotion. Affective findings in patients with schizophrenia may be, in some cases, unreliable because of the parkinsonian effects of the neuroleptic drugs and to cultural differences in body language. Affective disturbances in schizophrenia include **blunted affect, flat affect,** and **inappropriate affect** (see Chapter 1).

E **Sense of self** is the perception of one's individuality, separateness from others, and continuity in space and time. The erosion of the sense of self may lead to the delusions of reference and influence found in schizophrenia.

1. **In normal individuals,** a solid sense of self is thought to be the basis of good self-esteem and an ability of the individual to weather losses, disappointments, and slights from others.

2. **In schizophrenia,** as well as in other conditions, a disrupted sense of self may manifest as:
    a. Loss of self-esteem
    b. Confusion about sexual identity
    c. An inability to separate oneself from events in the environment (i.e., feeling that one's thoughts have harmed another person)
    d. Projection of one's own fears or suspicions onto others
    e. Experiencing the self and others as dichotomous opposites (i.e., all good or all bad) with little integration of the opposing features

F **Volitional symptoms** are among the most persistent and intractable features of schizophrenia. Difficulties initiating and maintaining purposeful and goal-directed activity and interest in the environment may account for the difficulties many patients with schizophrenia experience in maintaining stable work and living situations.

1. **Interest** in the environment may be difficult to generate and maintain for schizophrenic patients. This difficulty may be related to ambivalence or to an inability to generate interest internally. It may result from conflicting wishes or desires.

2. **Initiative,** or the ability to begin a goal-directed activity, is often lacking in advanced cases of schizophrenia. Patients may experience difficulty finding housing, financial support, and other

needs as a consequence of this symptom. They may also be unable to initiate spontaneous movement without direction from others.

3. **Drive** is the ability to pursue a goal-directed activity after it has been started. Difficulties in maintaining goal-directed behavior appear to be common in, although not unique to, schizophrenia. These difficulties may be a result of the cognitive symptoms experienced by these patients or the inability to sustain thoughts amid the perceptual and cognitive disturbances of schizophrenia.

4. **Ambition** may be preserved in the absence of drive and initiative, as in patients whose grandiose wishes are to be film or music stars, or ambition may be absent. Unrealistic ambitions combined with the patients' delusions may be an organizing principle for complex dysfunctional patterns of behavior.

G **Relationship to the external world** may change. Patients with schizophrenia tend to become increasingly preoccupied with internal events and decreasingly influenced by external events. Preoccupation with delusional and hallucinatory symptoms and difficulty in communicating with others may lead to withdrawal from the world, which is called autism in its extreme form.

H **Motor activity** may change. Some alterations in motor activity and behavior may be associated with the pharmacologic treatment of schizophrenia.

1. **Quantitative changes.** The amount of activity and its "driven" quality ranges from the extremes of agitation in excited catatonic states and acute psychotic exacerbations to the withdrawn and inactive states associated with catatonic stupor and chronic institutionalization. **Akathisia, bradykinesia,** and **tardive dyskinesia** are commonly associated with the effects of neuroleptic medications rather than with schizophrenia (see VII G 1 e).

    a. **Catatonic stupor** is a state of dramatic motor inactivity in which patients may, if untreated, be immobile for weeks or months at a time. Patients may be unable to initiate eating, drinking, or elimination. As patients recover, it is clear that they have been aware of events in the environment. Patients in a catatonic state may require aggressive medical care to avoid dehydration, electrolyte disturbances, and infections. In some cases, catatonic stupor may change abruptly to catatonic excitement. Medical illnesses and affective disorders are the most common causes of catatonia.

    b. **Catatonic excitement,** a hypermetabolic state, is a psychiatric emergency. A patient's activity and speech may be excessive, driven, and purposeless. Patients in this state may be violent. Before pharmacologic treatment and electroconvulsive therapy (ECT) were available, patients in this state frequently died of acute hyperthermia. Organic conditions (e.g., use of phencyclidine) and mania may also cause catatonic excitement.

2. **Qualitative changes.** Psychopharmacologic interventions frequently confuse the clinical picture of movement abnormalities by adding features of parkinsonian movement difficulties and the choreoathetotic movements of tardive dyskinesia. Even without pharmacologic treatment, patients with schizophrenia may exhibit a variety of movement abnormalities (e.g., increased flexor muscle tone, unusual mannerisms, bizarre gestures).

    a. **Catatonic posturing** is demonstrated by patients who assume strange postures and hold them for long periods.

    (1) In **catatonic rigidity,** patients resist being moved from their unusual rigid postures.

    (2) In **waxy flexibility,** patients' limbs may be moved like wax, and they hold the newly assumed position for long periods.

    b. **Echopraxia** is the behavioral equivalent of echolalia. Patients involuntarily mimic the movements of another person.

    c. **Automatic obedience** refers to the following of directives in an unquestioning, robot-like manner.

    d. **Mannerisms and grimacing** refers to patients' artificial and stilted appearance. Inappropriate silliness is evident, particularly in hebephrenic patients and patients with frontal lobe damage, and is frequently accompanied by unusual mannerisms. Particular mannerisms may have special meanings that are connected to delusions or hallucinations. Grimacing movements may be subtle or pronounced but may be mistaken for the orofacial dystonias of tardive dyskinesia.

e. **Stereotyped behaviors** (stereotypy) involves the purposeless repetitive movements (or verbalizations) seen in a variety of conditions. These movements may involve the entire body such as rocking or may involve repetition of complex gestures. The movements may have magical significance or may be purposeless to the patient.

f. **Perseveration** is involuntary repetition of a task. For example, patients who are asked to copy a series of circles may continue to copy the figures until they run off the page. Patients may repeat an answer to a question until asked to stop. Perseveration is also seen in patients with organic mental syndromes, particularly those with damage to premotor areas.

[I] **Social behavior** may be impaired. In early and severe cases of schizophrenia, patients may display a loss of the social skills, body language, and empathic abilities that permit successful interaction with others and pursuit of social and vocational functioning. Frequently, normal individuals perceive schizophrenic persons as bizarre, hostile, or socially inept. Impairment of social skills; disturbances of thought, perception, speech, and behavior; or long-term institutionalization may result in schizophrenic patients who are severely socially debilitated and who may live on the fringe of society as severely dysfunctional "street people." In the past, these same individuals may have been long-term institutionalized patients.

V COURSE

The course of schizophrenia may be highly variable, ranging from the presence or absence of a prodromal phase, remission or lack of symptoms between episodes, a downward deteriorating course, or full or social recovery. Course and prognosis vary widely depending on a variety of social, economic, and treatment factors as well as the diagnostic criteria used to define the population.

[A] **Onset**   The **peak time of onset** of schizophrenia is late adolescence and early adulthood, a time of multiple stresses related to leaving home, choosing a career, and developing relationships. Onset tends to be earlier for men than women, and a smaller peak occurs in the fourth decade, particularly among women.

1. It has been proposed that separation from parents unmasks psychotic features that have been present since childhood.

2. Other studies suggest that these intense stresses are responsible for activating the processes that result in schizophrenia.

3. A third explanation for the late adolescent time of onset involves the final maturation of the brain in the late teenage years. This final stage of neurodevelopment may leave the brains of persons with schizophrenia more vulnerable to stress.

4. Patients with **early onset** tend to have more disorganized features and a worse prognosis for recovery and preservation of function than do patients with late onset.

5. Patients with **late onset** tend to have more paranoid features and a better prognosis and preservation of function than do patients with early onset.

[B] **Precipitating events**   Initiating factors are now viewed as stressors that may activate a predisposition to the development of schizophrenia. They can also occur in other psychiatric illnesses such as bipolar disorder.

1. **Psychosocial stressors.** Cultures experiencing social and economic stress are associated with high rates of schizophrenia. However, it cannot yet be determined which stressors produce schizophrenia in vulnerable individuals.

2. **Traumatic events.** On a case-by-case basis, specific traumatic events that appear to precipitate schizophrenic symptoms can be isolated. However, it is not clear that either the level of stress or loss for schizophrenic individuals is different than might be experienced by normal individuals.

3. **Drug and alcohol abuse.** Certain drugs (e.g., amphetamines, cocaine, hallucinogens, phencyclidine, anticholinergics) and alcohol may precipitate psychotic symptoms. Whether these drugs cause schizophrenia-like syndromes or precipitate the development of schizophrenia in vulnerable individuals is not clear. Some patients use substances as self-medication to dispel unwanted

symptoms. For example, nicotine, which is frequently used by patients with schizophrenia, may alleviate negative symptoms by stimulating dopaminergic neurons in the frontal lobes. Anxiolytic substances may be used to combat side effects of neuroleptics such as akathisia.

C **Clinical course**

1. **Initial presentation.** The onset of schizophrenia is variable and has prognostic significance.
   a. Schizophrenia may present abruptly with confusion, agitation, affective involvement, hallucinations, and delusions occurring after an identifiable stressor. This clinical picture may develop in a period as short as 1 or 2 days; however, relatively few of these patients develop schizophrenia with the chronic course required for a *DSM-IV* diagnosis. Instead, they meet the criteria for **brief psychotic disorder** or **schizophreniform disorder,** which has a less than 6-month course.
   b. **Trema** (German for "stage fright") is characterized by anxious, irritable, and depressed feelings that may last from a few days to 1 month or longer. These feelings may be a reaction to perceptions that something is going wrong. As this condition progresses, patients may feel as though the environment is odd and ominous. Such a trema may progress to frank psychosis or may resolve as if a discrete episode.
   c. An **insidious prodromal phase** portends a bad prognosis when psychotic features eventually appear. In general, the prognosis is worse if patients experience substantial deterioration in functioning without ever having achieved a high level of psychosocial functioning before the onset of psychotic symptoms. This course may be associated with subsequent high levels of negative symptoms. Symptoms observed in patients with this pattern of onset include:
      (1) Social withdrawal
      (2) Impairment in role functioning (e.g., as a student, parent, spouse)
      (3) Peculiar behavior
      (4) Neglect of grooming and personal hygiene
      (5) Blunted or inappropriate affect
      (6) Vague, digressive, overelaborative, or circumstantial speech, or poverty of speech or content of speech
      (7) Odd beliefs that are inconsistent with the cultural group of which the patient is a member, or magical thinking that influences behavior
      (8) Unusual perceptual experiences such as recurrent illusions, "telepathy," or recurrent déjà vu experiences
      (9) Marked lack of initiative, drive, ambition, interest, or energy
      (10) Diminished ability to correctly perceive social cues, particularly abstract social cues

2. **Acute phase.** Schizophrenia cannot be diagnosed without an acute phase involving worsening psychotic symptoms such as positive symptoms of delusions, hallucinations, catatonia or agitation, and the possible worsening of negative symptoms.

3. **Stabilization phase.** This period, which may last as long as 6 months or more, involves gradually decreasing severity of symptoms (usually positive symptoms) from the acute phase.

4. **Stable phase.** This phase, which can last months to years, is characterized by little variation in symptom severity. Significant resolution of positive symptoms from the acute phase may occur, with some patients appearing asymptomatic. Negative symptoms may be more evident with attenuation of positive symptoms. Most patients recover some social function but continue to experience some symptoms.

5. **Deterioration from a previous level of functioning** is a key feature of schizophrenia. Role performance in relationships, work, self-care, or school performance is impaired. Patients often do not return to their previous level of functioning. Residual symptoms may interfere with social functioning. However, some recent studies challenge the assumption that this deterioration is uniform and lifelong.
   a. **Patterns of long-term courses.** Onset may be acute or insidious. The course may involve a single continuous episode of symptoms, be episodic, or evolve from episodic to continuous. The outcome may range from eventual severe impairment to complete recovery. Almost all combinations of these elements are possible. About 25% of schizophrenic patients experience the insidious onset of symptoms, continuous course, and eventual severe impairment.

b. Patterns of recovery. It should be noted that much of the data on the prognosis of schizophrenia are based on observations of patients who have recognized disease of less than 10 years or of patients whose behaviors may represent adaptations to institutionalized life. In addition, the prognosis may depend on socioeconomic factors and the availability of adequate psychosocial interventions. Many of the factors following may be viewed as intermediate-term prognostic factors. Different measures of recovery produce different outcome estimates.

   (1) **Social recovery** is often defined as economic and residential independence with little disruption in social relationships. Social recovery is often more common than complete remission of symptoms because many patients still suffer from negative symptoms. Several studies suggest that over a period of 15 years or longer, more than two-thirds of schizophrenic patients experience either complete, or "social," recovery with adequate treatment.

      (a) Errors in this measurement are possible because it is tied to the status of the economy and to the level of tolerance for social deviance in the culture.

      (b) Rates of social recovery tend to be higher than those for complete recovery.

   (2) **Complete recovery** implies complete remission of psychotic symptoms and a return to previous levels of social and occupational functioning.

   (3) **Hospitalization rates** have been used to measure recovery failures. Although these values are the easiest to determine, they are probably the least accurate measure of the course of schizophrenia. Rates of rehospitalization may depend on a variety of factors, ranging from the available health care resources and service delivery systems to community acceptance of deviant behavior.

D **Prognostic variables**   Early in the course of schizophrenia, a number of variables have been identified that predict a short to intermediate course of schizophrenia. Long-term prognostic factors have not been identified. Positive symptoms (see I A 1) carry much less ominous prognostic implications than do negative symptoms (see I A 2).

1. **Separation of good from poor prognostic factors.** Patients currently fitting *DSM-IV* diagnostic criteria for schizophrenia are a group that has been selected for poor prognostic features in the short or intermediate term.

   a. Acute psychotic disorders are now considered to be **schizophreniform disorder** or **brief psychotic disorder** if they do not continue for the 6-month course required for a diagnosis of schizophrenia.

   b. Patients with mood disorders in addition to psychotic symptoms are now diagnosed as having **schizoaffective disorder, major depression with psychotic features,** or **bipolar disorder.**

   c. Many patients previously considered to be schizophrenic are now included in diagnostic categories of **delusional disorder** and **borderline personality disorder.**

2. **Poor prognostic factors.** Patients with a predominance of negative symptoms, poor cognitive performance on neuropsychological testing, and abnormalities on computed tomography (CT), MRI, and PET scans are reported to have poor outcomes.

E **Quality of life**

1. **Social network.** Compared with normal individuals, patients with chronic schizophrenia tend to have small social networks. Whereas the social networks of normal individuals may be composed of 20 to 30 individuals, chronic schizophrenic patients may have networks as small as three to five people. The networks of people with chronic mental illnesses also tend to be highly interconnected.

   a. Before the onset of illness, schizophrenic patients have fewer and less satisfactory social relationships than people with affective disorders or normal subjects.

   b. The existence of social connections outside the family is associated with a good prognosis.

   c. In contrast to affective psychosis, family involvement can have positive or negative prognostic significance.

2. **Impaired educational achievement.** Despite normal or high intelligence, many schizophrenic patients are unable to complete educational plans after the onset of illness.

3. **Impaired work performance.** Employment appears to improve the prognosis of schizophrenic patients. However, these patients may have significant difficulties finding employment, particularly

during economic depressions. Schizophrenic patients often have jobs that require less skill than their education and intelligence suggest.

4. **Marital relationships.** Marriage rates for individuals with schizophrenia are lower than rates for the general population. Schizophrenic men tend to be married less frequently than schizophrenic women.

5. **Crime.** Most individuals with schizophrenia are no more violent than average persons, except for a small subset of persons with a history of violent actions when experiencing psychosis. The publicity of some violent crimes committed by persons with schizophrenia can exaggerate the public perception of dangerousness. There is evidence that when services are not provided to schizophrenic persons through the mental health system, they may enter the criminal justice system, usually for minor, nonviolent crimes.

6. **Premature death.** The risk of death in young schizophrenic patients is several times higher than in the general population. As schizophrenic individuals become older, their risk of mortality approaches that of the general population.
   a. Schizophrenic patients risk premature death from suicide, homicide, and medical illnesses (e.g., cardiovascular disease, infectious diseases, cancer).
   b. Another particular risk factor for people with schizophrenia is smoking. Some evidence suggests that smoking briefly "normalizes" some average evoked potential abnormalities associated with schizophrenia, leading to the hypothesis that schizophrenic patients may smoke heavily as a form of self-treatment of symptoms. The neoplasms that are common in patients with schizophrenia are those associated with smoking.

7. **Homelessness.** An estimated 5% to 8% of people with schizophrenia are homeless. Many more live in substandard housing or depend on relatives to maintain their standard of living, including housing.

8. **Psychiatric comorbidity.** Patients with schizophrenia are reported to suffer from other psychiatric symptoms, including anxiety, depression, and obsessive-compulsive symptoms. It is not clear in all cases that these reports represent carefully screened populations (e.g., excluding autistic people from the sample) or that depressive symptoms have been differentiated from deficit symptoms.

VI DIFFERENTIAL DIAGNOSIS

The diagnosis of schizophrenia is made after a complete clinical and historical evaluation of an individual patient. **Symptoms must be present for at least 6 months** to make the diagnosis of schizophrenia. If the duration is less than 6 months, a variety of other diagnoses are appropriate, including schizophreniform disorder, brief psychotic disorder, psychotic disorder not otherwise specified, and acute psychotic symptoms in borderline personality disorder.

A Organic mental disorders and syndromes (psychotic symptoms attributable to a medical condition)

1. An acute medical illness that affects the brain, with psychotic symptoms, is called a **delirium.**

2. Long-term, supposedly irreversible, medical or neurologic syndromes with cognitive and psychiatric features are called **dementias.** Dementias often mimic the negative symptoms of schizophrenia.

3. To differentiate schizophrenia from organic mental syndromes, psychiatrists must rely on a high index of suspicion, an exacting mental status examination, physical and neurologic examinations and sometimes a neuropsychological examination.
   a. Localized brain illnesses and injuries may produce **focal abnormalities,** resulting primarily from localized damage to the brain that can mimic a variety of cognitive, behavioral, and even linguistic findings found in schizophrenia.
   b. **Nonfocal,** or generalized, **alterations** in brain function can manifest as acute confusion and psychotic symptoms suggestive of schizophrenia. Visual hallucinations are somewhat more common, and auditory hallucinations are less common in organic mental syndromes.

4. **Medical disorders** known to cause psychiatric symptoms should be considered when evaluating patients (Table 3–4).

TABLE 3–4 Medical Disorders that Can Mimic Schizophrenia

Disorders	Comments
Vascular disorders	Vascular disorders must be considered in older patients. Cerebral vasculitis is particularly apt to mimic schizophrenia.
Autoimmune diseases	SLE is notorious for mimicking schizophrenia. Steroids used in treatment of autoimmune disease may cause organic mental syndromes.
Nutritional deficiencies	Overdoses of vitamins are also part of the differential diagnosis.
Metabolic disturbances	
Alcoholism	Delirium tremens and alcoholic hallucinations are frequently mistaken for acute schizophrenia.
Sleep disorders	Patients with narcolepsy are more likely to present with symptoms of depression than schizophrenia.
Sleep apnea	
Kleine-Levin syndrome	
Narcolepsy	
Hydrocephalus	
Obstructive hydrocephalus	
Normal-pressure hydrocephalus	
Epilepsy	
Complex partial seizures	
Absence seizures	
Degenerative diseases	Degenerative diseases occur more often in older people, who have a low probability of developing schizophrenia.
Congenital disorders	The development of schizophrenia is associated with the smaller of a pair of twins who has poor motor function and slow development, theoretically as a result of intrauterine insult. Children and adolescents who demonstrate symptoms of minimal brain dysfunction may develop schizophrenia.
A subclinical form of PKU	
Smaller twin	
Minimal brain dysfunction	
Infections	Bacterial infection, particularly associated with meningitis, may be the cause of an organic mental syndrome. Although rare, parasitic infection may result in a dramatic organic mental syndrome.
Bacteria	
Fungi	
Viruses	
Parasites	
Toxicity	
Drug abuse	
Abuse of gasoline and toluene-based inhalants	
Carbon monoxide	
Lead	
Agricultural and industrial chemicals	
Prescribed medication	
Digitalis	
Anticholinergics	
Antihypertensives	
CNS depressants	
Steroids	
Traumatic insults to the brain	Left temporal lobe damage is particularly likely to produce schizophrenia-like symptoms.
Acute subdural hematomas	
Chronic subdural hematomas	
Direct trauma	
Postconcussion syndrome	
Left temporal lobe damage	
Endocrine disorders	
Thyroid problems	
Parathyroid problems	
Pituitary adenomas	
Pheochromocytoma	
Neoplasms	In addition to primary and metastatic tumors of the brain, tumors in other parts of the body may cause psychiatric symptoms and cognitive deficits through paraneoplastic effects.

CNS = central nervous system; PKU = phenylketonuria; SLE = systemic lupus erythematosus.

B Mood disorders   These conditions are often accompanied by symptoms that are confused with those of other psychotic illnesses, including schizophrenia. For example, depression with severe melancholic features is, in some studies, a more common cause of the catatonic syndrome than schizophrenia. Mood-congruent delusions and hallucinations are a common feature of severe mood disorders.

1. **Manic episodes**
   a. Manic patients who present with irritability, suspicions of persecution, delusions, and hallucinations may be indistinguishable from patients with schizophrenia. At the height of a manic episode, patients may demonstrate bizarre behaviors, incoherence, and other features thought to be pathognomonic of schizophrenia. Careful family histories and longitudinal observations may be required to differentiate among these conditions.
   b. If organic causes for the manic syndrome and personality disorder have been ruled out, a manic episode by definition implies that the patient suffers from **bipolar disorder.** Patients with bipolar disorder usually suffer from both manic and depressive episodes at some time in their lives. However, only mania is present in a few patients.

2. **Major depressive episodes** (including those associated with bipolar disorder). Patients with severe depression may present with paranoid symptoms, social withdrawal, and severely restricted affect, all of which are suggestive of schizophrenia. Patients who develop melancholic features and delusions concerning cancer—a rotting body, guilt, and other mood-congruent delusions—particularly resemble schizophrenic individuals. Likewise, indecisiveness, slowing of thoughts, and lack of spontaneity in speech and behavior may resemble the negative symptoms of schizophrenia. Recent studies suggest that depression, at least in the first episode of psychosis, may be part of the overall illness pattern, which remits along with other acute symptoms and without additional treatment. This implies that separating depressive symptoms from acute psychotic symptoms may be unwarranted.

3. **Postpsychotic depression.** There is some controversy regarding whether postpsychotic depression represents a true depression with the same biologic features as a major depressive episode or if it represents a phase of predominant negative symptoms of schizophrenia. Likewise, oversedation and parkinsonian symptoms may resemble the clinical picture of depression.
   a. During a first psychotic episode, different criteria reveal that up to 75% of patients suffer from depressive symptoms. However, 98% of these symptoms remit with the resolution of psychosis. This suggests that antidepressant treatment should not be initiated except in patients for whom depression persists after the resolution of the psychotic episode.
   b. Since the introduction of the atypical neuroleptics, some patients have had dramatic recoveries from psychosis only to realize that they have lost out on many things. Depression related to life circumstances is best addressed through psychotherapy.

4. **Schizoaffective disorder** (Table 3–5). Patients present with either a manic episode or a major depressive episode with acute psychotic symptoms suggestive of schizophrenia or as an episode of psychotic symptoms without mood symptoms (in an individual in whom a mood disorder has been previously diagnosed). Criteria for diagnosing this disorder are:
   a. A family history that is more positive for mood disorder than for schizophrenia
   b. A prognosis intermediate between mood disorders and schizophrenia
   c. Response to combinations of medications and treatments used for both schizophrenia and mood disorders

C Other psychoses
1. **Brief psychotic disorder** (Table 3–6). Similar to schizophreniform disorder, this diagnostic category describes patients who were considered schizophrenic under previous diagnostic criteria but whose good prognosis differentiates them from the patients diagnosed as schizophrenic under current criteria. The illness of a brief psychotic disorder lasts **between 1 day and 1 month.** Clearly, the differential diagnosis for acutely psychotic persons is very large, with a need to rule out medical conditions, substance abuse, and mood disorders.

2. **Schizophreniform disorder** (Table 3–7). This diagnostic category was created to differentiate those who were previously regarded as "good prognosis" schizophrenic patients from "poor prognosis" schizophrenic patients. Patients with symptoms suggestive of schizophrenia for

TABLE 3–5 *DSM-IV* **Diagnostic Criteria for Schizoaffective Disorder**

A. An uninterrupted period of illness during which there is either a major depressive episode or manic episode concurrent with symptoms that meet criteria A for schizophrenia.

B. During the same period of illness, there have been delusions or hallucinations for at least 2 weeks in the absence of prominent mood symptoms.

C. Symptoms meeting criteria for a mood episode are present for a substantial portion of the total duration of the active and residual periods of the illness.

D. Not caused by the direct effects of substance abuse.

Specify type:
Bipolar type: If manic episode or both manic and major depressive episodes
Depressive type: If major depressive episode only

TABLE 3–6 *DSM-IV* **Diagnostic Criteria for Brief Psychotic Disorder**

A. Presence of at least one of the following symptoms:
1. Delusions
2. Hallucinations
3. Disorganized speech (e.g., frequent derailment or incoherence)
4. Grossly disorganized or catatonic behavior

B. Duration of an episode of the disturbance is at least 1 day and no more than 1 month, with eventual return to premorbid level of functioning. (When the diagnosis must be made without waiting for the expected recovery, it should be qualified as "provisional.")

C. Not better accounted for by a mood disorder (i.e., no full mood syndrome is present) or schizophrenia and not caused by the direct effects of a substance or general medical condition

Specify if:
With marked stressor(s) [brief reactive]: If symptoms occur shortly after and apparently in response to events that, singly or together, would be markedly stressful to almost anyone in similar circumstances in the person's culture
Without marked stressor(s): If psychotic symptoms do not occur shortly after or are not apparently in response to events that, singly or together, would be markedly stressful to almost anyone in similar circumstances in the person's culture
With postpartum onset: If onset within 4 weeks' postpartum

TABLE 3–7 *DSM-IV* **Diagnostic Criteria for Schizophreniform Disorder**

A. Meets criteria A, D, and E for schizophrenia
B. An episode of the disorder lasts at least 1 month but less than 6 months.

Prognostic features should be specified in the diagnosis:
With good prognostic features (at least two of the following):
1. Onset of prominent psychotic symptoms within 4 weeks of the first noticeable change in usual behavior or functioning
2. Confusion or perplexity at the height of the psychotic episode
3. Good premorbid social and occupational functioning
4. Absence of blunted or flat affect
Without good prognostic features:
Should be specified if good prognostic features are absent

whom no organic cause for psychotic symptoms has been found and who meet the diagnostic criteria for schizophrenia, except that their symptoms have lasted less than 6 months, are appropriately diagnosed as having schizophreniform disorder. A few patients with schizophreniform disorder eventually meet the criteria for schizophrenia. However, the majority of patients with schizophreniform disorder recover without ever having met the diagnostic criteria for schizophrenia.

3. **Delusional disorder** (Table 3–8). Without an accurate history and attempts to corroborate the patient's complaints, delusional disorder may be easily mistaken for schizophrenia. Although the delusions may be quite elaborate, they must not be bizarre.

   a. If persons have negative symptoms, hallucinations, disorganized speech, or disorganized or catatonic behavior for more than a few hours, the diagnosis of schizophrenia should be made. The delusions may be plausible (e.g., being under surveillance, being poisoned or contaminated, being in love with someone famous, having a serious illness). Patients lack the deterioration of global functioning generally seen in schizophrenia, and many of them are able to maintain employment throughout much of their illness.

   b. Because patients are convinced of the validity of their complaints, they may not seek treatment for their condition, which often develops later in life than schizophrenia. Initial physician contact and treatment may occur as part of evaluation for commitment or a forensic evaluation after arrest. Patients with delusional disorder can be highly resistant to treatment with psychotherapy or medications.

4. **Psychotic disorder not otherwise specified.** This diagnosis of exclusion is reserved for patients who have some diagnostic features of schizophrenia but who do not meet all the diagnostic criteria. This diagnosis is appropriate for patients with nonorganic psychotic presentations, which, after exhaustive examination, do not fit another diagnostic criterion for classification of psychotic symptoms.

D **Other disorders** If there is **no episode of acute psychosis,** other diagnoses may be appropriate. Patients who fit the current diagnostic criteria for schizophrenia are unlikely to be confused with other diagnostic groups. However, symptoms suggestive of schizophrenia may be found in a number of conditions, which must be ruled out (see Table 3–4).

1. **Personality disorders.** With the decline of the use of such terms as "process schizophrenia" and "pseudoneurotic schizophrenia," there has been less diagnostic confusion between schizophrenia and personality disorders. However, in the case of several specific personality disorders, features of the clinical presentation may be confused with those of schizophrenia. Personality disorders most likely to be confused with schizophrenia include the following (using *DSM-IV* nomenclature):

   a. **Paranoid personality disorder** involves interpreting the actions of others as deliberately demeaning or threatening. Behavior is characterized by questioning the loyalty of others, holding grudges about insults or slights, and lacking trust in others. This disorder can be differentiated from paranoid schizophrenia in that it lacks acute psychotic episodes and extreme deterioration.

TABLE 3–8 *DSM-IV* **Diagnostic Criteria for Delusional Disorder**

A. Nonbizarre delusions (i.e., involving situations that could occur in real life such as being followed, poisoned, infected, having a disease, loved at a distance) of at least 1 month's duration

B. Has never met criteria A for schizophrenia (for more than a few hours)

C. Apart from the impact of the delusion(s) or its ramifications, functioning is not markedly impaired, and behavior is not odd or bizarre

D. If mood episodes have occurred concurrently with delusions, total duration has been brief relative to the duration of the delusional periods

E. Not caused by the direct effects of a substance (e.g., drugs of abuse, medication) or a general medical condition

Specify type:

   Erotomanic type: Delusions that another person, usually of higher status, is in love with the individual

   Grandiose type: Delusions of inflated worth, power, knowledge, identity, or special relationship to a deity or famous person

   Jealous type: Delusions that one's sexual partner is unfaithful

   Persecutory type: Delusions that one (or someone to whom one is close) is being malevolently treated in some way

   Somatic type: Delusions that the person has some physical defect or general condition

   Mixed type: Delusions characteristic of more than one of the above types but no one theme predominates

   Unspecified type

b. **Schizoid personality disorder** is often found among biologic relatives of schizophrenic patients, which suggests that these disorders share some undetermined genetic commonality. The lack of social interests of affected patients results in a restricted lifestyle, which may be confused with the social deterioration of schizophrenia. However, the lack of hallucinations and delusions differentiates these individuals from schizophrenic patients.

c. **Schizotypal personality disorder** is also frequently found among biologic relatives of schizophrenic individuals. Because of the odd beliefs, magical ideation, and eccentric behavior and appearance of these patients, this disorder may be confused with schizophrenia. However, it can be differentiated from schizophrenia because of the lack of a history of an acute phase (see V C 2).

   (1) Phenomenologic investigations suggest that extreme social anxiety may be the genetic link between schizophrenia and schizotypal relatives.

   (2) Further refinements of this diagnosis and its relationship to genetic factors in schizophrenia may involve differentiation of affective versus nonaffective subtypes of this disorder (which may be more appropriately assigned to borderline personality disorder).

   (3) Some evidence suggests that people who suffer from schizotypal personality disorder may suffer from similar sensory gating problems as do people with schizophrenia.

d. **Borderline personality disorder** is characterized by suffering from a lifelong pattern of unstable relationships, rapid mood swings, and an unstable self-image. In severe cases, psychotic features may appear in response to stress, but they are rarely of sufficient duration or intensity to make a diagnosis of schizophrenia. The intense reexperience of trauma that occurs in some cases of this disorder may be mistaken for psychosis.

e. **Other personality disorders** exhibit symptoms of sufficient severity that they may sometimes be misdiagnosed as schizophrenia by incautious clinicians.

   (1) **Dependent personality disorder** may be mistaken for exhibiting schizophrenic ambivalence, lack of drive, and fear of being alone.

   (2) **Obsessive-compulsive personality disorder** may demonstrate such restrictions of affective expression that it is mistaken for the flattened affect described in former diagnostic systems for schizophrenia. In addition, ambivalence, circumstantial speech, and other features may give the impression of schizophrenia without a diagnostic evaluation.

2. **Developmental disabilities.** Asperger syndrome (a high-functioning form of autism), in particular, may be mistaken for schizophrenia if *DSM-IV* criteria are not used. Patients suffering from this disorder are often eccentric, emotionally labile, and anxious, and they demonstrate poor social functioning, repetitive behavior, and fixed habits. Affect may be interpreted as bizarre or flat. Social interactions are severely impaired by a lack of empathy or understanding of other people, and motor performance is clumsy and poorly coordinated. Because these patients do not generally have positive symptoms, they may be most easily mistaken for "simple schizophrenics" by casual diagnosticians.

E **Religious and cultural subgroups** Diagnosticians from one culture may confuse beliefs and behavior patterns associated with another culture with symptoms of schizophrenia. A member of one group or culture who evaluates members of another religious group must not consider the religious beliefs of the other person to be psychotic if the beliefs are held by a group of people of which the patient is a member. Likewise, physicians from another culture must not interpret cultural differences in body language and acceptable affective expression as bizarre. To best avoid this diagnostic confusion, individuals should consult physicians from their own culture or clinicians experienced with that culture.

VII **TREATMENT**

Schizophrenia is not currently considered curable, and most patients experience symptoms off and on for the rest of their lives. Recovery rates are better for the following schizophrenic patients: those with a late onset of illness, those from developing countries, and those recovering in times of economic prosperity. Perhaps because of a later onset, women tend to have a better prognosis for schizophrenia in many parts of the world.

A **Overview**

1. Treatment programs for persons with schizophrenia must be individualized and comprehensive, taking into account the biologic, psychological, and social needs of each patient. Attention must also be paid to the continuity of care. The care setting should be as nonrestrictive as possible, and every attempt should be made to reintegrate patients into the community.

2. Modern treatment methods in the United States make it possible for about 90% of schizophrenic patients to recover sufficiently to live outside the hospital most of the time. Some studies suggest that about 75% of individuals who meet the diagnostic criteria for schizophrenia experience substantial or complete recovery 20 to 25 years (or longer) after the onset of illness.

3. Guidelines for the modern treatment of schizophrenia are now available from several sources.
   a. Treatment guidelines published by the American Psychiatric Association in 2004 are part of a series of practice guidelines in psychiatry.
   b. The *Expert Consensus Guidelines,* first published in *The Journal of Clinical Psychiatry* in 1997 and revised in 1999, make specific recommendations on the uses of antipsychotic medications.
   c. The *Texas Medication Algorithm* published by the State of Texas Department of Mental Health and Mental Retardation presents a concise guide to medication choices in the treatment of schizophrenia.
   d. The recommendations of the *Schizophrenia: Practice Outcomes Research Team* published in *Schizophrenia Bulletin* present multidisciplinary treatment guidelines and provide a comprehensive look at treatment of persons with schizophrenia in the community.

B **Hospitalization** Hospitals were once the primary treatment setting for persons with schizophrenia; at one time, it was not uncommon for affected individuals to spend the rest of their lives in hospitals. Hospitalization now usually focuses on more acute issues, with a minority of patients in long-term hospitalization.

1. **Indications.** Hospitalization is indicated because of specific problems associated with a person's illness rather than because of the appearance of symptoms (Table 3–9).
   a. First episodes of psychosis and unusual presentations of psychotic conditions in patients with more chronic forms of schizophrenia may warrant hospitalization.
   b. Hospitalization is not necessarily indicated for an exacerbation of psychotic symptoms if adequate community alternatives are available.

2. **Goals**
   a. **Protection.** The hospital should be a safe environment where physical needs can be met, stresses can be minimized, and impulses can be controlled.
   b. **Diagnosis.** Twenty-four–hour care allows for extensive observation and evaluation of a patient's problems, strengths, history, support, and response to treatment. In addition, access to sophisticated diagnostic laboratory and neuroradiologic tests gives physicians the opportunity to differentiate schizophrenia from psychotic disorders resulting from medical conditions.
   c. **Therapy.** Various kinds of treatments, including neuroleptic medication, vocational and psychosocial rehabilitation, and family education, which are all designed to return the patient to

TABLE 3–9 Hospitalization of Patients with Schizophrenia

Problems Requiring Short-term Hospital Care	Problems Requiring Long-term Hospital Care
Risk of suicidal and homicidal ideation	Lack of appropriate community mental health resources
Command hallucinations of a threatening nature, with the clinician's assessment that the patient may act on these hallucinations	Provision of rehabilitative services before discharge to community programs
Extreme fear	Care for a severely debilitated schizophrenic patient
Significant confusion	Treatment of significant comorbidity from medical illnesses, substance abuse, medication complications
	Protection from self-inflicted harm or danger to others

the community, can be started in the hospital. Atypical neuroleptics, cognitive and behavioral treatments, and structured schedules may help decrease negative symptoms. There is no evidence that inpatient psychotherapy without medication is of any benefit.

3. **Side effects of hospitalization**
   a. Possible loss of self-esteem and social stigmatization as a result of being on a "mental ward"
   b. Possible loss of social supports in the community
   c. Loss of social and living skills required to live in the world outside the hospital (i.e., institutionalism) with prolonged hospitalization

4. **Changing role of the hospital.** Changing views concerning the importance of hospitalization in the treatment of patients with schizophrenia result from economic pressures and increasing beliefs about the superiority of community treatment over hospitalization.
   a. **Current trends.** Where adequate community treatment systems exist, it is presumed that community programs will assume many of the treatment functions of the inpatient unit. Present trends include major reductions in length of stay and frequency of hospitalization, with a focus on acute stabilization and discharge as well as an emphasis on diagnostic clarification rather than on psychotherapeutic treatment.
   b. **Alternatives to hospitalization.** Particularly in the public sector, attempts are being made to provide community-based alternatives to hospitalization. Some of these alternatives involve houses in the community where physicians, nurses, and others provide acute stabilization of psychotic symptoms and rapid reintegration into the community. In other cases, motels and therapeutic foster homes have been used for these purposes.
      (1) In general, these settings are not as well set up to handle violence and to deal with a medical evaluation as hospitals, but they provide less disruption for shorter periods of time.
      (2) These facilities are probably most appropriate for patients whose illnesses are well known, not for first-episode psychotic patients.

5. **Therapeutic milieu.** The therapeutic environment of the inpatient ward is known as the "therapeutic milieu." Inpatient psychiatric wards frequently use the therapeutic milieu as a major treatment modality for schizophrenic patients. Formal milieu therapy depends on attention to the social structure of the ward and on adequate numbers of well-trained staff. Interactions between staff, patients, and formal social organizations (e.g., the patient's ward government) are tools regularly used in milieu therapy. Trends are away from emphasis on milieu therapy because of decreasing lengths of hospital stay and a change of the focus of the hospital stay to diagnosis, rehabilitation programs, and psychoeducational activities.
   a. **Structure.** One aspect of the staff's role in the therapeutic milieu is to support the patient's impaired reality testing, impulse control, and modulation of environmental stimulation. The staff works to reduce the patient's anxiety and control injurious behavior. The structure of the ward should contain regular, structured activities; time alone; and help with personal hygiene and self-care. Milieu therapy avoids intense probing and anxiety-provoking psychotherapeutic interventions, which can be overwhelming for psychotic patients.
   b. **Flexibility.** The milieu should be flexible enough to respond to the changing needs of individuals with regard to length of stay, extent of restrictions, contact with family, group involvement, and activity levels. For example, as a patient's positive symptoms resolve, efforts may be initiated to increase the patient's socialization with other patients, engage the patient in structured recreational and vocational activities, and encourage the patient's participation in the ward government.
   c. **Ward community.** The other patients, as individuals and as a group, are used as therapeutic agents in the therapeutic milieu. Open, direct communication and individual responsibility are encouraged. The more organized and improved patients can provide hope and act as models for patients in earlier stages of recovery. As a group, patients are encouraged to make decisions about daily activities of the ward and to help change the maladaptive behavior of patients through open feedback.
   d. **Side effects.** Target-symptom–oriented treatment plans and posthospitalization care plans that involve all staff, including staff from programs outside the hospital, may remedy the side effects of milieu treatment.
      (1) Premature and harsh confrontation from staff and other patients or too much pressure for recovery may exacerbate psychotic symptoms or delay recovery.

(2) A structured, tolerant atmosphere may promote dependence on the ward, making it difficult to return to the community.

(3) Excessive demands for participation may cause overstimulation and disorganization.

(4) Patients who are in more advanced recovery stages may take advantage of those who are not doing so well, unless interactions between patients are monitored carefully.

(5) Staff may retain patients in the ward milieu longer than is desirable, creating a tendency for patients to return prematurely to the ward without ever developing a relationship with community services. This appears to be a problem with neophyte therapists who become enmeshed with patients and their social networks, believing that only they really understand the patient. This may result in a fragmentation of team efforts and poor communication with outpatient therapists. Good supervision can reduce this risk to the continuity of care.

    e. **Organizational continuity.** With shorter lengths of stay and an increasing reliance of treatment systems on community-based treatment, hospitals need to be a more highly integrated member of the overall mental health treatment system. Case managers from the community are increasingly involved in ward treatment. Diagnostic and treatment information must be relayed between community and hospital staff, and inpatient treatment objectives must be jointly negotiated between systems. Survival of inpatient, hospital-based treatment programs for patients with schizophrenia may increasingly depend on the ability of the inpatient units to respond to needs of the community mental health system.

C **Group therapy**   Group therapy has long been a mainstay of the treatment of schizophrenic patients in both inpatient and outpatient settings. It is best used in conjunction with other forms of therapy, particularly medications.

1. Although there is a paucity of well-controlled studies of group therapy in schizophrenia, the studies that do exist support the contention that group therapy focused on communication, alleviation of symptoms, and social skills produces improvements in social integration. Patients in such group therapy also have fewer readmissions to the hospital than do patients who receive only social skills training.

2. There is little evidence that open-ended, insight-oriented group therapy is effective in the treatment of schizophrenic patients. Some physicians believe that unstructured, confrontational group techniques may exacerbate psychotic symptomatology.

D **Individual psychotherapy**   Supportive and adaptive therapeutic techniques that are oriented to helping patients adapt to the details of daily life are far more effective in the management of schizophrenic patients than are insight-oriented techniques that focus on patients' inner experiences. Cognitive and behavioral therapies may reduce deficit symptoms in schizophrenia.

1. **Therapeutic relationship**
   a. **Supportive psychotherapy** is characterized by warm, open relationships that focus on promoting patients' self-esteem and helping them learn about their real strengths and limitations. Effective therapy focuses on practical and concrete issues.
   b. Attempts to establish a **close or intense therapeutic relationship** may exacerbate symptoms in patients who are highly suspicious or who feel overwhelmed by interpersonal relationships.
   c. **Nondirective and affectively restricted therapeutic styles** may also cause patients to experience anxiety and exacerbations of symptoms. Insight-oriented psychotherapy alone has not proved to be effective in individuals with schizophrenia.

2. **Therapeutic techniques.** The principles of psychotherapy of schizophrenic patients are as follows:
   a. **Education.** One of the main techniques of the therapist is to teach patients about their illness. The therapist should teach techniques of managing stress, understanding symptoms, and the knowing value of compliance with pharmacologic treatments. This approach encourages patients to assume responsibility for their own treatment.
   b. **Focusing on problem solving.** The therapist focuses on helping patients solve concrete problems that arise in daily life. The therapist may offer possible solutions to problems presented by patients, including an analysis of possible positive and negative outcomes of each solution. The therapist attempts to develop problem-solving skills for patients in financial, interpersonal, residential, and other areas of patients' daily lives.

    c. **Setting reasonable expectations for change.** Therapists who have unreasonable expectations for a "cure" may convey these expectations to patients in a counterproductive manner. Therapists who have generally positive expectations for improving functioning and life satisfaction appear to be correlated with good patient outcomes.

    d. **Expressing emotions effectively.** Therapies that encourage expression of emotion for its own sake or for "cathartic" value may trigger exacerbations in some patients. The therapist should encourage a discussion of private feelings and how to deal with these feelings but not encourage full-blown expressions of anger and hostility.

    e. **Crisis intervention.** The therapist may be able to intervene in crises in patients' lives to prevent serious escalations. Unlike the passive roles in other forms of therapy, the therapist may need to become active in working with patients' families, landlords, or social agencies to reduce the escalation of crises into psychotic episodes.

    f. **Concrete limit setting.** The therapist may need to set concrete limits such as avoiding substance abuse and violence. These discussions frequently include discussions of consequences of harmful behaviors.

    g. **Managing dependence.** One of the functions of the therapy of schizophrenic patients is to increase patients' appropriate socialization with other people in the community. In meeting this goal, therapists encourage patients to rely on a large network of people in the community rather than on only the therapist.

    h. **Illness self-management.** The therapist and a patient construct "experimental" designs intended to help the patient observe factors that may make both the positive and negative symptoms of illness better or worse. Patients may learn how to initiate activity, reduce social isolation, control symptoms with medications, and many other self-management skills.

    i. **Cognitive remediation.** In contrast to rehabilitation, which focuses on relearning concrete social and functional skills, cognitive remediation attempts to reverse neuropsychological performance deficits that are characteristic of schizophrenia. This approach involves the use of behavioral techniques and education to improve outcome, which is assessed by methods such as the Wisconsin Card Sort Test. This approach has produced improvements in patients with brain injury and autism but is new in its application to individuals with schizophrenia.

E **Community treatment** The majority of patients with schizophrenia now receive most of their treatment in the community. This was not the case 50 years ago, when many state-run hospitals served as warehouses for people with an illness then considered untreatable. With the development of psychiatric medications and modern treatment methodologies, it is now possible to treat some persons with schizophrenia without ever having to resort to hospitalization.

1. The cornerstone of modern treatment of schizophrenia is **case management.** For community treatment to work, the sometimes disparate goals of multiple public and private agencies must be managed to provide an individualized treatment plan for a particular patient. Although physicians sometimes play the role of case manager, social workers, nurses, or rehabilitation counselors usually assume this role. Sometimes even patients who are trained to help others negotiate their way through the often complex treatment system may serve as case managers.

    a. **Linkage.** The primary role of the case manager is to help patients establish and maintain access to various community resources. This can be a significant challenge because some patients' cognitive difficulties make it impossible for them to successfully apply for and obtain services such as housing, disability benefits, and vocational rehabilitation. Case managers often provide transportation to help patients keep appointments and commitments with various community programs. Case managers also maintain lines of communication to help ensure that the involved agencies efficiently share information.

    b. **Treatment planning and monitoring.** Case managers are frequently the clinicians responsible for maintaining the treatment record and ensuring that services are delivered appropriately. In some settings (e.g., high-caseload clinics), this is primarily a paperwork-related task to ensure quality assurance and availability of treatment history. In more effective clinical settings (e.g., low-caseload clinics), the case manager is the clinician who is most involved in case of a particular patient, maintaining contact on a frequent basis and checking for signs of relapse, noncompliance, and adverse effects.

    c. Intensive case management. This treatment approach can help persons with severe schizophrenia stay in the community. In this type of program, case managers serve only a few clients (e.g., eight to 12 per caseload) and often assess and work with their clients on a daily basis. Some intensive programs provide access to members of the treatment team 24 hours a day, 7 days a week. This enables more effective monitoring of treatment response and can allow for rapid response to crisis, in hopes of reducing the need for expensive hospitalization. Intensive treatment can involve such methods as monitored medication administration.

    d. Advocacy. The case manager may need to seek resources and services for schizophrenic patients. **Case-specific advocacy** is aimed at gaining resources for the individual patient, and **class-specific advocacy** is aimed at gaining services, resources, or access to services for a group of patients.

2. Because returning patients to productive lives in the community has become a priority, **psychosocial rehabilitation** has become a significant part of treatment programs. Goals of these programs are to reduce symptoms, remediate disabilities, and overcome handicaps associated with schizophrenia. In the past, patients who left inpatient institutions had insufficient skills necessary for independent living; they lacked the skills in social interactions required to gain or retain employment and to form social support networks needed for survival. Preliminary data suggest that patients who participate in psychosocial rehabilitation programs suffer relapse at a lower rate than control subjects. These programs focus on the following issues:

    a. Social skills training. Patients require the skills necessary to communicate with both strangers and familiar people involved in their lives. More effective social skills can reduce the socially inappropriate behavior and symptom-based communications that can lead to patients' becoming social outcasts in their own communities.

    b. Living skills acquisition. Patients who have become ill before establishing independence and those who have lived in institutions for much of their lives may be unable to shop for themselves, prepare food, or maintain their own living space.

    c. Housing. Many persons with schizophrenia have difficulty finding and maintaining housing. Modern community mental health programs offer supervised housing during the transition period between hospitalization and residential living while patients try to establish independence.

    d. Managing finances. The management of money, even if it is received monthly, may pose substantial problems for some patients. In extreme cases, patients may spend or lose an entire monthly check in a few days or weeks. To better ensure patients do not go without food, housing, or medications because of mismanaged finances, modern treatment programs may offer financial management assistance. This frequently takes the form of **designated payee** services in which a patient's disability check is received and distributed by a third party or agency.

    e. Managing the illness. Patients are taught to manage medication administration, watch for side effects, and report potentially dangerous developments in the treatment system in an appropriate and assertive manner.

    f. Recreational activities. Patients are taught to pursue recreational and physical activities to reduce stress and promote general health.

F Self-help programs

1. Consumer clubhouses. Some persons with schizophrenia receive the majority of their treatment and support from consumer-operated self-help organizations. Programs for mentally ill people such as the internationally known Fountain House are a source of support and self-esteem for persons suffering form major mental illness. Psychosocial rehabilitation, vocational training, housing assistance, and financial management services are offered by some consumer-operated, not-for-profit organizations. Such programs are the chief source of specially trained persons with mental illness, who in turn, become providers of services to persons with schizophrenia.

2. Illness self-management. The objective of this treatment method is to train patients with persistent schizophrenic symptoms to manage their own illnesses to a greater extent than previously encouraged by the mental health treatment system. Several forms of this training exist, but most encourage the development of skills in several specific areas.

    a. Symptom control includes learning to recognize and respond to signs of relapse, differentiating relapse from medication side effects, and working with persistent symptoms.

b. **Substance avoidance** focuses on avoiding alcohol abuse and the use of street drugs.

c. **Medication management** requires an understanding of how medications work; how they are taken; and how different side effects should be managed, including when to seek medical help.

d. **Learning to work with the health care system** involves education about how to communicate with health care providers, navigate the service delivery system, and advocate for oneself.

3. **Advocacy movement.** Advocacy groups have brought about significant changes in the amount of attention paid to the struggles of persons with schizophrenia. The **National Alliance for the Mentally Ill (NAMI)** has brought much attention to the need for more research into effective treatments for severe and persistent mental illnesses. NAMI is also a major voice of parents, siblings, and children who care for persons with illnesses such as schizophrenia. The organization offers valuable educational programs to help dispel the stigma associated with schizophrenia and help families better understand the symptoms of schizophrenia.

G Pharmacologic treatment

1. **Typical neuroleptics.** Since the 1960s, the typical neuroleptics (e.g., chlorpromazine, thioridazine, and haloperidol) have been the mainstay of the pharmacologic treatment of schizophrenia. All typical neuroleptics exert primary effects by blocking dopamine receptors, particularly D-2 receptors.

a. **Efficacy**

(1) **Acute treatment.** Therapy with typical neuroleptics is frequently successful, with amelioration of symptoms such as hallucinations, delusions, and agitation. Typical neuroleptics are less effective with chronic or well-organized delusions, and they have little effect on negative symptoms such as apathy, anhedonia, and amotivation.

(2) **Maintenance treatment.** Dopamine blockers have a proven record in reducing the risk of relapse, particularly when used in conjunction with a comprehensive treatment plan.

(a) Within 1 month of discharge, 7% of patients with schizophrenia have relapsed, and nearly 50% relapse within 1 year of discharge.

(b) Two groups of schizophrenic patients may not be effectively treated with maintenance neuroleptics:

(i) Patients who have had a single acute psychotic episode

(ii) Very deteriorated chronic schizophrenic patients who may be refractory to treatment

b. **Choice of agent.** At least nine typical neuroleptics are readily available in the United States, and more agents are available in other nations (Table 3–10). The choice of the proper agent is more of an art than a science, and as both the physician and patient gain experience, the job becomes easier.

(1) Route of administration is an important consideration, particularly when the patient's presentation or history suggests the need for acute parental administration or use of longer-acting depot injections.

(2) Side-effect profile is also important. Matching the potential side effects to the patient's presentation or history may be effective. For example, more sedating drugs may be chosen for more agitated patients, or drugs with more adrenergic blockade may be avoided in older patients or in those with cardiac histories.

c. **Dosage**

(1) **Acute psychosis.** The equivalent of 200 to 400 mg chlorpromazine initially given in divided doses is adequate. In most patients, significant effects are reached in 3 to 10 days, but some patients may require 30 or more days to respond. Massive doses of 1,000 to 2,000 mg are sometimes used, but controlled studies indicate that this approach is no more effective than standard dosing. However, a small subset of patients apparently responds only to very high doses.

(2) **Stabilization phase.** After patients with acute symptoms have begun to respond to treatment, the dosage is frequently titrated toward a maintenance level. This may involve a titration phase that attempts to balance symptoms control and possibly incapacitating side effects (e.g., sedation, orthostatic hypotension).

(3) **Maintenance phase.** The goal of the maintenance phase is to keep patients as free from symptoms as possible while avoiding any potentially incapacitating side effects. Physicians

TABLE 3-10 Typical Neuroleptics

Generic Name	Trade Name(s)	Approximate Equivalent Oral Dose (mg)	Usual Inpatient Oral Dosage Range (mg/day)
Phenothiazines			
Aliphatic			
	Thorazine	100	50–1500
Chlorpromazine			
Piperidine			
Thioridazine	Mellaril	100	50–800
Piperazine			
Fluphenazine	Prolixin, Permitil	2–4	2–60
Trifluoperazine	Stelazine	5	5–80
Perphanazine	Trilafon	10	16–64
Butyrophenones			
Haloperidol	Haldol	2–4	2–60
Thioxanthenes			
Thiothixene	Navane	5	5–80
Dihydroindolones			
Molindone	Moban, Lidone	10	20–225
Dibenzoxazepines			
Loxapine	Loxitane, Daxolin	10	20–225

may recommend that patients who are prone to violent outbursts or self-destructive behavior tolerate a higher level of side effects to minimize risk of harm. At this point, once-a-day administration is sufficient for almost all patients. In some patients, weekly dosage adjustments may be necessary, depending on the severity of their illness. In other individuals, no dosage adjustments are necessary for months at a time.

(4) **Nonresponse.** It is not uncommon to see relapses in patients whose schizophrenia was once under control because they no longer respond to an agent.

(a) The choice of medication should be reassessed. Several alternative drugs are available. Use of an agent in another chemical class may help, or the addition of augmenting medication may be indicated.

(b) Incapacitating side effects (e.g., akathisia, severe parkinsonism) may interfere with response to typical neuroleptics. The occurrence of tardive dyskinesia may necessitate the switch to another drug such as an atypical neuroleptic (see VII G 1 e [1] [e]).

(c) Blood levels should be obtained. The results may indicate if an effective therapeutic blood level has been reached or exceeded. Noncompliance can sometimes also be identified.

(d) Although waiting weeks to months to ascertain response is not inappropriate, this approach can rarely be implemented in this day of reduced hospital length of stay and community treatment.

d. **Route of administration**

(1) **Oral forms.** Almost all neuroleptics are available in pill, capsule, or elixir preparations for ease of administration. However, many patients with schizophrenia may have trouble adhering to an orally administered regimen.

(2) **Parenteral forms.** Intramuscular and intravenous preparations of most typical neuroleptics are available. The parenteral route is necessary for patients who are too agitated or incapacitated to comply with treatment.

(3) **Long-acting injections.** Depot formulations of two typical and one atypical neuroleptics (fluphenazine, haloperidol, and risperidone) are available that are generally effective for 2 weeks (fluphenazine and risperidone) and 4 weeks (haloperidol). Patients who prefer not to have to take medication on a daily basis may seek this route of administration. Physicians should also consider using this route in patients with a history of dangerous behavior and established noncompliance.

e. **Adverse effects**

(1) **Extrapyramidal syndromes (EPS)** result from blockade of dopamine receptors in the basal ganglia and occur more commonly with the high-potency neuroleptics.

(a) **Acute dystonic reactions,** which are more common in young male patients early in treatment, involve sudden tonic contractions of the muscles of the tongue, neck (**torticollis**), back (**opisthotonos**), mouth, and eyes (**oculogyric crises**). As well as being extremely frightening, such reactions can be dangerous if the patient's airway is compromised. These patients can be effectively treated with benztropine (1 to 2 mg intramuscularly) or diphenhydramine (25 to 50 mg intramuscularly or intravenously). Prophylaxis is accomplished with regular, orally administered anticholinergic medication.

(b) **Drug-induced parkinsonism** is characterized by cogwheel rigidity, bradykinesia, tremor, loss of postural reflexes, mask-like facies, and drooling. It is more common in elderly patients, and although it usually occurs in the first weeks of treatment, it may appear at varying times with varying doses. It can be effectively treated with any of the antiparkinsonian medications (Table 3–11) and may also respond to a decrease in neuroleptic dosage. Antiparkinsonian agents can often be tapered off after 4 to 8 weeks of maintenance treatment for about half of patients taking typical neuroleptics. If these EPS remain unresponsive, a trial of an atypical neuroleptic is indicated.

(c) **Akathisia** is a syndrome of motor restlessness, which may involve the entire body but is often most obvious in patients' inability to keep their legs and feet still. It can be mistaken for anxiety, agitation, or an increase in psychotic symptomatology. The akathisia may respond to antiparkinsonian agents, but if the patient responds poorly, a decrease in dosage or change to another neuroleptic is indicated. In some cases, akathisia can be successfully treated with propranolol, benzodiazepines, or vitamin E.

(d) **Neuroleptic-induced catatonia,** which occurs more commonly with the high-potency agents, is characterized by withdrawal; mutism; and motor abnormalities, including rigidity, immobility, and waxy flexibility. Although it can be mistaken for a worsening of patients' psychotic symptoms, it is a complication of neuroleptic therapy. It may represent a variant of the neuroleptic malignant syndrome (see VII G 1 e [2]). It should be treated by temporarily discontinuing neuroleptic therapy and, on resolution, changing to a different class of neuroleptic. Amantadine, 100 mg orally three times daily, may also be helpful.

(e) **Tardive dyskinesia** is a late-onset movement disorder that is thought to result from a disturbance in the dopamine–acetylcholine balance in the basal ganglia. Mechanisms theorized to account for this phenomenon include an increase in the numbers or sensitivity of dopamine receptors in certain parts of the brain after chronic blockade with neuroleptics. However, these theories do not fit all the data about the physiology of this condition.

(i) **Fasciculations of the tongue** may be the earliest symptom, followed by **lingual–facial hyperkinesias,** which are persistent involuntary chewing, smacking, or grimacing movements.

(ii) **Choreoathetotic movements of the extremities and trunk,** including the respiratory muscles, can be extremely disabling in severe cases. The symptoms are

TABLE 3–11 Antiparkinsonian Medications

Generic Name	Trade Name(s)	Usual Oral Dosage Range (mg/day)
Benztropine	Cogentin	1–8
Trihexyphenidyl	Artrane, Tremin	2–10
Biperiden	Akineton	2–6
Amantadine	Symmetrel	100–300
Diphenhydramine	Benadryl	25–200

often noticeable when there is a dosage reduction or discontinuation of neuroleptic medication, but they can usually be detected by close examination between neuroleptic doses.

(iii) The syndrome can usually be reversed if it is detected early and neuroleptics are discontinued.

(iv) In severe cases, tardive dyskinesia may be irreversible and can progress with continued neuroleptic treatment.

(v) Symptoms are worsened by anticholinergic medication, which should be discontinued if possible.

(vi) Increased doses of neuroleptics may cause apparent temporary improvement by increasing the dopamine-receptor blockade. However, this ultimately causes further progression of the movement disorder.

(vii) Patients should be screened every 6 months for early signs and should be maintained on the lowest possible dose to minimize this serious complication of long-term neuroleptic use.

(viii) Patients withdrawn abruptly from neuroleptics sometimes demonstrate a **withdrawal–emergent dyskinesia** with transient features of tardive dyskinesia that lasts for several days. It is unclear whether this syndrome is an early form of tardive dyskinesia or has another pathophysiologic mechanism.

(2) **Neuroleptic malignant syndrome,** a potentially life-threatening complication of neuroleptic therapy, is characterized by muscular rigidity, fever, autonomic instability, and an altered level of consciousness. Onset of the full-blown syndrome is rapid over 1 to 2 days after a period of gradual progressive rigidity. Treatment involves immediate discontinuation of the neuroleptic medication and support of respiratory, renal, and cardiovascular functioning and possibly treatment with dantrolene or bromocriptine.

(3) **Anticholinergic effects occur with low-potency neuroleptics at a higher rate than with the high-potency neuroleptics.** Anticholinergic effects are often seen as a direct result of treatment with a combination of drugs, including neuroleptics, anticholinergic agents used to treat parkinsonian side effects of the neuroleptics, and the inappropriate use of medications from other classes such as the tricyclic antidepressants. In extreme cases of polypharmacy, combinations (e.g., a low-potency neuroleptic, a tricyclic antidepressant, and one or more anticholinergic agents) may produce a **life-threatening anticholinergic delirium.** Clinicians must watch for the development of increasing psychotic symptoms with the addition of more or different medications to a patient's treatment plan and should suspect anticholinergic delirium in these circumstances. **Anticholinergic side effects include the following:**

(a) **At low doses.** Effects include blurred vision when changing from close to distant objects, dry mouth, urinary retention in men with enlarged prostate glands, and constipation.

(b) **Anticholinergic poisoning** occurs at **high doses.** Signs and symptoms include restless agitation; confusion; disorientation; hallucinations; delusions; hot, flushed, dry skin; pupil dilation; tachycardia; decreased bowel sounds; and urinary retention. Central anticholinergic poisoning may occur without obvious physiologic signs, making iatrogenic anticholinergic poisoning a particularly insidious risk of polypharmacy.

(c) **Anticholinergic abuse.** Because of the ability of anticholinergic agents to alter consciousness, patients sometimes abuse prescriptions for anticholinergic agents. Clinicians should treat parkinsonian symptoms with drugs with low antimuscarinic effects (e.g., amantadine) in at-risk patients.

(4) **Cardiovascular effects** of neuroleptics most commonly include orthostatic hypotension, particularly in elderly patients, which results from adrenergic blockade. This symptom is most commonly associated with the low-potency neuroleptics. In rare cases, neuroleptics may be associated with serious ventricular arrhythmias with electrocardiographic (ECG) abnormalities (i.e., T-wave changes, prolonged QT intervals) and with cardiac repolarization abnormalities. Risks of all cardiovascular complications are greatest with the low-potency neuroleptics.

(5) **Hypothalamic effects** may include changes in libido, appetite, and temperature regulation. Hypersecretion of prolactin by the hypothalamus can be induced by dopaminergic

blockades. Hyperprolactinemia may result in loss of sexual functioning, amenorrhea, breast enlargement, and galactorrhea.

   (6) **Jaundice** and elevation of liver enzymes may occur with any of the neuroleptics. Physicians should monitor patients for signs of hepatic problems and consider testing of liver enzyme and bilirubin levels when indicated.

   (7) **Agranulocytosis** is a rare and unpredictable reaction to neuroleptics and many other types of medications. Patients should be told to report spontaneous bruises, infections that do not resolve, or cuts that do not heal. Agranulocytosis can usually be reversed when detected early enough but has caused death in patients who are taking neuroleptics.

   (8) **Dermatologic effects** include allergic rashes, which respond to discontinuation of the drug, and photosensitivity, which can be treated with sunscreen.

   (9) **Ophthalmologic effects** include a pigmentary retinopathy associated with thioridazine in doses greater than 800 mg/day. Rarely, lens and corneal pigmentation has been reported with chlorpromazine, thioridazine, and thiothixene after long-term treatment. Blurred vision and worsening of narrow-angle glaucoma secondary to anticholinergic effects are more common.

2. **Atypical neuroleptics.** The newest drugs for the treatment of schizophrenia are sometimes referred to as the atypical neuroleptics. Clozapine, risperidone, olanzapine, quetiapine, ziprasidone, and aripiprazole have opened a new era in the treatment of schizophrenia, helping some patients who were previously thought to be resistant to treatment and decreasing the risk of EPS and tardive dyskinesia. Atypical neuroleptics are thought to be more effective through more selective blockade of dopamine receptor subtypes than typical neuroleptics. By definition, atypical neuroleptics affect serotonin receptors, particularly blockade of the 5-HT2A receptor. Atypical neurolpetics are associated with an increased risk of metabolic syndrome and increased risk of death in elderly patients (Table 3–12).

   a. **Efficacy**

      (1) **Acute treatment.** Therapy with atypical neuroleptics is frequently successful, with amelioration of symptoms such as hallucinations, delusions, and agitation. Atypical neuroleptics can also be effective with negative symptoms such as apathy, anhedonia, and amotivation.

      (2) **Maintenance treatment.** Atypical neuroleptics also decrease the risk of relapse and may be more effective than the older typical neuroleptics when patients are more adherent to treatment attributed to fewer negative symptoms and less uncomfortable side effects.

   b. **Clozapine.** This agent was the first novel antipsychotic in general use in the United States.

      (1) **Cost and special issues.** Because of potentially lethal side effects (see VII G 2 b [6]), clozapine is available in the United States under a unique prescribing arrangement. Clozapine is prescribed as a part of a system of care that initially includes mandatory weekly blood counts and other monitoring. When first approved, the Food and Drug Administration required that this blood work be performed by a specific laboratory system, which drove the cost of the treatment to between $8,000 and $9,000 per year per patient. About 30% of treatment-resistant schizophrenic patients may benefit significantly from clozapine, but the many significant side effects still limit the clinical use of the medication to patients who have more severe schizophrenia or who have failed trials of other atypical neuroleptics.

TABLE 3–12 Atypical Neuroleptics

Generic Name	Trade Name(s)	Usual Oral Dosage Range (mg/day)
Clozapine	Clozaril	150–300 bid
Risperidone	Risperdal	2–3 bid
	Risperdal Consta	25–50 IM q 2wks
Olanzapine	Zyprexa	10–30
Quetiapine	Seroquel	100–400 bid
Ziprasidone	Geodon	80–240
Aripiprazole	Abilify	10–30

(2) Pharmacology

(a) Structurally, clozapine is a dibenzodiazepine, similar to the neuroleptic loxapine.

(b) The specific mechanism of action is not yet understood. To a small extent, it blocks D-1 receptors in the mesolimbic and cortical areas of the brain but has little effect on dopamine receptors in the striatum, possibly accounting for some of its unique properties. Clozapine also affects serotonergic, adrenergic, histaminergic, and cholinergic pathways, and any one of these mechanisms could possibly explain its antipsychotic properties (see III D).

(3) Clinical effects. The effects of clozapine differ significantly from those of earlier antipsychotic agents. In addition to reducing the positive symptoms of schizophrenia, clozapine reduces negative symptoms in some patients. It appears to have a markedly reduced propensity to produce neuroleptic malignant syndrome, EPS, and tardive dyskinesia (although a very small group of studies reports the occurrence of each of these conditions with clozapine). Clozapine also appears to convey particular benefits in psychotic patients with tendencies to attempt suicidal or aggressive behaviors.

(4) Use. Prescribing clozapine is not easy. The physician must register with the drug manufacturer and be a part of the system of care, which includes a pharmacist and a clinician to perform monitoring functions. Initially, weekly blood tests must be performed, and patients must be located if they fail to report for tests. Clearly informing patients of all the risks is quite complicated, both before starting the medication (if they can legally give consent) and after starting the medication (if they regain the ability to consent to the treatment as a result of the clozapine).

(5) Dosage and administration. It is recommended that clozapine be initiated at 12.5 mg once or twice a day, increasing to an average of 300 to 600 mg/day over a 2-week period. In severe cases, doses may be gradually titrated up to 900 mg/day. It should be emphasized that some patients do not respond to clozapine. After an adequate therapeutic trial, maintaining nonresponsive patients on clozapine makes little sense.

(6) Side effects. Significant adverse effects may occur.

(a) The risk of life-threatening **agranulocytosis** requires intensive monitoring of the patient's complete blood count (CBC) and state of health. Patients may not be started on clozapine if their initial weight count is below 3,500/mm^3. White blood cell count and absolute neutrophil count must be done weekly for the first 6 months and then possibly less frequently if counts have been stable. **Febrile conditions** occur in the first few weeks after initiation of the drug. However, febrile conditions may represent infections secondary to agranulocytosis. Therefore, any fever in a patient taking clozapine must receive an aggressive and expert workup.

(b) **Seizures** may occur with clozapine treatment, particularly at higher dosages.

(c) Cardiovascular adverse events with clozapine have included **myocarditis and respiratory or cardiac arrest,** necessitating the slow titration of dosage.

(d) **Sedation** can be excessive, particularly in the early stages of treatment. **Excessive salivation,** especially at night, may be a serious problem for some patients. Unlike sedation, excessive salivation seems to be a more persistent side effect. Although some treatments (e.g., anticholinergic drugs) are available, each treatment carries its own risks.

(e) **Weight gain** may occur in more than 50% of patients taking clozapine. Development of **metabolic syndrome** with hyperglycemia and hyperlipidemias must be monitored on a regular basis.

(f) **Other side effects** such as nausea and gastrointestinal (GI) disturbances are fairly common. Headache occurs fairly often, and many other side effects are found with lesser frequency. Patients who have experienced therapeutic benefit from clozapine often prefer to live with these substantial side effects.

c. Risperidone. This agent has been in use since the 1990s for the treatment of schizophrenia. The major advantage of risperidone over clozapine is the low risk of agranulocytosis.

(1) Mechanism of action. With blockade of both dopamine and serotonin receptors, risperidone can improve both the positive and negative symptoms of schizophrenia.

(2) Dosage and administration. Risperidone is usually administered in twice-daily doses, starting at 1 mg twice daily, and increasing to 3 mg twice daily over the first few days.

Convenient dosage forms (as low as 0.25 mg) have made this drug popular for treating patients requiring only minimal dosages of antipsychotics. A rapidly dissolving sol-tab is available for patients who have difficulty taking tablets. Risperidone is also the only atypical neuroleptic currently available in a long-acting (2 weeks) depot neuroleptic formulation.

(3) Side effects. Unfortunately, at higher dosages, risperidone begins to exert less specific blockade of dopamine receptors and can cause EPS in some patients.

(a) Because **increased prolactin secretion** is common (as with older dopamine-blocking agents), galactorrhea, gynecomastia, amenorrhea, and sexual performance dysfunction can be expected in some patients.

(b) QTc prolongation may occur but is rarely clinically significant.

(c) Weight gain is not common with risperidone use, but patients must be monitored for weight, hyperglycemia, and hyperlipidemias.

(d) Other side effects include insomnia, agitation, dizziness, and constipation.

d. Olanzapine. The third atypical neuroleptic approved for treatment of schizophrenia in the United States, olanzapine can be very effective for treating negative symptoms, and it is not commonly known to cause EPS.

(1) Mechanism of action. Blockade of both dopamine and serotonin receptors can improve both the positive and negative symptoms of schizophrenia. Blockade of histamine receptors may be responsible for sedation known to occur with olanzapine.

(2) Dosage and administration. Usually olanzapine is administered in once-daily doses, starting at 5 to 10 mg/day and increasing up to 20 mg/day over the first few days. An orally disintegrating tablet is available for patients who have difficulty taking oral medications. Olanzapine is one of only two atypical neuroleptics currently available in an intramuscular injectable formulation.

(3) Side effects. Unfortunately, at higher doses, weight gain becomes a concern with olanzapine. Up to 50% of olanzapine patients experience weight gain and worrisome rates of hyperglycemia and hyperlipidemias.

(a) Other side effects include sedation, dry mouth, and constipation.

e. Quetiapine. This agent is the fourth atypical neuroleptic approved for treatment of schizophrenia in the United States. Quetiapine can be very effective for treating negative symptoms, and some patients report decreased symptoms of anxiety.

(1) Mechanism of action. Blockade of both dopamine and serotonin receptors can improve both the positive and negative symptoms of schizophrenia. Rapid dissociation from the D2 receptor may account for the striking lack of EPS with quetiapine.

(2) Dosage and administration. Quetiapine is usually administered in twice-daily doses, starting at 100 to 200 mg/day and increasing up to 800/day over the first week.

(3) Side effects. Sedation is the most commonly reported side effect of quetiapine.

(a) Weight gain is known to occur with quetiapine, and patients must be monitored for weight, hyperglycemia, and hyperlipidemias.

(b) Other side effects include dizziness, dry mouth, GI effects, and lightheadedness.

f. Ziprasidone. This agent is the fifth atypical neuroleptic approved for treatment of schizophrenia in the United States. Ziprasidone can be very effective for treating both the positive and negative symptoms, and some patients report improvement in depressed moods.

(1) Mechanism of action. Blockade of both dopamine and serotonin receptors can improve both the positive and negative symptoms of schizophrenia. Ziprasidone uniquely provides partial agonist activity at the 5HT-1a receptor and reuptake inhibition of serotonin and norepinephrine.

(2) Dosage and administration. Ziprasidone is usually administered in once-daily doses, starting at 40 to 80 mg daily and increasing up to 240 mg/day over the first week. Ziprasidone is one of only two atypical neuroleptics currently available in an intramuscular injectable formulation.

(3) Side effects. Agitation is the most commonly reported side effect of ziprasidone, with some patients developing akathisia.

(a) QTc prolongation is known to occur with ziprasidone, requiring electrocardiographic clearance in patients with cardiac histories.

       (b) Weight gain is not common with ziprasidone, but patients must still be monitored for weight, hyperglycemia, and hyperlipidemias.

       (c) Other side effects include dizziness, GI effects, sedation, and lightheadedness.

    g. Aripiprazole. This agent is the most recent atypical neuroleptic approved for treatment of schizrenia in the United States. Aripiprazole can be very effective for treating negative symptoms.

      (1) Mechanism of action. Although blockade of some dopamine and serotonin receptors occurs, partial agonist activities at D3 and 5HT-1a make aripiprazole unique among the atypical neuroleptics.

      (2) Dosage and administration. Aripiprazole is usually administered in once-daily doses, starting at 10 to 15 mg/day and increasing up to 30 mg/day over the first few weeks.

      (3) Side effects. Agitation, anxiety, and insomnia are reported side effects of aripiprazole, and some patients find these side effects difficult to tolerate.

       (a) Patients rarely gain weight while taking aripiprazole, but weight, hyperglycemia, and hyperlipidemia must be monitored with all atypical neuroleptics.

       (b) Other side effects include GI effects, and lightheadedness.

    h. Zotepine. This atypical neuroleptic has been approved for treatment of schizophrenia in Europe but is not yet available in the United States.

    i. Ritanserin and mianserin. These two drugs, which are already available in Europe, are primarily 5-HT2 antagonists without dopamine blockade. In the next few years, these agents or similar drugs may be available in the United States.

  3. Other pharmacologic agents. Although neuroleptics are the drugs of choice in the treatment of schizophrenia, it is sometimes necessary to turn to other classes if patients are nonresponsive or intolerant of side effects of neuroleptics. Augmentation strategies for nonresponse are covered in some of the schizophrenia treatment algorithms.

    a. Anticonvulsants and lithium. The addition of a mood stabilizer is recommended for the treatment of patients who have not achieved a satisfactory response to trials of neuroleptics alone.

      (1) Valproate can be effective. This agent can be added to clozapine to treat clozapine-induced seizures without substantially increasing the risk of agranulocytosis.

      (2) Carbamazepine can also be effective but should never be used with clozapine.

      (3) Newer anticonvulsants such as **gabapentin, topiramate,** and **lamotrigine** may also be useful in adjunctive treatment.

      (4) In patients with significant affective symptoms, including signs of mood swings, **lithium** has also been found to be an effective adjunctive agent.

    b. Antidepressants. Patients with a history of schizophrenia may develop full diagnostic criteria of depression. All classes of antidepressants are worth trying for patients with signs of **significant schizophrenia and depression.**

      (1) Newer antidepressants. Some of the newer agents, such as the selective serotonin reuptake inhibitors (SSRIs), may be useful in patients in whom **panic attacks** are evident.

      (2) SSRIs. These agents are useful when **obsessive-compulsive disorder (OCD)–like syndromes** occur in individuals with schizophrenia. According to some reports, atypical neuroleptics may precipitate OCD symptoms.

    c. Anxiolytics and sedatives. Agitation in schizophrenia can be severe and life threatening.

      (1) Benzodiazepines are frequently used in the short-term treatment of agitation in schizophrenia. These agents, particularly lorazepam, are also the drugs of choice in adjunctive management of catatonic schizophrenia. However, although patients with both akathisia and tardive dyskinesia may respond to benzodiazepines, long-term use of these drugs can be problematic; as many as 50% of all patients with schizophrenia have had substance abuse problems. Benzodiazepines should be avoided when clozapine is used, and they should never be used when the clozapine dose is being titrated initially.

      (2) Barbiturates are no longer commonly used in the therapy of schizophrenia, but they are sometimes used as a treatment of last resort in agitated psychotic patients who do not respond to high doses of neuroleptics and benzodiazepines.

    d. β-blockers. These agents are effective in the treatment of akathisia, and they may be effective against some medication-induced tremors. Propranolol is frequently used for this purpose, and longer acting, less lipophyllic agents may be more convenient in long-term treatment. In addition, propranolol has shown promise in treating some cases of severe psychosis and cases of severe aggression. Pindolol, which actually has some serotonergic activity, may have other uses in psychiatry (e.g., as an adjunct treatment with antidepressants).

H **Electroconvulsive therapy (ECT)** Until modern medications for use in schizophrenia treatment were developed, ECT was the only effective treatment option available. ECT still plays an important role in the therapy of treatment-resistant schizophrenia. Current treatment algorithms indicate that ECT should be considered after three or four drug trials. ECT is likely most effective in patients with affective symptoms and in catatonia.

1. **Indications**
    a. When life-threatening circumstances such as severe catatonia or extreme suicidal ideation are present
    b. When massive doses of neuroleptics become disabling and patients can be maintained on standard doses of neuroleptics after ECT
    c. When patients are clearly refractory to standard treatments and augmentations

2. **Difficulties.** The negative public perception of ECT and risks of anesthesia make this a difficult course when treating schizophrenia outside of academic centers. It can be very difficult to establish informed consent to use ECT in patients with schizophrenia.

Study Questions

Directions: *Each of the numbered items or incomplete statements in this section is followed by answers or by completions of the statement. Select the ONE lettered answer or completion that is BEST in each case.*

1. Which of the following brain regions appears abnormal in schizophrenia?

 (A) Medulla oblongata
 (B) Optic chiasm
 (C) Prefrontal cortex
 (D) Reticular activating system (RAS)
 (E) Third ventricle

2. A 34-year-old woman complains that she is gaining weight since she started taking chlorpromazine for chronic undifferentiated schizophrenia. A complete review of systems and history shows evidence of breast enlargement and lactation. However, a serum pregnancy test is negative. Which of the following neuroleptics would be a good choice for a treatment change?

 (A) Fluphenazine
 (B) Haloperidol
 (C) Risperidone
 (D) Thioridazine
 (E) Ziprasidone

3. A 21-year-old man is brought to the emergency department by his family. They report that he has been acting strangely for the past 2 weeks since coming home abruptly from college in the middle of the semester. In addition, they mention his rapid speech. The man states that he has been hearing voices and seeing small creatures out the corner of his eye. He presents with an agitated and restless manner. Which of the following is the next appropriate treatment step?

 (A) Send the patient to the nearest state hospital for treatment.
 (B) Order psychological testing.
 (C) Interview the family to complete a genogram.
 (D) Perform a complete physical examination and consider laboratory tests.
 (E) Start a depot neuroleptic agent.

4. A 40-year-old man presents to a mental health center complaining that his neighbors have been spying on him. He reports a complicated delusion: the Internal Revenue Service is conspiring to take away his home. He denies any hallucinations or mood changes, and he has been able to work as a truck mechanic without loss of function. Which of the following diagnoses is most appropriate?

 (A) Delusional disorder
 (B) Major depression with psychotic features
 (C) Schizoaffective disorder
 (D) Schizophrenia
 (E) Schizophreniform disorder

5. A 29-year-old man who lives in a group home and takes fluphenazine on a daily basis develops a high fever and muscle rigidity. The man undergoes examination and testing at the local emergency department, where a creatine phosphokinase value comes back as 10,000. Which of the following therapeutic steps should be taken next?

 (A) Send the patient home with instructions to take acetaminophen every 4 hours.
 (B) Send the patient home on an atypical antipsychotic.
 (C) Admit the patient to an intensive care unit.
 (D) Admit the patient to a state hospital.
 (E) Send the patient home on benztropine (1 mg tid).

6. The patient described in Question 5 has been hospitalized but plans to return to the community. The treating psychiatrist recommends which of the following changes in the medication regimen?

- [A] Changing to fluphenazine decanoate
- [B] Changing to haloperidol
- [C] Changing to olanzapine
- [D] Adding benztropine
- [E] Adding lithium

7. Which of the following neurotransmitters is believed to play the most critical role in the development of and treatment of schizophrenia?

- [A] Acetylcholine
- [B] Norepinephrine
- [C] Phospholipid
- [D] Protein G
- [E] Serotonin

8. A disheveled 27-year-old man presents with bizarre movements, agitated behavior, and rapid and unintelligible speech. The patient has had signs of psychosis for much of the past few months, and the family reports that the patient twice spent a month in state psychiatric hospitals. Which of the following schizophrenic subtypes can most appropriately be applied to this patient?

- [A] Catatonic
- [B] Chronic undifferentiated
- [C] Paranoid
- [D] Residual

9. A 45-year-old woman with no psychiatric history presents with disheveled appearance, almost mute speech, and thought blocking of several months' duration. She also fears that her internal organs have been stolen by a transplant surgeon to be used in a military robot. Which of the following diagnoses is most appropriate?

- [A] Bipolar disorder
- [B] Borderline personality disorder
- [C] Delusional disorder
- [D] Schizoaffective disorder
- [E] Schizophrenia

10. A 24-year-old man is discharged from the psychiatric ward with a diagnosis of paranoid schizophrenia. Four weeks after discharge, he tells his psychiatrist that he stopped taking his medications 2 days ago. Which of the following interventions is most appropriate?

- [A] Hospitalize the patient in a psychiatric ward.
- [B] Switch to a depot antipsychotic.
- [C] Refer for psychotherapy.
- [D] Inquire about side effects from the medication.
- [E] Discharge the patient from the clinic.

11. The patient described in Question 10 reports that although he receives Social Security Disability Income (SSDI), he has not been able to afford all of his medication. Which of the following interventions is most appropriate?

- [A] Rehospitalize the patient in a psychiatric ward.
- [B] Switch to a less expensive antipsychotic.
- [C] Refer the patient for psychotherapy.
- [D] Inquire into how he has budgeted his money.
- [E] Discharge the patient from the clinic.

12. The patient described in Question 10 reports that he has been giving much of his money away to panhandlers. Which of the following interventions is most appropriate?

- Ⓐ Rehospitalize the patient in the psychiatric ward.
- Ⓑ Refer the patient for case management,
- Ⓒ Refer the patient for psychosurgery.
- Ⓓ Inquire into how he can get a larger disability check.
- Ⓔ Discharge the patient from the clinic.

13. Schizophrenia may develop as a result of which of the following factors?

- Ⓐ Schizophrenigenic fathers
- Ⓑ Expressed emotions
- Ⓒ Living in rural areas as opposed to cities
- Ⓓ Schizophrenigenic mothers
- Ⓔ Polygenic transmission

14. What is the most consistent finding in brain structural abnormalities in schizophrenia?

- Ⓐ Enlargement of the third ventricle
- Ⓑ Loss of cerebrospinal fluid (CSF)
- Ⓒ Enlargement of the lateral ventricles
- Ⓓ Increased size of the thalamus
- Ⓔ Abnormalities in the cell architecture in the prefrontal cortex

15. The increase in the risk of developing schizophrenia for persons born after the Dutch hardship winter (1945–1946) is explained by which of the following factors?

- Ⓐ Poor prenatal malnutrition
- Ⓑ Expressed emotions
- Ⓒ Living in industrial areas as opposed to rural areas
- Ⓓ Good obstetric care
- Ⓔ Polygenic transmission

Directions: *The response options for items 16–19 are the same. Select one answer for each question in the set. Match the clinical picture with the type of drug that could change the situation.*

- Ⓐ Anticholinergics
- Ⓑ Atypical neuroleptics
- Ⓒ Barbiturates
- Ⓓ Benzodiazepines
- Ⓔ Depot haloperidol

16. A patient who is sometimes agitated has been tried on several different typical and atypical antipsychotics with little success

17. A patient on thiothixene who develops a pill-rolling tremor and shuffling gait

18. A patient who has a positive response to antipsychotic medication in the hospital but becomes noncompliant shortly after five discharges in 1 year

19. A patient whose hallucinations respond to haloperidol but severe negative symptoms prevent successful discharge from the state hospital

Directions: *The response options for items 20–23 are the same. Select one answer for each question in the set. Match the following diagnostic criteria with the most likely diagnosis.*

- Ⓐ Brief psychotic disorder
- Ⓑ Delusional disorder
- Ⓒ Schizoaffective disorder
- Ⓓ Schizophrenia
- Ⓔ Schizophreniform disorder

20. A patient presents with hallucinations and bizarre delusions lasting 8 weeks.

21. A patient presents with periods of mood disturbance with psychosis and periods of psychosis without mood disturbance over the past 3 years.

22. A patient presents with a second lifetime episode of hallucinations and bizarre delusions that again lasts only a few days.

23. A patient who otherwise appears normal presents with a 5-month belief that a champion race car driver has fallen madly in love with her; she believes he demonstrates his love by painting the patient's age as the number on his car.

Directions: *The response options for items 24–26 are the same. Select one answer for each question in the set. Choose the best neuroleptic for the clinical scenario.*

- A. Aripiprazole
- B. Chlorpromazine
- C. Clozapine
- D. Olanzapine
- E. Ziprasidone

24. A patient presents with persistent suicide attempts after treatment with fluphenazine, risperidone, and quetiapine.

25. A severely overweight patient presents with cardiac conduction abnormalities after myocarditis from clozapine.

26. A patient reporting an allergy to ziprasidone requires intramuscular administration of a neuroleptic in the emergency department.

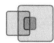 *Answers and Explanations*

1. The answer is C [*III D 2 d*]. Abnormalities in the cell architecture have been reported in the prefrontal cortex. All other regions appear normal.

2. The answer is E [*VII G 2 e*]. Ziprasidone does not cause hyperprolactinemia, which can occur with fluphenazine, haloperidol, risperidone, and thioridazine.

3. The answer is D [*VI A 3*]. Acute medical causes of psychotic symptoms must be ruled out through a complete physical examination and any indicated medical tests.

4. The answer is A [*VI C 3 a, b*]. Delusional disorder often occurs later in life and lacks the global functional deterioration seen in individuals with schizophrenia and schizophreniform disorder. Diagnosis of schizoaffective disorder or psychotic depression requires substantial mood changes.

5. The answer is C [*VII G 1 e 2*]. Neuroleptic malignant syndrome is potentially life threatening and requires admission to an intensive care unit for support of respiratory, renal, and cardiovascular functioning.

6. The answer is C [*VII G 2 d*]. Switching to an atypical neuroleptic would reduce the risk of another episode. Olanzapine would be the best choice of a neuroleptic. Lithium is not indicated by this history. Benztropine will not help neuroleptic malignant syndrome.

7. The answer is E [*III D 1 b, 4, a, b*]. Serotonin plays the more prominent role in the pathophysiology of schizophrenia. Acetylcholine has no role in the development of or treatment of schizophrenia. Anticholinergic medications are only used to treat side effects. Phospholipids and G proteins are found in membranes and are not neurotransmitters.

8. The answer is A [*IV H 1 a, b*]. Catatonia is distinguished by either dramatic increase or dramatic decrease in motor activity. Chronic undifferentiated, paranoid, and residual subtypes do not involve significant changes in movements.

9. The answer is E [*V A*]. In women, the onset of schizophrenia can occur much later than in men. Individuals with bipolar disorder or schizoaffective disorder would normally have had prior episodes. This patient has deteriorated too much to have delusional disorder and has been psychotic too long to have psychosis in a personality disorder.

10. The answer is D [*VII G 1 b (2), (4) (b)*]. Side effects are a common cause of nonadherence to treatment. Consideration of side effects and their importance should be the first step in evaluation of nonadherence. Nonadherence to treatment is a common clinical challenge and must be managed in a way that keeps the patient in treatment.

11. The answer is D [*VII E 1 e*]. Nonadherence to a medication regimen for financial reasons may have a complex cause and must be thoroughly investigated. This patient does not meet current admission criteria for rehospitalization. Do not automatically switch to a cheaper medication because free drug programs or other psychosocial interventions may keep this patient on the correct regimen. Psychotherapy can help but cannot replace medication in most cases.

12. The answer is B [*VII E 1, 2 d*]. Financial management poses a substantial problem for many patients but can be improved through case management or psychosocial rehabilitation.

13. The answer is E [*III A 2*]. Polygenic transmission would be consistent with findings of differences in severity of the disease and the variable rates of pathology in some families. Expressed emotions may contribute to relapse rates, but not development, of schizophrenia. Living in industrialized areas as opposed to rural areas may increase the risk. The theory of schizophrenigenic mothers has been discredited, and fathers were not blamed at the time.

14. The answer is C [*III D 2 a, b, d*]. The most consistent finding in brain structural abnormalities in schizophrenia is enlargement of the lateral, not the third, ventricles. Several studies have found that the size of the thalamus decreases. Cerebrospinal fluid may expand to replace the lost volume. Abnormalities in the cell architecture may occur in the prefrontal cortex, not in the visual cortex.

15. The answer is A [*III B 1 b*]. Poor prenatal nutrition caused by hardships during World War II is thought to have increased the risk of developing schizophrenia. Expressed emotions may contribute to relapse rates but not to the development of schizophrenia. Residence in rural areas may be less stressful than living in urban areas. Obstetric problems may increase the risk of developing schizophrenia. Polygenic transmission would be consistent with findings of differences in severity of the disease and the variable rates of pathology in some families.

16. The answer is D [*VII G 3 c (1)*]. The agitation of akathisia can be treated with benzodiazepines. Anticholinergics rarely work to reduce akathisia. Barbiturates are used only in extremely rare cases of prolonged agitation. Depot neuroleptics could prolong the time at risk for akathisia.

17. The answer is A [*VII G 1 e (1) (a)*]. Anticholinergics are indicated for treating EPS that occur as a result of neuroleptic use. The pill-rolling tremor and shuffling gait of EPS often respond to anticholinergics. Use of an atypical neuroleptic is not always the best choice when a patient already responds to a typical neuroleptic. Benzodiazepines and barbiturates are not the primary choice for treating EPS. Depot neuroleptics could also cause EPS.

18. The answer is E [*VII G 1 d (3)*]. Depot neuroleptics are a proven way to better ensure compliance in such a "heavy-dose" patient. Compliance cannot be assured with the other options.

19. The answer is B [*VII G 2*]. Atypical antipsychotics are the best treatment for negative symptoms. Negative symptoms are the primary indication for use of the more expensive atypical neuroleptics. There is no reason to expect a response to anticholinergics, benzodiazepines, barbiturates, or depot haloperidol.

20. The answer is E [*VI C 2*]. Schizophreniform disorder involves psychotic symptoms lasting longer than 2 weeks but less than 6 months.

21. The answer is C [*VI B 4*]. Schizoaffective disorder involves both periods of mood disturbance with psychosis and periods of psychosis without mood disturbance.

22. The answer is A [*VI C 1*]. Brief psychotic disorder involves periods of psychosis lasting less than 1 month. This disorder can recur later in life.

23. The answer is B [*VI C 3*]. Delusional disorder lacks the global functional deterioration seen in schizophrenia and schizophreniform disorder. In the erotomanic type of delusional disorder, patients believe someone (usually of a higher status) has fallen in love with them. Brief psychotic disorder involves periods of psychosis lasting less than 1 month.

24. The answer is C [*VII G 2 b*]. Clozapine appears to convey particular benefits in psychotic patients with tendencies to attempt suicidal or aggressive behaviors.

25. The answer is A [*VII G 2 f, g*]. Aripiprazole and ziprasidone have the lowest weight gain risk, but ziprasidone can cause QTc prolongation.

26. The answer is D [*VII G 2 d, f*]. Only olanzapine and ziprasidone have currently available intramuscular formulations.

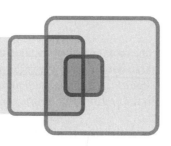

chapter 4

Mood Disorders

JOSHUA T. THORNHILL IV

I   DEFINITION

The prominent feature of mood disorders is a **disturbance of mood** along the happy–sad axis. Disorders featuring anxious mood are described in Chapter 5. The *Diagnostic and Statistical Manual of Mental Disorders*, 4th edition (*DSM-IV*) classifies mood disorders to include **major depressive disorder, bipolar I disorder, bipolar II disorder, dysthymic disorder, cyclothymic disorder, mood disorder caused by a general medical condition, and substance-induced mood disorder.**

II   HISTORY

Serious investigation into the etiology and classification of mood disorders began in the middle of the nineteenth century. As in other areas of psychiatry and medicine, prevailing theories have continually shifted, particularly regarding the tendency to view mood disorders as a problem with the brain (a biologically based illness) or a problem with the mind (a psychologically based illness).

A **Nineteenth century**   In the **mid-to-late nineteenth century,** a number of clinicians began to see the possibility of differentiating forms of "insanity."

1. Rather than lumping all such patients together, **Emil Kraepelin** noted that some psychotic patients had a cyclical pattern and prominent mood symptoms (manic depression) and others had a more chronic pattern that also featured cognitive impairment (i.e., **dementia praecox,** now called **schizophrenia**).

2. At the turn of the twentieth century, neuropathologists found abnormal brains in patients with Alzheimer's disease and neurosyphilis. Many assumed that brain disease was also the cause of schizophrenia and depression.

B **Twentieth century**   In the twentieth century, particularly in the United States, psychoanalytic theorists believed that many mood disorders stemmed from the psychological response to loss. Experts often differentiated between **endogenous** (caused by biologic factors) and **exogenous** (caused by loss or other environmental stresses) depression.

1. During the **first half of the century,** the emphasis on psychological factors meant fewer research efforts into the neurochemical and neuroanatomic aspects of mood disorders.

2. In the **1950s,** the serendipitous observation that two drugs affect depression stimulated appreciation of the biologic underpinnings of mood disorders.
   a. **Iproniazid,** which was being studied as a treatment for tuberculosis, elevated the mood of (often depressed) patients. Knowledge that this drug acted as a **monoamine oxidase (MAO) inhibitor** led to speculation that low levels of monoamines (e.g., norepinephrine [NE], serotonin [5-HT], dopamine) might play a role in the etiology of depression.
   b. **Reserpine,** an antihypertensive drug that **depletes monoamines** presynaptically, caused depression in some patients.

C **Twenty-first century**   As studies into the neurochemical and neuroanatomic aspects of the brain continue, experts currently believe that the interaction of biologic and psychosocial factors determines which individuals will develop mood disorders. The exogenous–endogenous dichotomy is no longer seen as a critical distinction because patients with and without obvious environmental causes of depression can have similar prognoses and treatment responses.

III DIAGNOSIS

[A] **Identification of mood episodes** Diagnosis of a mood disorder requires the identification of mood episodes, which are not the actual diagnoses in themselves. Rather, they are the building blocks clinicians use in making the diagnosis of a mood disorder (see III B). The *DSM-IV* defines **four types of mood episodes:** major depressive episode, manic episode, mixed episode, and hypomanic episode. The criteria for each type require that the mood symptoms lead to serious distress or dysfunction and that they are not caused by the effects of drugs, alcohol, or a medical condition.

1. **Major depressive episode (MDE).** The criteria for MDE are shown in Table 4–1. Symptoms must represent a change from baseline and must persist for at least 2 weeks to be characteristic of MDE.
   a. Patients must exhibit **either depressed mood or a notable decrease in interest or pleasure.** Another name for the inability to experience pleasure is **anhedonia.** Loss of interest commonly extends to **loss of libido.**
   b. Patients typically exhibit **neurovegetative symptoms** of depression such as changes in sleep and appetite. Sleep impairment may involve initial insomnia (trouble falling asleep), middle insomnia (awakening during the night), or terminal insomnia (early morning awakening). Whereas sleep and appetite usually decrease in MDE, patients with **atypical depression** note oversleeping and increased appetite with weight gain.
   c. **Fatigue** and **impaired concentration** are common.
   d. **Psychomotor activity** may be increased (agitation, including pacing and hand wringing) or decreased (retardation, including soft speech, lack of eye contact, immobility).

TABLE 4–1 *DSM-IV* **Diagnostic Criteria for a Major Depressive Episode**

A. At least five of the following symptoms have been present during the same 2-week period and represent a change from previous functioning; at least one of the symptoms is either (1) depressed mood or (2) loss of interest or pleasure.
   1. Depressed mood most of the day, nearly every day, as indicated by either subjective report (e.g., feels sad or empty) or observation made by others (e.g., appears tearful); in children and adolescents, irritable mood suffices
   2. Markedly diminished interest or pleasure in all, or almost all, activities most of the day, nearly every day (as indicated either by subjective account or observation made by others)
   3. Significant weight loss or weight gain when not dieting (e.g., >5% of body weight in 1 month) or decrease or increase in appetite nearly every day; in children, consider failure to make expected weight gains
   4. Insomnia or hypersomnia nearly every day
   5. Psychomotor agitation or retardation nearly every day (observable by others, not merely subjective feelings of restlessness or being slowed down)
   6. Fatigue or loss of energy nearly every day
   7. Feelings of worthlessness or excessive or inappropriate guilt (which may be delusional) nearly every day (not merely self-reproach or guilt about being sick)
   8. Diminished ability to think or concentrate, or indecisiveness, nearly every day (either by subjective account or as observed by others)
   9. Recurrent thoughts of death (not just fear of dying); recurrent suicidal ideation without a specific plan; or a suicide attempt or a specific plan for committing suicide
B. The symptoms cause clinically significant distress or impairment in social, occupational, or other important areas of functioning.
C. The symptoms are not caused by the direct effects of a substance (e.g., drugs of abuse, medication) or a general medical condition (e.g., hypothyroidism).
D. The symptoms are not better accounted for by bereavement (after the loss of a loved one, the symptoms persist for longer than 2 months or are characterized by marked functional impairment, morbid preoccupation with worthlessness, suicidal ideation, psychotic symptoms, or psychomotor retardation).

    e. Feelings of **worthlessness** and **guilt** are often present. The guilt may be **delusional** (i.e., a fixed, false belief such as thinking that one has committed a great crime or caused a natural disaster).

    f. **Thoughts of death** or **suicidal ideation** are also common. Suicidal ideation can range from passive ideas (e.g., wishing one would develop cancer) to active plans.

2. Manic episode. This features a distinct period of elevated or irritable mood that lasts at least 1 week. *DSM-IV* criteria are given in Table 4–2. Features of mania include the following:

    a. **Grandiosity** involves an elevated opinion of one's features and accomplishments. Manic patients may feel extraordinarily attractive, engage in name dropping, exaggerate educational and career achievements, and feel superior to other people. **Grandiose delusions** may also be seen. For example, a patient may believe that he has achieved world peace or owns a billion-dollar company.

    b. During a manic episode, **most patients need little sleep.** Whereas depressed individuals complain about their short nights, patients with mania feel well rested after only 2 or 3 hours of sleep.

    c. **Pressured speech,** as observed by clinicians, may reflect a **flight of ideas** or **racing thoughts.**

    d. Manic patients are **easily distracted** and become interested in various environmental stimuli. This can lead to difficulty in engaging such a patient during an interview. During mental status testing, vigilance tests such as the continuous performance task (CPT) show evidence of this dysfunction.

    e. An **increase in goal-directed activities** as well as participation in **potentially dangerous activities** such as gambling, sexual promiscuity, or reckless driving often occurs.

3. Mixed episode. This describes a period during which patients satisfy criteria for **both manic episode and MDE over a 1-week period.** Such patients might exhibit pressured speech, irritability, and the need for little sleep, while feeling worthless and suicidal.

4. Hypomanic episode. This is similar in many ways to a manic episode but is less severe. Differences in the criteria include the following.

    a. The episode need only last 4 days.

    b. The episode must not lead to hospitalization, must not include psychotic features (e.g., delusions), and must not cause severe social or occupational impairment.

B **Diagnosis of mood disorders** Differentiation of the mood disorders listed below depends on the presence or absence of the mood episodes discussed in III A 4. Table 4–3 may help clarify the various diagnoses.

TABLE 4–2 *DSM-IV* Diagnostic Criteria for a Manic Episode

A. A distinct period of abnormally and persistently elevated, expansive, or irritable mood lasts at least 1 week (or any duration if hospitalization is necessary)

B. During the period of mood disturbance, at least three of the following symptoms have persisted (four if the mood is only irritable) and have been present to a significant degree:
1. Inflated self-esteem or grandiosity
2. Decreased need for sleep (e.g., feels rested after only 3 hours of sleep)
3. More talkative than usual or pressure to keep talking
4. Flight of ideas or subjective experience that thoughts are racing
5. Distractibility (i.e., attention too easily drawn to unimportant or irrelevant external stimuli)
6. Increase in goal-directed activity (e.g., socially, at work or school, or sexually) or psychomotor agitation
7. Excessive involvement in pleasurable activities that have a high potential for painful consequences (e.g., the person engages in unrestrained buying sprees, sexual indiscretions, or foolish business investments)

C. The mood disturbance is sufficiently severe to cause marked impairment in the occupational functioning or in usual social activities or relationships with others or to necessitate hospitalization to prevent harm to self or others or psychotic features are present.

D. The symptoms are not caused by the direct effects of a substance (e.g., drugs of abuse, medication) or a general medical condition (e.g., hyperthyroidism).

Note: Manic episodes that are clearly precipitated by somatic antidepressant treatment (e.g., medication, electroconvulsive therapy, light therapy) should not count toward a diagnosis of bipolar I disorder.

TABLE 4-3   Differentiation of Mood Disorders

Diagnosis	Major Depressive Episode	Milder Depression	Manic or Mixed Episode	Hypomania
Major depressive disorder	+	±	−	−
Dysthymic disorder	−*	+	−	−
Bipolar I disorder	±	±	+	±
Bipolar II disorder	+	±	−	+
Cyclothymia	−	+	−†	+

+ = This syndrome must be present to make the diagnosis; − = this syndrome must be absent to make the diagnosis; ± = this syndrome may be present or absent.
*A major depressive episode must not occur during the first 2 years of the illness.
†A manic episode must not occur during the first 2 years of the illness.

1. **Major depressive disorder**
   a. **Diagnostic criteria.** The diagnosis requires the presence of one or more MDE and the absence of any manic, hypomanic, or mixed episodes.
   b. **Associated clinical features**
      (1) **Psychotic features.** These conditions, which are seen in some patients, are most often **mood congruent** (i.e., the content of the delusion or hallucination reflects depression). A mood-congruent delusion might be the belief that one has committed terrible crimes or sins. A mood-congruent hallucination might be a voice that tells one to die or says that one is a loser.
      (2) **Melancholia.** A more severe subtype of major depression, melancholia features more profound anhedonia and neurovegetative symptoms. Early morning awakening and significant weight loss are common (see III C).
      (3) **Mortality and morbidity.** In addition to the risk of suicide, affected patients have a higher risk of illness or death from medical causes.
      (4) **Psychiatric comorbidity.** Patients are at risk for several other psychiatric conditions (e.g., alcohol or other substance abuse, anxiety disorders).
   c. **Epidemiology**
      (1) **Risk and prevalence.** The lifetime risk of developing major depressive disorder is about 15% overall; the prevalence in women is roughly twice the prevalence in men. The risk is similar in different countries and across races.
      (2) **Age of onset.** The age of onset can range from childhood to old age; the mean age of onset is about 40 years old.
      (3) **Recurrence.** Approximately 50% of people who have one episode of major depression will have one or more additional episodes. After two episodes, the recurrence rate is about 70%, and after three episodes, it is about 90%.
   d. **Differential diagnosis.** The symptoms of major depressive disorder can overlap with symptoms of many other illnesses.
      (1) **Other psychiatric disorders.** Conditions with symptoms that are similar to major depressive disorder include dysthymic disorder, adjustment disorder with depressed mood, schizoaffective disorder, dementia, anxiety disorders, and personality disorders.
      (2) **Substance-induced mood disorders.** Causes may include intoxication with depressant drugs (e.g., alcohol, opiates, barbiturates); withdrawal from stimulants (e.g., cocaine, amphetamines); or treatment with medications such as steroids, some antihypertensives (i.e., reserpine, propranolol), and cimetidine.
      (3) **Mood disorders caused by a general medical condition.** Depression has been associated with a number of medical illnesses, including hypothyroidism, stroke, anemia, pancreatic cancer, Parkinson's disease, sleep apnea, and tuberculosis.
      (4) **Normal bereavement.** Many symptoms of a major depressive episode may be features of normal bereavement. In such cases, a diagnosis of major depressive disorder is not usually made unless the MDE criteria are still met 2 months after the loss. Some symptoms such as hallucinations unrelated to the loss and prolonged functional impairment are

atypical of normal bereavement and more suggestive of major depression. One must recognize that the symptoms and duration of "normal" bereavement vary among cultures.

2. **Dysthymic disorder**
   a. **Diagnostic criteria**
      (1) Patients present with a **chronic depression** (at least 2 years in duration for adults and 1 year for children and adolescents) that has **not** been **severe enough to meet the criteria for MDE.** Instead of the five symptoms required of MDE, patients must have two of the following: increased or decreased appetite, increased or decreased sleep, low energy, low self-esteem, poor concentration or decision-making ability, and hopelessness.
      (2) If patients experience an MDE after 2 years of having a dysthymic disorder, more than one diagnosis is made (dysthymic disorder and major depressive disorder).
      (3) In addition, patients must never have met criteria for manic episode, mixed episode, or hypomanic episode.
   b. **Associated clinical features.** Dysthymic disorder is associated with social impairment, health problems, alcohol and other drug abuse, and major depressive disorder. Coexistence of dysthymic disorder and major depression is sometimes referred to as **double depression.**
   c. **Epidemiology.** The lifetime risk of dysthymic disorder is about 5% overall; the prevalence rate in women is about twice that in men. Patients who develop dysthymic disorder before age 21 years are more likely to develop major depressive disorder later.
   d. **Differential diagnosis.** The possible diagnoses are similar to those of major depressive disorder (see III B 1 d).

3. **Bipolar I disorder.** Bipolar is a misnomer for this illness because a single manic episode is sufficient for the diagnosis (i.e., one only needs one "pole"). However, most patients experience both manic and depressive symptoms, and the first episode may be manic, hypomanic, depressed, or mixed. Of course, if the first episode is hypomanic or depressed, the proper diagnosis will not be made until the later emergence of mania.
   a. **Diagnostic criteria.** Patients have experienced **at least one manic or mixed episode** unless the symptoms were caused by a substance (including antidepressants) or a general medical condition. MDEs may or may not have ever been present.
   b. **Associated clinical features**
      (1) **Psychotic features.** Delusions, hallucinations, and disorganization can be seen during manic episodes, with severity similar in degree to that in schizophrenia. These are most often **mood congruent.** A mood-congruent delusion in mania might be the belief that one has found a cure for cancer or won an Academy Award. A mood-congruent hallucination might involve hearing the voice of God.
      (2) **Morbidity and mortality.** Attempted and completed suicide are both common. Comorbid medical problems can deteriorate because of poor compliance stemming from grandiosity or generally impaired judgment. Reckless behavior can increase the risk of sexually transmitted diseases and injuries.
      (3) **Psychiatric comorbidity.** Alcohol and other forms of drug abuse frequently complicate manic episodes and can carry into other phases of this disorder. Eating disorders, anxiety disorders, and attention deficit hyperactivity disorder (ADHD) are also associated with bipolar illness.
   c. **Epidemiology.** The lifetime risk of bipolar I disorder is about 1%, and it is similar in men and women and across racial groups. The mean age of onset is 30 years. More than 90% of people who have a manic episode will have additional episodes of mania or major depression.
   d. **Differential diagnosis**
      (1) **Other psychiatric disorders.** Similar symptoms are seen in bipolar II disorder and cyclothymic disorder. When psychotic symptoms exist, it can be difficult to differentiate bipolar I disorder from schizophrenia or schizoaffective disorder. However, if a patient has ever had delusions or hallucinations for at least 2 weeks in the absence of mania or major depression, then a psychotic disorder (rather than a mood disorder with psychotic features) must be diagnosed. Narcissistic personality disorder also has overlapping features.
      (2) **Substance-induced mood disorder.** Intoxication with stimulants such as cocaine or amphetamine can mimic mania. Antidepressant drugs can occasionally cause patients

to "switch" from depression to mania. Other prescription medications (e.g., corticosteroids, dopamine agonists, anticholinergics, cimetidine) can also precipitate manic symptoms.

    (3) **Mood disorder caused by a general medical condition.** Manic symptoms can be seen with infectious diseases, acquired immunodeficiency syndrome (AIDS), endocrinopathies (e.g., Cushing disease, hyperthyroidism), lupus, and a variety of neurologic disorders (e.g., epilepsy, multiple sclerosis [MS], Wilson disease).

4. **Bipolar II disorder.** This disorder is officially recognized for the first time in the *DSM-IV*.
   a. **Diagnostic criteria.** Patients have had **at least one MDE and one hypomanic episode** in the absence of any manic or mixed episodes.
   b. **Associated features.** Suicide is a risk, particularly during depressive episodes. As with major depression and bipolar I disorder, comorbidity with substance abuse or anxiety disorders is common.
   c. **Epidemiology.** The lifetime risk is approximately 0.5% and is higher in women than in men. There do not appear to be racial differences.
   d. **Differential diagnosis.** The possible diagnoses are similar to those of bipolar I disorder (see III B 3 d).

5. **Cyclothymic disorder.** This disorder could be described as dysthymic disorder with intermittent hypomanic periods. Similar to dysthymic disorder, it is a chronic rather than episodic illness.
   a. **Diagnostic criteria.** A patient who, over at least 2 years (1 year in children and adolescents), experiences **repeated episodes of hypomania and depression (not severe enough to meet criteria for major depressive disorder)** is diagnosed with cyclothymic disorder. During the first 2 years, a patient may not have an MDE, manic, or mixed episode. If such episodes occur after 2 years, more than one diagnosis may be made (e.g., cyclothymic disorder and bipolar I disorder).
   b. **Associated features.** Substance abuse and social and occupational dysfunction are common.
   c. **Epidemiology.** The lifetime risk of cyclothymic disorder is about 1%; it is slightly higher in women than in men. The age of onset is usually in the teens or early adulthood, and the course tends to be chronic. Up to 50% of people with cyclothymic disorder may ultimately develop bipolar disorder.
   d. **Differential diagnosis.** Possible diagnoses are similar to those for bipolar I disorder (see III B 3 d). In addition, the features of cyclothymic disorder must be differentiated from the mood swings seen in borderline personality disorder.

6. **Mood disorder caused by a general medical condition** and **substance-induced mood disorder.** These conditions are two other mood disorder diagnoses in the *DSM-IV*. As noted previously, other mood disorder diagnoses (e.g., major depressive disorder) are not made if medical illness or drug use appears to be the cause of the symptoms. Clinical examples include the following:
   a. A 69-year-old man recently suffered a left anterior stroke and now has the symptoms of an MDE. The appropriate diagnosis is mood disorder caused by a cerebrovascular accident, with a major depressive-like episode.
   b. A 32-year-old woman who presents to an emergency department with manic behavior has traces of amphetamine in her urine. The symptoms clear over several days without pharmacologic treatment. The diagnosis is amphetamine-induced mood disorder with manic features, with onset during intoxication.

C **Mood disorder specifiers**   The *DSM-IV* provides a number of specifiers that better describe a current or most recent mood episode.

1. **Severity or remission status (with or without psychosis).** Mood episodes can be described in two ways: as mild, moderate, or severe and as partial or full remission. When symptoms are severe, the **presence or absence of psychotic features** should be noted. When psychotic features are present, they should be described as mood congruent or mood incongruent.

2. **Catatonic features.** This specifier is used when a mood episode features two of the following: immobility; excess purposeless activity; negativism or mutism; posturing, mannerisms, or stereotypic behaviors; and echolalia or echopraxia.

3. **Melancholia.** This more severe presentation of depression is more common in inpatients and those with psychotic features. This specifier describes patients who exhibit (during the worst of the episode) a **loss of almost all pleasure** and three of the following:
   a. A distinct quality to the sad mood (e.g., it does not resemble normal grief or sadness)
   b. Symptoms that are worse in the morning
   c. Early morning awakening
   d. Marked psychomotor changes
   e. Marked anorexia or weight loss
   f. Excessive guilt

4. **Atypical features** of depression. Symptoms that are opposite to what is commonly observed, particularly increased weight or sleep, occur. Affected patients exhibit mood brightening in the face of positive events and can also report heaviness in their limbs and chronic rejection sensitivity.

5. **Other specifiers. Postpartum onset** (onset within 4 weeks postpartum; a nonpsychotic depression may occur in 10% to 20% of women. Note: Postpartum psychosis occurs in about one per 1,000 births), **seasonal pattern** (two seasonally linked MDEs in the past year, with full remission also occurring seasonally), and **rapid cycling** (four or more mood episodes in the past 12 months, with remission or a polarity switch between episodes) may occur.

IV ETIOLOGY

Over the years, experts have debated whether mood disorders represent brain disease or reflected intrapsychic conflicts. Most recently, they have returned to the belief that the conditions represent a biologic process. The etiology is probably multifactorial.

A Genetic factors Both major depressive and bipolar disorders run in families, which does not necessarily indicate genetic transmission. However, a variety of research techniques has shown the etiology of mood disorders to be at least partly genetic.

1. **Family studies**
   a. **Major depressive disorder.** Approximately 50% of individuals with major depressive disorder have a first-degree relative with a mood disorder, which is more often depression than bipolar disorder. Whereas concordance for identical twins is approximately 50%, siblings (including fraternal twins) have an approximate 15% risk. When one twin of a concordant pair has major depression, the other twin usually has depression rather than bipolar illness.
   b. **Bipolar disorder.** Approximately 90% of people with bipolar illness have a first-degree relative with a mood disorder, either bipolar or depressive. Estimates of concordance range between 33% and 90% for monozygotic twins and between 5% and 25% for other siblings. If the twin of a bipolar patient becomes ill, the twin will usually have a bipolar disorder.

2. **Adoption studies** in both major depression and bipolar disorder have supported a genetic etiology.

3. **Linkage studies.** This research is difficult because investigators are unsure whether to expect genetic patterns for particular mood disorders (e.g., pure major depression) or for a spectrum of diseases (e.g., major depression and dysthymic disorder, major depression and bipolar disorder).
   a. Studies have suggested that bipolar disorder is inherited in some families in an **X-linked pattern.**
   b. **Other linkage sites may be on chromosomes 4, 11** (the site of the gene for tyrosine hydroxylase), **18, and 21.** As of yet, no single chromosomal site seems to play a dominant role in the development of bipolar disorder, but several genes may interact to confer risk.

4. **Expanding triplet repeats.** This factor (i.e., repeating nucleotide bases), seen in the genetic basis of Huntington disease, may account for the finding that bipolar illness has earlier onset and more severe symptomatology in subsequent generations of some families.

B Neurochemical factors A number of neurotransmitters have been implicated in mood disorders, particularly **NE** and **5-HT**.

1. **NE** is associated with mood disorders, based on a variety of findings.
   a. Many effective antidepressant medications (e.g., desipramine, nortriptyline) block **NE** reuptake immediately and **downregulate β-receptors** after several weeks. Because the latter effect

correlates with the onset of action, it has been speculated that **adrenergic function may be abnormal in depression.**

    b. Measurements of NE or its metabolites in cerebrospinal fluid (CSF), plasma, and urine are variable. Metabolites of NE are generally diminished in depression.

    c. Increased NE activity has been speculated to be involved in mania.

2. 5-HT has been of more interest since the primarily serotonergic antidepressants were introduced.

    a. The **selective serotonin reuptake inhibitors (SSRIs)** such as fluoxetine have proved to be effective antidepressants.

    b. Some studies have found 5-HT and 5-hydroxyindoleacetic acid (5-HIAA, a serotonin metabolite) in low levels in depressed patients; 5-HT depletion (e.g., by a tryptophan-depleted diet) can worsen depression.

3. Dopamine is less solidly linked to depression, but there is some suggestive evidence.

    a. Bupropion is an effective antidepressant that is dopaminergic without directly affecting 5-HT or NE transmission.

    b. Parkinson's disease, which involves dopaminergic dysfunction, often leads to depressive symptoms.

    c. Dopaminergic agents such as the stimulant methylphenidate can be effective antidepressants in some patients.

4. Other neurotransmitters, including γ-aminobutyric acid (GABA) and neuropeptides, have also been implicated in mood disorders.

C Other biologic factors

1. Neuroendocrine regulation appears to be related to mood disorders.

    a. The hypothalamic–pituitary–adrenal (HPA) axis may be disrupted in depression, as the dexamethasone suppression test (DST) demonstrates. Normally, administration of dexamethasone (a synthetic corticosteroid) suppresses the HPA axis, and serum cortisol levels decrease. However, depressed patients have been found to exhibit **nonsuppression** (cortisol remains elevated). The DST is not sufficiently selective or specific to be used in routine clinical care, but it points to endocrine involvement.

    b. **Hypothyroidism** may mimic depression, and **hyperthyroidism** may mimic mania. In addition, a subset of depressed patients release a low amount of thyroid-stimulating hormone (TSH) after being given thyrotropin-releasing hormone (TRH).

2. Sleep and circadian rhythm

    a. Problems with sleep are common in individuals with mood disorders. Depressed patients may experience insomnia or hypersomnia, and manic patients typically have a decreased need for sleep.

    b. **Polysomnography** shows that many depressed patients have **shortened rapid eye movement (REM) latency** (i.e., the time from falling asleep to the first REM period is about 60 minutes rather than 90 minutes). Other abnormalities of sleep architecture are also found.

    c. **Sleep deprivation** is an effective treatment for depression, although depression returns after the next night's sleep.

3. Kindling is a phenomenon observed when repeated, subthreshold stimulation of the brain eventually results in seizure activity. It has been postulated that bipolar illness follows a similar paradigm. The temporal pattern may be suggestive: some patients have a first episode of illness in response to stress (e.g., a loss), with subsequent episodes following lower-grade stress, and spontaneous episodes eventually occurring.

D Psychological and social factors

1. Stress commonly precedes the first episode of both major depression and mania. It has been speculated that such stress can precipitate brain changes, which make an individual more vulnerable to future mood episodes.

2. Loss of a parent before the age of 11 years has been linked to depression in adulthood.

3. Some psychodynamic theorists have proposed that depression represents **anger turned inward;** that is, a person becomes angry at a loved one (often one who was lost), but because such anger is intrapsychically unacceptable, the patient experiences depression and self-hatred.

4. Animal studies have led to the model of depression as **learned helplessness.** An animal exposed to inescapable shock will, over time, fail to escape the shock even when given the opportunity. Antidepressant medications reverse this behavior.

5. Depressed individuals often express inaccurate, negative cognitions (e.g., "I've never done anything right"). **Cognitive therapy** aimed at changing these cognitions can improve depressive symptoms in many individuals.

V TREATMENT

A Overall treatment planning   Despite some variation in symptoms and severity, some general guidelines are appropriate in most cases.

1. **Treatment setting**
   a. **Type of clinician.** Most patients with mood disorders are treated by clinicians other than mental health professionals.
      (1) **Primary care physicians** provide much of the care for disorders that respond well to medication. However, this can present several problems, including:
         (a) Inadequate diagnosis
         (b) Limited time for supportive therapy (which improves compliance and treatment response)
      (2) **Psychiatrists** are able to provide both medication and psychotherapy.
      (3) Psychologists, psychiatric social workers, and other mental health professionals often provide assessment and psychotherapy.
   b. **Location of treatment.** Patients with mood disorders are most often treated in **outpatient settings,** although dangerous or disorganized patients and those who have failed outpatient treatment may require **hospitalization.** Patients receive daytime support, supervision, and therapy at a **psychiatric day hospital,** an intermediate setting in which patients return home at night.

2. **Diagnostic evaluation.** The various mood disorders are treated quite differently. Therefore, it is important to establish, for instance, if a patient with a current MDE has a history of mania. Comorbid psychiatric and medical problems must also be identified or ruled out. Such an evaluation can be performed in either an inpatient or outpatient setting.

3. **Assessment of safety.** Mood disorders carry a risk of suicide. All clinicians who deal with these patients must be familiar with assessment of suicidal risk so that appropriate steps can be taken (e.g., **voluntary or involuntary hospitalization**) when needed to ensure patients' safety. In addition, bipolar patients may engage in behavior that, although not suicidal, is dangerous to themselves or others. Evidence of such behavior (e.g., spending sprees) requires similar steps to protect the patient.

B Treatment of major depressive disorder

1. **Hospitalization.** Whereas most patients with major depression can safely be treated as outpatients, a subset of patients requires hospitalization, which can serve several functions.
   a. **Safety** for a suicidal or severely psychotic patient can often be best ensured in a hospital.
   b. **Treatment** can, at times, be more rapidly instituted in the hospital setting.
      (1) Medication doses can be advanced more rapidly in a setting where side effects can be rapidly identified and alleviated.
      (2) Electroconvulsive therapy (ECT), at times an outpatient procedure, is more commonly performed on inpatients.
   c. **Support** in the form of individual and group therapies, as well as general staff availability, is intensive in a hospital setting.

2. **Outpatient treatment.** Various levels and modalities of outpatient treatment are available.
   a. A **combination of psychotherapy and medication** is optimum for some patients with major depression, particularly those who have chronic conditions, have psychiatric comorbidity, or are refractory to pharmacotherapy alone. One clinician (e.g., a psychiatrist) or different clinicians (e.g., an internist and a social worker) may provide this treatment.

b. Several **models of psychotherapy** for depression have been used.
   (1) **Psychodynamic** (psychoanalytically oriented) **psychotherapy** is commonly used with depressed patients, although it is also the least well studied.
   (2) Two forms of psychotherapy, **cognitive therapy** (most studied; focuses on cognitive distortions) and **interpersonal therapy** (focuses on patient's interpersonal problems), have been found in controlled studies to be effective treatments for depression.

c. Because **support** appears to be an important variable both in treatment and safety, a number of supportive measures (in addition to individual therapy) are often used.
   (1) **Family or friends** are often involved in some phase of treatment.
   (2) **Day hospitalization** may be used instead of or as a transition from inpatient hospitalization.
   (3) **Supportive living arrangements** (group homes) may be recommended for patients with more refractory symptoms, more limited social supports, or comorbid factors.

3. **Somatic therapies.** All of the somatic therapies listed have proved similarly effective in treating patients with MDEs. Response to all of the antidepressant medications takes time, with full response usually seen within 4–6 weeks. When choosing a treatment for an individual patient, the clinician must consider prior treatment response in the patient or a family member, potential adherence issues, comorbid psychiatric or medical problems, and factors that might make side effects of a particular drug more problematic.
   a. **Tricyclic antidepressants (TCAs)** were the standard drug treatment for several decades, and they are still used for some patients. All TCAs are hepatically metabolized, renally excreted, and have a narrow therapeutic index. Relatively long half-lives allow once-daily dosing. Cardiotoxicity shared by these drugs leads to the lethality of overdose.
      (1) **Tertiary tricyclics** (e.g., imipramine, amitriptyline) are the oldest members of this class. A side effect profile that includes prominent sedative and anticholinergic effects limits their use.
      (2) **Secondary tricyclics** (e.g., nortriptyline, desipramine) tend to be less anticholinergic, less sedating, and less likely to cause orthostatic hypotension.
   b. **MAO inhibitors,** which were discovered in the 1950s, have not been popular because of the **hypertensive crisis** that these drugs may precipitate when they interact with sympathomimetic agents (including a diet high in tyramine, which is found in ripe cheese, for example). Other side effects include orthostatic hypotension, weight gain, and insomnia. A new class of **reversible inhibitors of monoamine oxidase A,** which may be as effective as the standard MAO inhibitors but much safer, is being clinically tested and not yet available in the United States.
   c. **SSRIs,** which were introduced in the 1980s, have the advantages of once-daily dosing and a wide therapeutic index. **Fluoxetine, sertraline, paroxetine, fluvoxamine, citalopram,** and **escitalopram** are currently available. Limitations include side effects (e.g., nausea, insomnia, anxiety, sexual dysfunction) and drug interactions:
      (1) SSRIs affect the hepatic P_{450} system, but each drug inhibits the isoforms (such as 2D6 or 2C19) to different degrees. To avoid a particular drug interaction, clinicians may choose one SSRI over another.
      (2) Combination with other serotonergic drugs can precipitate a potentially lethal **serotonin syndrome** featuring restlessness, confusion, diaphoresis, and myoclonus.
   d. **Triazolopyridines** include **trazodone** and **nefazodone.** Both of these agents have a short half-life (necessitating multiple daily dosing) and a wide therapeutic index. Whereas trazodone is very sedating, nefazodone is not; neither drug has prominent anticholinergic effects. Male patients taking trazodone run a risk of developing **priapism.** Nefazodone has been associated with liver failure and is contraindicated in those with liver disease.
   e. **Bupropion,** an aminoketone, blocks the reuptake of dopamine rather than 5-HT or NE. Although it is rarely lethal in overdose, it has a narrow therapeutic index because of a dose-related tendency to cause **seizures.** Side effects include restlessness, sweating, tremors, and constipation. The incidence of sexual side effects is low. Bupropion is contraindicated in patients with comorbid eating disorders. Multiple daily dosing is usually required.
   f. **Venlafaxine,** which has been called a selective 5-HT-NE reuptake inhibitor, has a wide therapeutic index. An extended-release formulation allows once-daily dosing. Side effects are dose dependent and resemble those associated with SSRIs. **Duloxetine** is the newest medication in this class that also has a similar side effect profile to the SSRIs.

g. Mirtazapine, an antagonist of α_2 (i.e., adrenergic, inhibitory) autoreceptors, acts presynaptically but by a different mechanism. It also blocks some postsynaptic serotonergic and histaminergic receptors. Mirtazapine results in increased noradrenergic and serotonergic activity and is very sedating.

h. ECT, when performed with present-day equipment and anesthetic procedures, is a safe and effective treatment for major depressive disorder. Transcranial magnetic stimulation, magnetic seizure therapy, and vagal nerve stimulation are under study as alternative approaches but are not recommended for routine clinical practice.

   (1) The use of ECT remains limited because of bias remaining from the years when it was a much cruder procedure. Use of ECT is often reserved for patients with psychotic depressions and those who have failed or are unable to tolerate trials of antidepressant medications.

   (2) Common **complications** are confusion immediately after the procedure and memory loss, which usually resolves within 6 months. There is no evidence that ECT causes permanent brain damage.

C Treatment of bipolar I and bipolar II disorders

1. **Hospitalization.** As is the case with major depressive disorder, a subset of patients with bipolar disorder requires hospitalization, usually because of the risks of suicide during the depressed phase or out-of-control behavior during the manic phase.

   a. Containment of manic behavior can prevent potentially disastrous consequences for affected patients, including financial loss, arrest, and destroyed relationships.

   b. Initial or reinstituted treatment with antipsychotic medication and mood stabilizers can be accomplished rapidly in the hospital.

   c. Compliance is often an issue in the treatment of patients with bipolar disorder, so intensive psychoeducation and the involvement of family and friends are important goals of hospitalization.

2. **Outpatient treatment**

   a. A combination of psychotherapy and medication is important.

   (1) Compliance is a large problem, particularly because many patients with bipolar disorder prefer hypomania to euthymia. When manic symptoms begin, they believe that they know better than their physicians. A strong **treatment alliance** and frequent visits aid compliance and enable early intervention if signs of mania begin. **Family-focused therapy** (psychosocial program involving available family), **cognitive therapy,** and **psychoeducation** have been shown to decrease the number of relapses.

   (2) During a depressed phase, psychotherapeutic approaches as noted for major depression are appropriate.

   b. Approximately one-third of patients with bipolar disorder develop a degree of **chronic functional impairment.** These patients may benefit from programs such as **day hospitals, vocational rehabilitation,** or **supportive living arrangements.**

3. **Somatic therapies.** Several drugs have been found to possess **mood-stabilizing** properties (i.e., they are effective in treating both mania and depression) in bipolar patients. **ECT** is also effective for both phases of the illness.

   a. Lithium, traditionally the first-line treatment for bipolar disorder, has been found effective as an acute treatment for mania and depression and as a prophylactic agent.

   (1) During **acute mania,** approximately 80% of patients respond to lithium, although such response may take 1 to 2 weeks. Antipsychotic drugs are often coadministered during this initial period to control behavior and psychosis.

   (2) During **acute bipolar depression,** approximately 80% of patients also respond to lithium, although it may take 6 to 8 weeks to see the full effect.

   (3) Lithium is effective at preventing future episodes of depression and mania, with **relapse rates** reduced by approximately 50% compared with placebo.

   (4) Side effects of lithium include tremor, sedation, nausea, polyuria, polydypsia, memory problems, and weight gain. Hypothyroidism occurs in some patients.

   (5) Lithium is **renally excreted** (it is treated by the kidney like sodium), so impaired renal function can lead to toxicity.

       (6) Lithium has a **narrow therapeutic index,** and high serum levels can lead to seizures, confusion, coma, and cardiac dysrhythmia. In the case of severe overdose, dialysis is effective. The danger of lithium toxicity requires extra care for patients taking nonsteroidal anti-inflammatory agents (except sulindac) and thiazide diuretics because these drugs reduce lithium clearance.

    b. Valproate has been found in many studies to be as effective as lithium in treating bipolar illness.

       (1) In patients with **acute mania,** some evidence suggests that whereas valproate may be a more effective treatment than lithium for mixed episodes, lithium may be more effective for traditional manic episodes.

       (2) The role of valproate in **bipolar depression** is less clear.

       (3) As a **prophylactic agent,** valproate appears to have a role, particularly in the case of **rapidly cycling patients.**

       (4) Side effects include dose-related symptoms (e.g., nausea, tremor, sedation, hair loss, weight gain) and rare, idiosyncratic responses, including hepatic failure, pancreatitis, and agranulocytosis.

       (5) Valproate is **hepatically metabolized,** so patients who take it are vulnerable to pharmacokinetic drug interactions.

       (6) Valproate has a **wide therapeutic index,** although it can be fatal in overdose.

    c. Carbamazepine

       (1) Carbamazepine appears to be effective in patients with **acute mania** and **bipolar depression.**

       (2) When used for **prophylaxis,** it appears to reduce the frequency and severity of manic and depressive episodes.

       (3) Common, dose-related **side effects** include blurred vision, ataxia, nausea, fatigue, hyponatremia, and asymptomatic leukopenia. Rare, idiosyncratic effects include agranulocytosis, liver failure, Stevens-Johnson syndrome, and pancreatitis.

       (4) Carbamazepine is **hepatically metabolized** and induces its own metabolism (so dosage adjustment may be needed over time). Pharmacokinetic drug interactions are seen with other hepatically metabolized drugs.

       (5) Carbamazepine is **toxic at high doses** (serum levels must be monitored) and can be lethal in overdose.

    d. Second-generation antipsychotics

       (1) Olanzapine, risperidone, ziprasidone, aripiprazole, and **quetiapine** have all been shown in clinical trials to be effective as monotherapy for acute treatment of mania. Evidence suggests that quetiapine and the combination of olanzapine and fluoxetine to be effective for the treatment of acute depressive episodes in patients with bipolar disorder.

       (2) Each of these drugs has also been shown to be effective as adjunctive therapy.

       (3) In varying degrees, these medications are associated with an increased risk of developing **diabetes mellitus** and **dyslipidemia.** Weight, blood pressure, glucose and lipids should be monitored in patients taking these medications.

    e. Lamotrigine

       (1) Lamotrigine has been show to be clinical effective as a maintenance treatment for bipolar disorder.

       (2) Except for a rash, lamotrigine has minimal side effects compared with placebo.

       (3) Lamotrigine seems to prevent depressive episodes better than manic episodes.

    f. Several other drug classes also have a role in the treatment of bipolar disorder.

       (1) Benzodiazepines, particularly **clonazepam,** may be used to treat mania. Sedation and a full night's sleep can markedly improve symptoms in some patients.

       (2) Antidepressants are frequently used in the depressed phase of bipolar illness, either alone or in combination with an agent such as lithium. However, this practice is not well studied. Clinicians must be cautious because most antidepressant agents have been reported to precipitate mania in some patients.

D **Treatment of dysthymia and cyclothymia**   Evidence-based therapy for these disorders is less well established than that for treatment of mania and depression.

    1. Dysthymia. Traditionally, dysthymia was treated with psychotherapy. The condition was believed to be poorly responsive to antidepressant medication.

      a. It now appears that this disorder may respond to drug treatment; **SSRIs** and **MAO inhibitors** are more effective than TCAs.

      b. **Cognitive therapy** and **behavioral therapy** are the two kinds of psychotherapy with the best evidence-based treatment data.

    2. Cyclothymia. Therapy may involve mood-stabilizing drugs. Antidepressants frequently precipitate manic symptoms. Supportive psychotherapy is also important.

BIBLIOGRAPHY

American Psychiatric Association: *Guideline Watch: Practice Guideline for the Treatment of Patients with Bipolar Disorder,* 2nd ed. Washington, DC, American Psychiatric Association, 2005.

American Psychiatric Association: *Guideline Watch: Practice Guideline for the Treatment of Patients with Major Depressive Disorder,* 2nd ed. Washington, DC, American Psychiatric Association, 2005.

Study Questions

Directions: *Each of the numbered items in this section is followed by possible answers. Select the ONE lettered answer that is BEST in each case.*

1. The prevalence rate of which of the following mood disorders is similar in men and women?
- [A] Bipolar I disorder
- [B] Bipolar II disorder
- [C] Cyclothymic disorder
- [D] Dysthymic disorder
- [E] Major depressive disorder

2. Which one of the following individuals is most likely to have a first-degree relative with a mood disorder?
- [A] A woman with major depressive disorder
- [B] A man with major depressive disorder
- [C] A man with dysthymia
- [D] A woman with bipolar I disorder
- [E] A woman with cyclothymia

3. The dexamethasone suppression test (DST) is best described by which of the following statements?
- [A] DST is a sensitive screening tool for major depressive disorder.
- [B] DST is a selective screening tool for major depressive disorder.
- [C] DST explains why hypothyroidism is associated with depressive symptoms.
- [D] DST differentiates nonpsychotic, depressed patients from those with psychotic features.
- [E] DST usually shows nonsuppression of cortisol in depressed patients.

4. Common side effects of selective serotonin reuptake inhibitors (SSRIs) include which of the following?
- [A] Constipation and orthostatic hypotension
- [B] Sedation and priapism
- [C] Restlessness, tremors, and seizures
- [D] Nausea, insomnia, and sexual dysfunction
- [E] Confusion and memory loss

5. The diagnosis of cyclothymic disorder requires which one of the following criteria?
- [A] Repeated episodes of hypomania and depression
- [B] A minimum duration of 6 months
- [C] At least one prior major depressive episode (MDE)
- [D] At least one prior manic episode
- [E] Comorbid substance abuse

6. What is the approximate percentage of patients with cyclothymic disorder who ultimately develop bipolar disorder?
- [A] 10%
- [B] 25%
- [C] 50%
- [D] 75%
- [E] 90%

7. Which of the following noradrenergic effects of antidepressant drugs is thought to best correlate with the onset of clinical efficacy?
- [A] Acute blockade of norepinephrine (NE) reuptake
- [B] Acute increase of NE in the synapse

C Blockade of α_1-receptors
D Blockade of β-receptors
E Downregulation of β-receptors

8. A 50-year-old woman who has recently started taking a tricyclic antidepressant is likely to complain about which one of these side effects?

A Diarrhea
B Drooling
C Rash
D Sedation
E Slowed heart rate

QUESTIONS 9–10

A 64-year-old male accountant presents to his internist with a 6-week history of worsening depression, insomnia, weight loss, poor concentration, fatigue, and suicidal ideation. He believes that his evil thoughts caused the recent death of his mother.

9. At this time, which of the following diagnoses is most likely an explanation for his symptoms?

A Bipolar I disorder
B Dysthymic disorder
C Major depressive disorder
D Schizophrenia
E Somatization disorder

10. The patient's belief about his mother would best be described as which of the following?

A A mood-congruent delusion
B A mood-incongruent delusion
C A melancholic symptom
D Thought broadcasting
E Thought insertion

Directions: Each set of matching questions in this section consists of a list of five to nine lettered options followed by several items. For each numbered item, select the ONE lettered option that is most closely associated with it. To avoid spending too much time on matching sets with large numbers of options, it is generally advisable to begin each set by reading the list of options. Then, for each item in the set, try to generate the correct answer and locate it in the option list, rather than evaluating each option individually. Each lettered option may be selected once, more than once, or not at all.

QUESTIONS 11–13

Match each clinical feature with the associated drug.

A Carbamazepine
B Lamotrigine
C Lithium
D Olanzapine
E Valproate

11. This drug is effective for maintenance treatment of bipolar disorder. Side effects may include a rash.

12. This agent may be particularly effective in bipolar patients who exhibit rapidly cycling illness.

13. Side effects of this agent include tremor, nausea, polyuria, and weight gain.

QUESTIONS 14–16

For each of the following patients, select the most likely diagnosis.

    [A] Adjustment disorder with depressed mood
    [B] Bipolar I disorder
    [C] Bipolar II disorder
    [D] Cyclothymic disorder
    [E] Dysthymic disorder
    [F] Major depressive disorder
    [G] Mood disorder caused by a general medical condition
    [H] Normal bereavement
    [I] Substance-induced mood disorder

14. A 23-year-old woman reports an almost 2-year history of poor sleep, low energy, and a general feeling of hopelessness. Three weeks ago, she stopped going to work because she could not concentrate and felt so run down that she could hardly get out of bed. She began to feel suicidal. She denies any significant medical history and use of any drugs or medications. Every weekend, she drinks two to three beers.

15. A 30-year-old man has spent the past 6 weeks in a rehabilitation hospital, recovering from multiple fractures and internal injuries he received in a motorcycle accident. He suffered no apparent head trauma. The man was treated with fluoxetine for 6 months for a major depressive episode at age 23 years. While he was in college, he twice experienced episodes that each lasted for a week or two in which he felt "on top of the world," needed little sleep, went out every night with friends, and ordered expensive electronic equipment that he later had to return. He did not seek or receive treatment for these episodes.

    Soon after the man's admission to the rehabilitation hospital, he began to feel agitated and restless. Since that time, he has had little appetite, has felt very guilty about the accident, has had trouble concentrating, and refuses to engage in any social activities on his unit, saying that he cannot enjoy anything or anyone. His pain medications were stopped several weeks ago, and his laboratory values are normal.

16. A 57-year-old woman with no psychiatric history has been feeling sad, anxious, and lonely since her husband died suddenly about 6 weeks ago. She has difficulty falling asleep almost every night and has a poor appetite. Although she has continued to work, she has become isolated from her friends and believes that she will never recover from the loss. She denies suicidal ideation and hallucinations. She is physically healthy and denies alcohol or drug use.

QUESTIONS 17–19

Choose the most appropriate treatment for each of the following psychiatric outpatients.

    [A] Bupropion
    [B] Cognitive therapy
    [C] Day hospitalization
    [D] Fluoxetine
    [E] Lithium
    [F] Nortriptyline
    [G] Trazodone
    [H] Valproate

17. A 25-year-old woman who has been diagnosed with major depressive disorder says that her most troubling symptom is insomnia, and she wants something to help her sleep. She was treated using medication for her first episode of depression at age 17, but she does not recall the name of the drug. At that time, she was briefly hospitalized because of an overdose attempt with her antidepressant.

18. A 30-year-old man has recently been diagnosed with major depressive disorder. He is able to work. Despite having a previously successful social life, he has become very isolated socially because he feels like such a hopeless "loser." Because he has a brother with bipolar disorder who has had repeated, troubling side effects from his medications, the man is very reluctant about taking antidepressant drugs.

19. A 65-year-old woman with a 30-year history of bipolar I disorder has just been discharged from a brief inpatient stay for mania. She has had frequent hospitalizations for agitation, grandiosity, and psychosis, which always responded well to lithium. However, it appears that she takes her medication erratically, and her poor treatment adherence contributes to the relapses. She was recently also diagnosed with hypertension, and her internist plans to start her on hydrochlorothiazide.

Answers and Explanations

1. The answer is A [*III B 1 c, 2 c, 3 c, 4 c, 5 c*]. Of the mood disorders listed, only bipolar I disorder has a similar prevalence in men and women. For cyclothymic disorder, there is only a slight increase in prevalence in women over men. Bipolar I disorder is equally common in men and women. Bipolar II disorder may be more common in women. Dysthymia is two to three times more common in women.

2. The answer is D [*IV A 1*]. Family studies have shown that whereas approximately 50% of patients with major depressive disorder have a first-degree relative with a mood disorder, 90% of patients with bipolar disorder have a first-degree relative with a mood disorder. Dysthymia and cyclothymia are also somewhat more common among first-degree relatives but not as strikingly as bipolar disorder. The gender of the patient is irrelevant to the answer.

3. The answer is E [*IV C 1 a*]. The dexamethasone suppression test (DST) involves the administration of a synthetic corticosteroid followed by measurement of serum cortisol levels. Whereas nondepressed individuals respond to the drug with decreased cortisol, many patients with major depressive disorder demonstrate nonsuppression and thus elevated cortisol levels. The DST is no longer used routinely because it lacks adequate specificity or selectivity for major depression. It does not differentiate psychotic patients and does not explain the association between thyroid disorders and mood symptoms. The DST does not help differentiate psychotic from nonpsychotic depression.

4. The answer is D [*V B 3*]. Common side effects of selective serotonin reuptake inhibitors (SSRIs) such as fluoxetine include nausea, insomnia, anxiety, and sexual dysfunction. Anticholinergic effects such as dry mouth, constipation, and orthostatic hypotension are commonly seen with tricyclic agents. Sedation is commonly seen with trazodone, and priapism also can occur with this drug. Restlessness and tremors are associated with bupropion, which can lead to seizures at high dosage. Confusion and memory loss are associated with electroconvulsive therapy (ECT).

5. The answer is A [*III B 5*]. The *Diagnostic and Statistical Manual of Mental Disorders,* 4th edition (*DSM-IV*) criteria for cyclothymic disorder require repeated episodes of hypomania and of depressive symptoms that are not severe enough to meet criteria for major depressive episode (MDE). The minimum duration for diagnosis is 2 years for adult patients (only 1 year is required in children and adolescents). Not only are prior major depressive or manic episodes not required, but their presence during the first 2 years of illness rules out a diagnosis of cyclothymic disorder. Although substance abuse is commonly associated with cyclothymic disorder, it is not required to make the diagnosis.

6. The answer is C [*III B 5 c*]. The onset of cyclothymia is usually in adolescence or early adulthood, and the course tends to be chronic. Up to 50% of affected individuals will ultimately have a manic or mixed episode and thus be diagnosed with bipolar disorder.

7. The answer is E [*IV B 1 a*]. Antidepressants are not β-blockers, or downregulation at the β-receptors would not occur. Downregulation of β-receptors takes several weeks, and the time course correlates well with the onset of antidepressant effect. Blockade of norepinephrine (NE) reuptake at the presynaptic membrane occurs shortly after noradrenergic antidepressants are administered, so NE increase in the synapse is similarly rapid. Likewise, α_1-blockade occurs shortly after dosing.

8. The answer is D [*V B 3 a*]. Tricyclic antidepressants have a variety of side effects, many of which are related to postsynaptic receptor-blocking effects. Blockade of muscarinic receptors causes anticholinergic symptoms such as dry mouth, constipation, blurred vision, and tachycardia. Blockade of histamine receptors produces sedation. Orthostatic hypotension is caused by adrenergic (α_1)-blockade. Diarrhea is not a common side effect of this drug class.

9–10. The answers are 9-C, 10-A [*III A 1, B 1 b (1)*]. The man meets all the criteria for major depressive disorder. Dysthymia alone could not account for his current symptoms, which are consistent with a major depressive episode (MDE). MDE can be a feature of several mood disorders, including major depressive disorder, bipolar I and bipolar II disorders, somatization disorder, and substance-induced mood disorder. To differentiate these, one would need a history of any prior mood episodes, concurrent medical problems, and drug and alcohol use.

Believing that thoughts can cause someone to die is delusional. Because the patient's symptoms are those of an MDE and the delusion has a depressing content (causing someone to die), the belief would be described as a mood-congruent delusion. Thought insertion is the belief that thoughts have been placed into the patient's head, and thought broadcasting is the belief that others can hear the patient's thoughts. Neither is related to this case. Delusions can occur in melancholic patients, but they are not a specific symptom of melancholia.

11–13. The answers are 11-B [*V C 3 e*], **12-E** [*V C 3 b*], and **13-C** [*V C 3 a*]. Although both lithium and lamotrigine have been shown to be effective for maintenance treatment of patients with bipolar disorder, lamotrigine can cause a rash as a side effect.

Valproate is a mood stabilizer that appears to be particularly effective in patients who have a pattern of rapid cycling illness (i.e., at least four episodes of mood disorder within a 12-month period).

Lithium, usually considered a first-line treatment for bipolar disorder, has side effects that include tremor, sedation, nausea, polyuria, polydipsia, memory problems, weight gain, and hypothyroidism.

14–16. The answers are 14-F [*III B 1*], **15-C** [*III B 4*], and **16-H** [*III B 1 d (4)*]. The 23-year-old woman has had the symptoms of dysthymia for almost 2 years. However, because she has developed a major depressive episode (MDE) within 2 years of symptom onset, the diagnosis is major depressive disorder. If she had remained dysthymic for 2 years or more before experiencing an MDE, then diagnoses of both dysthymic disorder and major depressive disorder would be appropriate (so-called "double depression"). Her reported alcohol intake, if accurate, would not account for her symptoms; however, this is worth pursuing further.

The man in the rehabilitation hospital is experiencing a major depressive episode (MDE), which can be seen in a number of disorders, including bipolar I, bipolar II, and major depressive disorder. In addition, substance use or a general medical condition can also induce an MDE. In this case, the patient appears to have a history of bipolar II disorder, with two hypomanic episodes, and one MDE. He is recovering from medical problems (fractures and internal injuries), but there is no evidence of a medical condition known to cause depressive symptoms physiologically (e.g., severe anemia, hypothyroidism, certain central nervous system conditions). In addition, although he recently experienced a severe psychosocial stressor (his accident), a diagnosis of adjustment disorder would not be appropriate because his symptoms meet criteria for another Axis I disorder (in this case, bipolar II disorder).

The recently widowed woman has many features of a major depressive episode (MDE), but this condition is consistent with normal bereavement. Her symptoms are not in excess of what one would expect to see after the loss of a husband, so a diagnosis of an adjustment disorder or major depressive disorder is not appropriate. Features that might lead to the diagnosis of major depressive disorder in a grieving individual include prominent psychotic features, serious or prolonged functional impairment, suicidal ideation, or the presence of a MDE for more than several months. Cultural factors regarding the severity and time course of normal bereavement should be considered.

17–19. The answers are 17-G [*V B 3*], **18-B** [*V B 2 b*], and **19-H** [*V C 3 b*]. Of the listed antidepressants, the 25-year-old woman with multiple depressive disorder and prominent insomnia would best be treated with trazodone, which is a sedating antidepressant with a wide therapeutic index. Nortriptyline is not very sedating and could be lethal if she overdosed on her medication again. Fluoxetine and bupropion can both cause restlessness and may worsen her insomnia. Fluoxetine has a wide therapeutic index, but bupropion can cause seizures in cases of overdose.

The 30-year-old man with major depressive disorder who is reluctant to take medication may do well with cognitive therapy. His belief that he is a "loser" is the sort of cognitive distortion seen in depressed patients and one that can respond to work with a cognitive therapist. If the man does later agree to take medication, bupropion might be a good choice because in view of his family history, this man is at risk for developing bipolar illness. Bupropion is less likely than many other antidepressants to precipitate mania. There is no indication that this man requires the level of support and supervision provided by a psychiatric day hospital, although if his condition deteriorated, this might be an option.

Of the choices given, valproate, with its wider therapeutic index and known efficacy in patients with bipolar disorder, would be the best option for the elderly woman with bipolar disorder. Although she is known to respond well to lithium, the addition of hydrochlorothiazide, a thiazide diuretic, to lithium could be dangerous in light of her difficulty with medication compliance. Thiazide diuretics decrease lithium clearance, resulting in higher serum levels. In compliant patients, the lithium dosage could be adjusted accordingly and maintained at a safe level. However, in this patient, there would be a risk of the lithium level's fluctuating downward (becoming ineffective) and upward (becoming toxic). Valproate may also be indicated because this patient might meet criteria for rapid cycling, as the clinical vignette suggests. Day hospitalization, although not effective alone in preventing relapses, might also provide support and improve compliance.

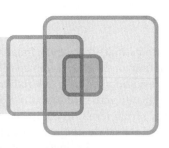

chapter 5

Anxiety Disorders

JOSHUA T. THORNHILL IV

I   **OVERVIEW**

Anxiety is abnormal fear out of proportion to any external stimulus. Significant anxiety is experienced by 10% to 15% of general medical outpatients and 10% of inpatients. Of the physically healthy population, 25% of individuals are anxious at some point in their lives. Approximately 7.5% of these people have a diagnosable anxiety disorder in any given month. Anxiety may be either a psychophysiologic response to a perception of internal or external danger or may be spontaneous.

A   Panic anxiety versus generalized anxiety

1. **Panic anxiety** arises spontaneously and does not have particular content associated with it. Panic anxiety may evolve gradually in nine stages:
   a. Spontaneous subclinical (limited symptom) anxiety attacks
   b. Gradual progression to full-blown panic attacks
   c. Hypochondriacal fears of occult disease
   d. Development of **anticipatory anxiety** about panic attacks
   e. Phobic avoidance of situations in which panic attacks occur or from which escape might be difficult if panic did occur
   f. Generalized avoidance (agoraphobia)
   g. Abuse of drugs or alcohol to control anxiety
   h. Depression
   i. Social limitations
2. **Panic attacks** are unprovoked, sudden episodes of anxiety that usually reach their peak within a few minutes and subside in less than 1 hour. Panic attacks may wake patients from sleep. A sense of dread, which is the most prominent psychological symptom, may be masked by or seem to be a reaction to the physical symptoms that frequently accompany panic attacks:
   a. Palpitations or rapid heart beat
   b. Sweating
   c. Tremor or shaking
   d. Dyspnea or feelings of smothering
   e. Feeling of choking
   f. Chest pain
   g. Dizziness or faintness
   h. Derealization (feelings of unreality) or depersonalization (feelings of detachment from oneself)
   i. Feelings of losing control or going crazy
   j. Fear of dying
   k. Paresthesias
   l. Chills or hot flashes
3. **Generalized anxiety** involves excessive worry about actual circumstances, events, or conflicts.
   a. Panic anxiety and generalized anxiety often accompany each other. Whereas subpanic anxiety may mimic generalized anxiety, anticipatory anxiety is a type of generalized anxiety.
   b. Whereas panic anxiety does not involve fear of any specific circumstance, generalized anxiety involves worry about specific circumstances.
   c. Symptoms of generalized anxiety fluctuate more than those of panic anxiety.

B Diagnostic categories of anxiety   Information about symptoms and diagnostic categories is taken from the *Diagnostic and Statistical Manual of Mental Disorders,* 4th edition (*DSM-IV*). In addition to the specific symptoms listed with each category, all *DSM-IV* categories of anxiety include significant distress or interference with normal functioning or routines caused by the symptoms.

1. **Panic disorder**
   a. **Symptoms.** Panic disorder consists of recurrent panic attacks characterized by sudden apprehension or fear (see I C 1 3) and usually accompanied by autonomic arousal that is not a reaction to physical exertion, a life-threatening situation, a substance, a medical factor, or another disorder (e.g., panic attacks occurring sporadically in depressed patients). To meet criteria for panic disorder, at least one panic attack must be followed by 1 month or more of persistent concerns about having more panic attacks, worries about the consequences or implications of the panic attack (e.g., that the patient is losing control or having a heart attack), or a change in behavior caused by the panic attacks (e.g., not leaving the house). Panic disorder seems to be associated with abnormal responsiveness to carbon dioxide, resulting in overreaction to a sense of suffocation. The disorder may be accompanied by agoraphobia (see I B 2).
   b. **Treatment.** Antidepressants (selective serotonin reuptake inhibitors [SSRIs], tricyclic antidepressants [TCAs], and monoamine oxidase [MAO] inhibitors), benzodiazepines, and cognitive behavior therapy have all been shown to be effective.

2. **Agoraphobia**
   a. **Symptoms.** Anxiety about being in situations from which escape might be difficult or embarrassing or for which help may not be available in the event of panic or other forms of discomfort or distress are characteristic of agoraphobia. Common agoraphobic situations include being away from home, sitting in the middle of a row of seats in a theater, being on a bridge or in an elevator, or traveling in a car or airplane. Such situations are either avoided or are endured only by having a companion nearby. Otherwise, remaining in the situation causes marked distress or panic.
   b. **Association with panic disorder.** If agoraphobia complicates panic disorder, the diagnosis is **panic disorder with agoraphobia.** If agoraphobia occurs in the absence of panic disorder, the diagnosis is **agoraphobia without a history of panic disorder.**

3. **Generalized anxiety disorder**
   a. **Symptoms.** At least 6 months of unrealistic worry about several life circumstances accompanied by at least three of six additional symptoms of anxiety, including restlessness or feeling keyed up, easy fatigability, difficulty concentrating or mind going blank, irritability, muscle tension, and insomnia characterizes panic disorder.
   b. **Treatment.** Benzodiazepines, buspirone, antidepressants, and sometimes β-adrenergic blockers are used to treat individuals with generalized anxiety disorder. Relaxation training, hypnosis, biofeedback, supportive and cognitive therapy, and related treatments are also useful.

4. **Obsessive-compulsive disorder (OCD)**
   a. **Symptoms**
      (1) **Obsessions.** Persistent intrusive, recurrent ideas, thoughts, feelings, images, or impulses, which are experienced as senseless or repugnant and which the patient tries to ignore or resist, may occur. When **poor insight** is present, patients do not view an obsession as absurd. If poor insight reaches **delusional** proportions, patients are convinced that their obsessions are realistic or justified.
      (2) **Compulsions.** Repetitive stereotyped physical or mental actions, which the patient recognizes as senseless and tries to resist, may also occur. Compulsions, which may be physical (e.g., handwashing) or mental (e.g., repeating a series of numbers to oneself), are performed with a subjective sense of necessity to prevent some future event or in response to an obsession or some rigid rule.
   b. **Treatment**
      (1) **Pharmacologic therapy.** The serotonergic TCA clomipramine and the selective SSRIs such as fluoxetine, paroxetine, sertraline, fluvoxamine, and citalopram are effective.
      (2) **Behavioral therapy.** Treatments involving exposure and response prevention are more effective than medications. In addition, whereas the benefit of behavior therapy has been

shown to persist for 6 years after completion, symptoms usually return rapidly after medication discontinuation. Cognitive behavior therapy and specialized techniques such as "stop thinking" can also be helpful (see III B 5).

   (3) **Other treatment modalities.** Combinations of pharmacotherapy and behavioral therapies are used in complicated and refractory cases, but an additive effect has not yet been demonstrated in simpler cases. Ablative neurosurgery is occasionally used for severe and very treatment-refractory OCD.

5. **Specific phobias**
   a. **Symptoms.** These phobias include excessive or irrational fear in response to the presence or anticipation of a specific object or situation (e.g., height, spiders, blood). Although the anxiety is recognized as inappropriate, the phobic stimulus is avoided or endured only with intense distress. Specific phobias often reflect universal reactions to stimuli that many people may find uncomfortable but evoke intense anxiety in a particular patient.
   b. **Subtypes**
      (1) **Animal type.** Fear of animals or insects usually begins in childhood.
      (2) **Natural environmental type.** This subtype, which also usually begins in childhood, is characterized by fear of storms, height, and other events in the environment.
      (3) **Blood–injection–injury type.** This phobia subtype, which is characterized by anxiety in response to seeing blood or injury or receiving an injection, is often familial and is associated with fainting (vasovagal syncope).
      (4) **Situational type.** This subtype is characterized by fear cued by specific situations such as elevators, bridges, and enclosed places but without panic disorder or other agoraphobic symptoms. However, situational phobia is similar to panic disorder with agoraphobia in its age of onset, familial aggregation, and gender ratios.
      (5) **Other type.** This category includes irrational fears of other stimuli, such as illness, or fears of falling if not near a wall or other means of physical support (**space phobia**).
   c. **Treatment.** Specific phobias are usually treated with behavioral therapies.

6. **Social phobia**
   a. **Symptoms.** A marked and persistent fear of humiliating oneself in social or performance situations that involve social scrutiny may be characteristic. Panic attacks may occur in social situations.
   b. **Treatment.** Social phobia is treated with SSRIs, monoamine oxidase (MAO) inhibitors, group therapy, cognitive behavior therapy, and occasionally with β-adrenergic blocking agents.

7. **Posttraumatic stress disorder (PTSD).** This syndrome of distress, reexperiencing, avoidance, and arousal develops after exposure to events or circumstances that involve actual death or injury or a threat to the physical integrity of oneself or others and that evoked intense fear, helplessness, or horror.
   a. **Symptoms.** Manifestations may appear immediately after the trauma, or they may be delayed for 6 months or more (**PTSD with delayed onset**). Symptoms include:
      (1) **Reexperiencing** the initial trauma occurs via intrusive memories of the event, dreams about the trauma, feeling as if the trauma were continuing to occur, and intense distress on exposure to cues that recall the event.
      (2) **Avoidance** of stimuli associated with the trauma and numbing of overall responsiveness occurs.
      (3) Symptoms of **excessive arousal** include insomnia, angry outbursts, hypervigilance, exaggerated startle response, and difficulty concentrating.
   b. **Treatment.** Discussion of the trauma as a means of achieving retroactive mastery may be effective. At times, confrontations with perpetrators can be helpful. Desensitization to situations that evoke reexperiencing or avoidance is often necessary. Group therapy and cognitive behavior therapy may be helpful. Adjunctive techniques (e.g., biofeedback) may be useful. Medications (SSRIs, benzodiazepines, atypical antipsychotics, and anticonvulsants) have been shown to reduce target symptoms.

8. **Acute stress disorder (ASD).** This diagnosis is new to the *DSM-IV*. A traumatic event, which is defined exactly as in PTSD, produces anxiety or arousal, avoidance, reexperiencing, and acute or delayed dissociative symptoms such as detachment or absence of emotional respon-

siveness, decreased awareness of surroundings, derealization, depersonalization, or dissociative amnesia. Three or more of these symptoms (including emotional numbing) must be present to make the diagnosis. Acute stress disorder begins within 1 month of the event and lasts 2 days to 4 weeks. The diagnosis is changed to PTSD (see I B 7) after acute stress disorder has been present for 1 month. Recent research suggests that because the presence of dissociation soon after a trauma does not identify a distinct subgroup of traumatized individuals, acute stress disorder may be just a variant or, at most, a precursor of PTSD.

9. **Anxiety disorder caused by a general medical condition.** This diagnosis, which replaces the *DSM-III-R* diagnosis of organic anxiety disorder, refers to anxiety caused by medical and surgical disorders (see I D 1–6).

10. **Substance-induced anxiety disorder.** This diagnosis is made when a psychoactive substance is responsible for anxiety symptoms (see I D 7). In the *DSM-III-R,* this diagnosis would have been included with organic anxiety disorder.

11. **Other primary psychiatric disorders.** Other conditions may be associated with anxiety, which may be the presenting complaint.
    a. **Depression.** Approximately 70% of depressed patients also feel anxious, and 20% to 30% of apparent cases of anxiety are caused by an underlying depression. Approximately 40% to 90% of patients with panic disorder become depressed, and 20% to 50% of depressed patients have panic attacks. A depressive diagnosis is changed to an anxiety disorder, and vice versa, in about 25% of patients initially diagnosed with a depressive or anxiety disorder. Depressed patients with blood relatives who are anxious are more likely to experience anxiety plus depression than those with a family history of depression only.
    b. **Psychosis.** As control of mental processes is lost, patients who experience psychotic disorganization caused by mania, schizophrenia, or brief psychotic disorders often display considerable anxiety, which may initially obscure the underlying severe disturbance of thinking, affect, or behavior.
    c. **Mania.** Bursts of overstimulation, excess energy, and racing thoughts may be experienced as panic attacks, especially in younger patients.
    d. **Delirium and dementia.** Anxiety is the most common emotion experienced by patients with acute organic mental syndromes (delirium) who are frightened by a sudden disruption of cognitive abilities, as well as by patients with dementia, whose mental syndromes are made worse by an intercurrent illness or by a sudden change in the environment (e.g., a change in the roommate of a hospitalized demented patient).
    e. **Adjustment disorder with anxiety.** Within 3 months of exposure to an obvious stress, patients experience anxiety or impairment in excess of that which would normally be expected. Anxiety and other symptoms appear soon after the onset of an event that most people would consider upsetting but not life-threatening, unlike with PTSD, and the symptoms are expected to resolve within 6 months of the stress' abating or the patient's achieving a new level of functioning.
    f. **Factitious disorder.** Rarely, individuals consciously simulate a mental disorder, including anxiety disorders, for the sole purpose of becoming a patient. The patient often relates an improbable history and has been hospitalized numerous times, often under different names.
    g. **Malingering** refers to the conscious simulation of a condition for some obvious gain (e.g., obtaining benzodiazepines). Malingering is more common in patients with a history of lying, drug abuse, and antisocial behavior.

C **Signs and symptoms**   A subjective state of anxiety may be obvious, or it may be masked by physical or other psychological complaints.

1. **Psychological symptoms**
   a. Apprehension, worry, fear, and anticipation of misfortune
   b. Sense of doom or panic
   c. Hypervigilance
   d. Irritability
   e. Fatigue
   f. Insomnia

     g. Predisposition to accidents

     h. Derealization (the world seems strange or unreal) and depersonalization (the patient feels unreal or changed)

     i. Difficulty concentrating

2. Somatic complaints

     a. Headache

     b. Dizziness and lightheadedness

     c. Palpitations and chest pain

     d. Upset stomach and diarrhea

     e. Frequent urination

     f. Lump in the throat

     g. Motor tension or restlessness

     h. Shortness of breath

     i. Paresthesias

     j. Dry mouth

3. Physical signs

     a. Diaphoresis

     b. Cool, clammy skin

     c. Tachycardia and arrhythmias

     d. Flushing and pallor

     e. Hyperreflexia

     f. Trembling, easy startling, and fidgeting

D Illnesses that cause anxiety Before investigating psychological causes of anxiety, it is important to exclude the possibility of physical disorders in which anxiety may be a presenting complaint even before other signs of disease become evident.

1. Cardiovascular disorders

     a. Arteriosclerotic heart disease

     b. Paroxysmal tachycardias

     c. Mitral valve prolapse

     d. Hyperdynamic β-adrenergic circulatory state

2. Pulmonary disorders

     a. Pulmonary embolism

     b. Hypoxemia

     c. Asthma

     d. Chronic obstructive lung disease

3. Disorders of the endocrine system and metabolism

     a. Hypoglycemia

     b. Hyperthyroidism or hypothyroidism

     c. Hypocalcemia

     d. Cushing's syndrome

     e. Porphyria

4. Tumors

     a. Insulinoma

     b. Carcinoid tumor

     c. Pheochromocytoma

5. Neurologic disorders

     a. Multiple sclerosis (MS)

     b. Temporal lobe epilepsy

     c. Delirium and dementia

     d. Ménière's disease

6. Infections

     a. Tuberculosis

     b. Brucellosis

7. **Drug-related disorders**
   a. Abstinence syndromes (e.g., withdrawal from central nervous system [CNS] depressants such as alcohol, tranquilizers, sleeping pills)
   b. Intoxication with sympathomimetics
   c. Akathisia
   d. Caffeinism
   e. Chinese restaurant syndrome, resulting from the ingestion of monosodium glutamate (MSG)
   f. Nicotine

E **Anxiety that mimics disease states** Anxiety may also mimic physical disease. For example, patients with **hyperventilation syndrome** complain of shortness of breath, weakness, paresthesias, headache, and carpopedal spasm. These patients are often unaware of feeling anxious about anything except being short of breath. Symptoms abate when the patient is calmed and the respiratory rate decreases. Treatment consists of instructing the patient to breathe into a paper bag, which is held over the nose and mouth. Carbon dioxide accumulates and reverses the respiratory alkalosis caused by hyperventilation.

II   PSYCHOLOGICAL COMPONENTS OF ANXIETY

A significant number of patients display anxiety symptoms that do not meet criteria for any specific *DSM-IV* diagnosis but still cause significant distress or disability. These forms of anxiety often reflect the meaning of the illness.

A **Situational anxiety** Severe stress may temporarily overwhelm any person's ability to cope. Even minor stress can have important symbolic meaning.

1. **Symptoms.** Even a relatively minor situation may feel overwhelming because it recalls other situations in which the individual was unable to cope or that aroused unresolved conflict. The intensity and nature of anxiety that evolves from a stressful situation depend on the meaning of the illness and the person's previous level of adjustment. Whereas a relatively well-adjusted patient may experience only transient symptoms, an underlying psychosis may be precipitated in a more marginally compensated patient.

2. **Treatment.** When patients must contend with acute, ongoing stress, antianxiety medication (when appropriate) and support should be offered. In addition, patients should be encouraged to talk about what the stress means to them. A greater sense of mastery, which is incompatible with the helplessness of anxiety, is facilitated by having the patient put the situation into words. The use of relaxation techniques and related therapies may also be effective (see III B).

B **Anxiety about death** Even nonfatal illnesses may remind individuals of their mortality.

1. **Symptoms.** Persistent fear of death, even in terminally ill patients, often symbolizes concern about loss of control, pain, isolation, helplessness, and the prospect of losing important relationships.

2. **Treatment.** Reassurance that patients will not be left alone and in pain often decreases the apparent fear of death.

C **Anxiety about mutilation, loss of prowess, or loss of attractiveness** is especially common in patients who feel that love, approval, and self-esteem depend on their strength or beauty.

1. **Symptoms.** Patients become anxious if an illness threatens their appearance or prowess. Such patients may attempt self-reassurance by demonstrating attractiveness (e.g., by behaving seductively) or strength (e.g., by exercising conspicuously) in inappropriate or even dangerous ways.

2. **Treatment.** Patients should be reassured that they still possess valued traits. The reaction of their families to the illness or surgery should be evaluated.

D **Anxiety about loss of self-esteem** Patients whose self-esteem is fragile are especially vulnerable to experiencing illness as an imperfection, weakness, or failure, which can lead to attempts to bolster a sense of self-worth by boasting about importance and superiority.

1. **Symptoms.** Patients may adopt a self-important air, insisting on being treated only by the most senior or well-known physicians and treating others as worthless inferiors. Attempts to convince these patients that they are not as important as they think they are only increase their insecurity, which is covered up with greater protestations of their own importance and, by comparison, the unimportance of others.

2. **Treatment.** Patients should be approached with appropriate deference and should be reassured that they are still important. Reasonable requests for special consideration (e.g., a telephone for a patient in the intensive care unit) during an acute illness should be granted.

E **Separation anxiety** Regressed adults (i.e., those who function psychologically more as children than as adults) may become frightened when they are separated from important caregivers. This state commonly is encountered in physically ill people, as well as in overly dependent individuals and some patients with psychotic and personality disorders.

1. **Symptoms.** Separation distress may be expressed directly as anxiety or indirectly as complaints of pain or, when left alone, by calls for assistance with trivial matters.

2. **Treatment.** Family and close friends should be encouraged to be with the patient as much as possible, and unrestricted visiting should be allowed. The nursing staff should be encouraged to visit the patient frequently for brief periods before the patient asks for help to avoid teaching the patient that the only way not to be left alone is to complain. The patient's room should be close to the nurse's station to facilitate frequent, brief visits. A roommate should be provided.

F **Stranger anxiety**

1. **Symptoms.** Patients who suffer from separation anxiety may also react adversely to unfamiliar people, including new physicians, nurses, and visitors. In hospitalized adults, this can lead to distress at shift changes or in other situations in which there are new caregivers.

2. **Treatment.** As much continuity in personnel as possible should be provided (e.g., the same nurse should be assigned to the patient every day). Unrestricted visiting by those familiar to the patient should be allowed, and unfamiliar visitors should be limited. Changes in roommates should be minimized. A careful mental status examination is necessary to be certain that patients are not reacting adversely to changes in the environment because of developing delirium.

G **Anxiety about loss of control**

1. **Symptoms.** Illness and hospitalization may be threatening to people who have a strong need to feel in complete control of their life and environment, especially when others must make decisions for them. Patients may attempt to gain a sense of control by refusing to comply with the physician's advice, becoming excessively demanding, making the physician feel helpless, or otherwise asserting control over those who are in a caregiving role or who are healthy.

2. **Treatment.** Patients should be allowed as much control as possible over their treatment. For example, the patient's opinion about therapeutic decisions should be solicited, and the patient should be consulted about which treatment schedules seem most reasonable to the patient.

H **Anxiety about dependency** Patients who fear loss of control also commonly have anxiety about being dependent on others, which is usually a necessary component of any serious illness. Fear of dependency is common in people whose normal dependency needs were not met in childhood (e.g., because of parental illness or unavailability).

1. **Symptoms.** Extremely strong dependency wishes, which have remained unchanged since childhood, threaten to break through when patients encounter a mild illness that could place them in a dependent position. Because patients are afraid that they will not be able to control their dependency needs, they reject attempts of others to be helpful and become hostile toward potential caregivers. Affected individuals may also assert their independence by being noncompliant, failing to keep appointments, or ignoring signs of increasing illness.

2. **Treatment.** When possible, patients should be reassured that the illness and the dependency required by it are temporary. They should be helped to maintain as much independent function as possible.

I Anxiety about intimacy

1. **Symptoms.** Patients with concerns about dependency may also be afraid of becoming too close emotionally to caregivers or loved ones. To protect themselves, they maintain a greater-than-normal emotional distance. They experience distress in response to expressions of friendliness or intimacy and may attempt to ward off (e.g., through hostility) people who are nice or express concern.

2. **Treatment.** Intimacy should not be forced. The patient's sense of formality (e.g., by always using the patient's last name) should be respected.

J Anxiety about being punished

1. **Symptoms.** Patients with an underlying sense of guilt about real or imagined transgressions may have a conscious or unconscious expectation of punishment. They may attempt to relieve guilt or avoid worry about when they will be punished by means of self-inflicted punishment (e.g., through an unhappy marriage, repeated accidents, not recovering from an illness, and other self-destructive behaviors.

2. **Treatment.** The suffering of these patients should be acknowledged, and attempts should be made to uncover the source of their guilt. Patients with a desire for insight may benefit from expressive psychotherapy.

K Signal anxiety

1. **Symptoms.** When awareness of a previously unconscious, unresolved psychological conflict is stimulated by some external occurrence (e.g., the patient had mixed feelings about a parent, and the patient's age is the same as that of the parent at the time of death), anxiety may signal the emergence of the conflict. This anxiety may call forth **psychological defenses (ego defenses),** which are unconscious mechanisms that avoid anxiety by keeping the conflict out of the patient's awareness.
   a. **Repression** (forgetting) is an automatic process by which memories, thoughts, and feelings are excluded from awareness.
   b. **Rationalization** is the act of explaining away psychologically meaningful data (e.g., "I'm anxious only because of a low blood sugar").
   c. **Reaction formation** is feeling the opposite of one's true emotion in order not to be aware of it (e.g., experiencing excessive affection toward someone who actually elicits hostility).
   d. **Isolation of affect** is experiencing the content of a thought without its associated emotions.
   e. **Denial** is remaining unaware of some aspect of reality (e.g., feeling that one does not have to be afraid of the consequences of an illness because one is not really sick).
   f. **Projection** is attributing one's own motives to someone else.
   g. **Projective identification** is incompletely projecting an intense emotional state, usually anger, onto another individual while inducing the emotion in the object of the projection through provoking behavior. Patients then experience the original emotion, but they feel that the only reason they have the emotion or thought is that they are attempting to protect themselves from the other individual's affect.

2. **Treatment.** When it is possible and practical, an attempt to resolve the underlying conflict should be undertaken. When patients cannot tolerate awareness of their motives, they should be helped to develop less disabling defenses against them (e.g., isolation of the affect rather than denial of it, or denial of anxiety rather than denial of the situation that causes it). Behavioral and adjunctive measures (e.g., relaxation training), which are useful for control of situational anxiety, may help lessen signal anxiety.

III TREATMENT OF ANXIETY

A **Psychotherapy**   This mode of treatment is effective for individuals with situational anxiety, generalized anxiety, and anxiety related to identifiable intrapsychic conflict. It is not effective for panic attacks and phobias. Psychotherapy may be facilitated by medication and behavioral techniques.

1. **Supportive therapy.** Psychotherapy that is primarily supportive is useful for acutely ill patients, patients under severe stress, and patients with limited emotional and psychosocial resources (e.g., because of social isolation or other psychiatric illness).

    a. Support of defenses. The principal therapeutic approach involves encouraging defenses that are as adaptive as possible. For example:

        (1) Patients with acute myocardial infarction should receive help minimizing the immediate danger because intense fear may contribute to the onset of lethal arrhythmias. However, when symptoms first appear, denial may lead to a fatal delay in seeking medical attention. Later in the course of the illness, denial of the need for treatment may cause noncompliance.

        (2) Marginally compensated schizophrenic patients might be encouraged to direct their attention to problems in everyday living that can be solved. They should not pay too much attention to psychotic thoughts that cannot be dealt with constructively.

        (3) People who are anxious because they feel out of control may gain a sense of mastery through intellectualization.

    b. Reality testing. With patients who tend to distort reality and misinterpret events, the physician may offer alternative explanations. Tactfully pointing out lapses in reality testing helps patients assess the situation more objectively.

    c. Advice. Help with problem solving is appropriate, especially when patients attempt to avoid anxiety through destructive or self-destructive behavior. For example, a patient might be advised to stop attempting to relieve anxiety by arguing with a spouse and to go for a walk instead.

    d. Adaptive behavior. Such patient behavior should be reinforced (encouraged).

2. Expressive (psychodynamic) psychotherapy. Patients whose anxiety reflects intrapsychic conflicts and who are able to understand and are interested in understanding themselves may gain more control of their symptoms by uncovering the psychological meaning of the anxiety and resolving conflict more effectively. Before applying expressive psychotherapy, it is important to assess a patient's ability to be aware of emotions without acting on or being overwhelmed by them. Components of expressive psychotherapy include:

    a. Clarification of the patient's statements in order to make them more comprehensible

    b. Confrontation of aspects of reality or the patient's emotions that the patient is ignoring (e.g., "You say that you are not anxious, but you look very nervous.")

    c. Interpretation of unconscious thoughts and feelings to bring them into the patient's awareness (e.g., "Do you think that you are anxious around your boss because he is so much like your father?")

B **Cognitive/behavior therapy** These treatment methods are effective for phobias, anticipatory anxiety, panic anxiety, generalized anxiety, situational anxiety, PTSD, acute stress disorder, and OCD.

1. In **systematic desensitization,** patients are taught deep muscle relaxation, which is incompatible with the tension of anxiety. Patients are then taught to visualize a scene involving thoughts that are the opposite of anxious thinking such as feeling safe, relaxed, and in control. Next patients imagine anxiety-provoking situations.

    a. As soon as anxiety begins to emerge, the scene that induces relaxation is reevoked until the anxiety ceases. Anxiety-provoking and comforting scenes are repeatedly paired until the thought of the former no longer causes anxiety.

    b. Beginning with the situation that provokes the least anxiety, patients gradually move up a hierarchy of situations to the ones that are most feared. Hypnosis may be used to facilitate the process.

    c. When patients can visualize the most anxiety-provoking scene while still feeling relaxed, less anxiety is experienced in the corresponding real-life situation.

    d. However, to consolidate this gain, "in vitro" desensitization in the physician's office must usually be followed by "in vivo" desensitization in actual situations by using a combination of relaxation and exposure while again progressing from the least to the most anxiety-provoking situation.

2. Graduated "in vivo" exposure places phobic patients (who are usually accompanied by a family member, friend, or physician for reassurance) in situations that evoke anxiety. Systematic desensitization may be necessary first if the patient becomes overwhelmingly anxious in the phobic situation. Relaxation techniques and hypnosis are used to change the association between phobic situations and anxiety to an association of those situations with relaxation and control.

3. **Panic control therapy** is a modification of cognitive behavior therapy, an established treatment for depression. Panic control therapy involves redefining symptoms of a panic attack such as dizziness or shortness of breath as harmless physiologic responses to anxiety rather than signs of a catastrophic illness. This kind of cognitive restructuring is facilitated by actual induction of panic symptoms (e.g., by spinning the patient around in a chair to produce dizziness). Patients are also taught to substitute relaxation of the anxiety that otherwise develops in response to physiologic triggers of a panic attack.

4. **Exposure and response prevention** are the cornerstones of the behavioral treatment of OCD. Patients are exposed to a stimulus that evokes rituals (e.g., touching a toilet seat) and are then helped to refrain from engaging in a compulsive behavior (e.g., handwashing) for increasing lengths of time while using adjunctive techniques to control the resulting anxiety. Response prevention for mental compulsions or obsessions is less effective in the absence of physical compulsions because the latter are easier for other people to restrain.

5. **"Stop thinking"** is a mental variant of response prevention in which patients repeat an obsessive thought until it seems overwhelming and then terminate the thought while saying "stop" out loud.

6. **Adjunctive behavioral techniques** may be useful for patients who suffer from any type of anxiety.
   a. **Relaxation techniques.** Because an individual cannot feel tense and relaxed at the same time, any method that decreases tension tends to relieve anxiety.
   b. **Hypnosis.** This altered state of consciousness permits heightened concentration and attention. Hypnosis helps patients concentrate on calming thoughts that are incompatible with anxiety. Patients who have excessive fear of loss of control or who have organic brain disease often cannot be hypnotized.
   c. **Biofeedback.** This technique is useful for patients who prefer to learn to relax with a machine or without anyone else present. It also has been used to treat migraine and tension headaches and mild essential hypertension. The level of muscular tension, usually in the forearm or frontalis muscles, is "fed back" through a visual or auditory stimulus to help patients learn to decrease motor tension and, with it, anxiety.

C **Psychopharmacology** Medication is indicated for the treatment of panic anxiety, acute situational anxiety, generalized anxiety disorder, agoraphobia, OCD, PTSD, and other anxiety disorders when these conditions are not responses to specific trauma or conflict. It is also indicated if a 3-month trial of psychotherapy and behavior therapy for treatment of exogenous anxiety is unsuccessful. Adjunctive use of antianxiety medication may facilitate psychotherapy and behavior therapy. Approximately 30% of patients with generalized anxiety disorder do not recover with appropriate pharmacotherapy. If complete recovery does not occur with appropriate drug therapy, the diagnosis may be incorrect (e.g., the patient may have anxiety secondary to a personality disorder, depression, or psychosis), or anxiety may be caused by a medical or substance-related disorder.

1. **Benzodiazepines** are effective antianxiety drugs. These agents are most useful for acute situational anxiety, anticipatory anxiety associated with panic attacks, generalized anxiety disorder, and panic disorder.
   a. **Uses**
      (1) **Panic anxiety.** The most widely used benzodiazepines for treating panic disorder are the triazolobenzodiazepine alprazolam (Xanax) and the anticonvulsant clonazepam (Klonopin).
         (a) Alprazolam has high potency (i.e., a small dose produces a large clinical effect), high lipid solubility, a short elimination half-life, and no active metabolites. Clonazepam has high potency, low lipid solubility, a long elimination half-life, and several active metabolites. As a result, alprazolam has a rapid onset and offset of action and requires frequent dosing, and clonazepam can be given less frequently but becomes more sedating with time as the parent drug and its metabolites accumulate.
         (b) Improvement should begin to be apparent within 1 month of treatment with a dosage of 2 to 10 mg/day of alprazolam or 1 to 5 mg/day of clonazepam. If improvement has not begun within 4 to 6 weeks, another medication (an antidepressant) should be tried (see III C 2).
         (c) Equivalently high doses of other benzodiazepines (e.g., 20 to 100 mg of diazepam) appear to be equally effective for panic disorder but are difficult to tolerate and require taking too many pills.

(2) Generalized and situational anxiety. Benzodiazepines are effective for generalized and situational anxiety. The benzodiazepine antianxiety drugs differ mainly in their elimination half-lives, potency, and lipid solubility. These properties vary for different preparations. For example, midazolam has a very short half-life, high potency, and high lipid solubility; diazepam has a long half-life, intermediate potency, and high lipid solubility; and chlordiazepoxide has a long half-life, low potency, and low lipid solubility.

    (a) Long-acting benzodiazepines include diazepam (Valium), chlordiazepoxide (Librium), clorazepate (Tranxene), and clonazepam (Klonopin). Long-acting preparations can be given less frequently during the day, although they are usually administered at least twice daily to minimize oversedating peaks in blood level. Discontinuation syndromes appear more gradually, last longer, and are often more attenuated than after discontinuation of shorter-acting benzodiazepines.

    (b) Short-acting benzodiazepines include midazolam (Versed), lorazepam (Ativan), oxazepam (Serax), and alprazolam (Xanax). Short-acting drugs must be given more frequently (as often as every 2 to 3 hours for some patients taking alprazolam). Discontinuation syndromes are more severe and abrupt than with longer-acting benzodiazepines, but these syndromes last a shorter period of time.

    (c) Clorazepate (Tranxene) is a **diazepam prodrug** that has no action of its own but is metabolized to diazepam after ingestion.

(3) Insomnia

    (a) Benzodiazepines such as flurazepam (Dalmane), temazepam (Restoril), triazolam (Halcion), and estazolam (ProSom) are used to treat acute insomnia associated with stress, jet lag, or a change in sleep phase.

    (b) Zolpidem (Ambien), a nonbenzodiazepine hypnotic, is selective for a subtype of the benzodiazepine receptor (type 1 receptor), which results in fewer side effects and withdrawal syndromes. Zaleplon (Sonata) and Eszopiclone (Lunesta) are also nonbenzodiazepine medications that act on the benzodiazepine type 1 receptor with a side effect profile similar to that of zolpidem.

    (c) The marketing strategy of the drug manufacturer determines the labeling of medications that act on benzodiazepine receptors as hypnotics; any benzodiazepine can be used to treat insomnia as well as anxiety.

b. Administration. Benzodiazepines are most effective when used to treat time-limited anxiety that occurs in response to clear-cut stress and when treatment lasts less than 8 weeks. However, chronically anxious patients or patients with limited intrapsychic or external resources may need long-term therapy. Because generalized anxiety disorder follows a relapsing course, repeated treatment episodes are often necessary.

c. Addiction. Benzodiazepine addiction is rare in medical patients. However, individuals with a history of alcohol or drug abuse, physician shopping, and antisocial behavior are at risk for abusing benzodiazepines. The most frequently abused benzodiazepines are diazepam, alprazolam, and lorazepam.

d. Abstinence syndromes. Withdrawal symptoms may appear up to 10 days after abrupt discontinuation of moderate doses of benzodiazepines that have been taken for more than 1 month. Signs and symptoms of withdrawal include anxiety, insomnia, irritability, and, at times, psychosis, delirium, and seizures. Some patients may experience prolonged, attenuated withdrawal symptoms lasting up to 1 year. Withdrawal is more abrupt and severe and seizures are more likely to occur after discontinuation of short-acting benzodiazepines.

e. Common side effects. Sedation, memory problems, and impaired psychomotor performance may occur. Tolerance develops to the sedative effects of benzodiazepines but not to the anxiolytic effects or impaired performance. Alcohol and benzodiazepines have additive effects that impair driving. Benzodiazepines may cause or aggravate depression. Because of drug accumulation, use of longer-acting benzodiazepines is a common cause of falls in the elderly.

2. Antidepressants

  a. Uses

    (1) Panic disorder. Antidepressants (SSRIs, TCAs, and MAO inhibitors) have been found effective for panic disorder.

(2) **Generalized anxiety disorder.** The TCAs have been noted to be as effective as the benzodiazepines in the treatment of generalized anxiety disorder, even if the particular antidepressant is not sedating and the patient is not also depressed. The SSRIs and nefazodone can also ameliorate generalized anxiety.

(3) **OCD.** In high doses, clomipramine and the SSRIs are effective for treatment of OCD. The overall response rate to serotonergic antidepressants is about 40% to 50%. Except in milder forms of OCD, these medications reduce symptoms but do not cure them.

(4) **PTSD.** Intrusive recall, depression, anxiety, and arousal may respond to SSRIs. Patients with arousal and recurrence of symptoms may respond to carbamazepine. Arousal may improve with antidepressants or benzodiazepines. However, high comorbidity with substance-related disorders necessitates caution with this class of medication.

(5) **Insomnia.** Sedating antidepressants (e.g., trazodone, nefazodone, amitriptyline, doxepin) often are effective as treatments for chronic insomnia. Tolerance to the hypnotic effect usually does not develop.

b. **Administration.** Standard antidepressant dosages (e.g., 150 to 300 mg/day of imipramine or its equivalent) are often necessary to treat anxiety, but lower dosages often suffice for insomnia. High dosages (e.g., 80 mg/day of fluoxetine) are usually needed to treat OCD. It is often recommended that antidepressants be discontinued after 6 to 12 months of having no symptoms, but chronic treatment is often required to prevent relapse.

3. **MAO inhibitors**
   a. **Uses.** MAO inhibitors are useful for panic disorder, social phobia, and depression accompanied by irreversible vegetative symptoms such as hyperphagia and hypersomnia, sensitivity to rejection, mood reactivity (i.e., being temporarily cheered up by positive interactions), prominent anxiety, and treatment resistance.
   b. **Administration.** Phenelzine (45 to 90 mg/day) and tranylcypromine (20 to 80 mg/day) are used most frequently in the United States. Because of a high prevalence of rapid metabolism, higher doses may be necessary. Additional MAO inhibitor antidepressants include isocarboxazid (Marplan; 20 to 60 mg/day) and selegiline (Eldepryl; 20 to 50 mg/day).
   c. **Side effects and interactions.** MAO inhibitors can be sedating or stimulating. These agents can produce hypertensive crises when administered with foods that are high in tyramine content (e.g., cheese) and with sympathomimetic substances. Fatal serotonin syndrome, which involves myoclonus, fever, headaches, nausea, seizures, and cardiotoxicity, may occur when MAO inhibitors are combined with SSRIs, dextromethorphan, and other serotoninergic compounds.

4. **Buspirone (BuSpar)**
   a. **Uses.** Buspirone is an azaspirone antianxiety drug with partial agonist effects at the serotonin 5-HT$_{1A}$ receptor that is used for generalized anxiety disorder. This agent can also ameliorate episodic aggressive outbursts and agitation in brain-damaged individuals. Unlike benzodiazepines, buspirone does not have a rapid onset of action.
   b. **Administration.** Buspirone must be given in divided doses (total: 10 to 60 mg/day) for 1 month before it is effective.
   c. **Side effects.** Buspirone does not cause sedation, physical dependence, psychomotor impairment, respiratory depression, or abstinence syndromes, and it does not raise the seizure threshold. It has few clinically important interactions other than serotonin syndrome when coadministered with MAO inhibitors. Because higher doses cause dysphoria, patients do not escalate the dose (as may occur with benzodiazepines). Because buspirone is not a CNS depressant, it does not suppress withdrawal from benzodiazepines and cannot be directly substituted for them.

5. **Barbiturates**
   a. **Uses.** Barbiturates should not be prescribed for anxiety or insomnia except in the very rare case of the patient who has been taking them for years and cannot be withdrawn.
   b. **Side effects.** Barbiturates (e.g., phenobarbital, secobarbital), propanediols (e.g., meprobamate), and related compounds (e.g., glutethimide) cause physical dependence, addiction, and severe abstinence syndromes. They are extremely dangerous if taken in overdose.

6. **Antihistamines** (e.g., hydroxyzine, diphenhydramine) are frequently used as antianxiety drugs and hypnotics for elderly patients and for those in whom addiction may be a problem. However,

these agents are not as predictably effective as other antianxiety drugs, and their anticholinergic and sedating side effects can aggravate memory loss and loss of coordination.

7. **Antipsychotic drugs**
    a. **Uses**
        (1) Antipsychotic drugs are indicated for anxiety associated with psychoses such as schizophrenia, mania, and psychotic depression. They are rarely useful for other forms of anxiety.
        (2) Low doses of antipsychotic may temporarily reduce self-destructive behavior in some patients with borderline personality disorder; however, continued benefit has not been demonstrated.
    b. **Side effects.** The danger of long-term side effects, especially tardive dyskinesia, precludes continued administration of neuroleptic medications to nonpsychotic patients. Atypical antipsychotic drugs (e.g., risperidone, olanzapine, quetiepine, clozapine) have a lower risk of tardive dyskinesia but are no more effective for nonpsychotic anxiety.

8. **β-blocking agents** (e.g., propranolol) are indicated for patients whose anxiety is accompanied by signs of adrenergic stimulation (e.g., sweating, tremor) and for patients with performance anxiety. These agents are not as predictably effective as the benzodiazepines or the antidepressants in relieving generalized anxiety. High doses can diminish agitation and assaultive behavior in brain-injured individuals. One dose may be useful in relieving stage fright. Atenolol may reduce social phobia in some patients, but findings have been inconclusive.

BIBLIOGRAPHY

American Psychiatric Association: *Diagnostic and Statistical Manual of Mental Disorders,* 4th ed. Washington, DC, American Psychiatric Association, 1994.

American Psychiatric Association: *Guideline Watch: Practice Guideline for Treatment of Patients with Panic Disorder.* Washington, DC, American Psychiatric Association, 2006.

American Psychiatric Association: *Practice Guideline for the Treatment of Patients with Acute Stress Disorder and Posttraumatic Stress Disorder.* Washington, DC, American Psychiatric Association, 2004.

Study Questions

Directions: *Each of the numbered items or incomplete statements in this section is followed by answers or by completions of the statement. Select the ONE lettered answer or completion that is BEST in each case.*

1. A patient with panic anxiety can become agoraphobic if
   - [A] phobic and anxious traits are inherited together.
   - [B] the patient becomes frightened of situations in which anxiety attacks were experienced.
   - [C] a stressful experience occurs.
   - [D] the patient has deep-seated conflicts.
   - [E] medication side effects predominate.

2. Posttraumatic stress disorder (PTSD) differs from adjustment disorder in that PTSD
   - [A] occurs in veterans.
   - [B] is characterized by impairment of social functioning.
   - [C] persists long after the stress has abated.
   - [D] is characterized by preoccupation with the stress.
   - [E] can be accompanied by depression.

3. A 25-year-old woman who recently had an extramarital affair believes that her physician disapproves strongly of her behavior, which she thinks is not really objectionable. This is an example of the defense of
   - [A] Denial
   - [B] Isolation
   - [C] Projection
   - [D] Reaction formation
   - [E] Repression

4. Soon after admission to the coronary care unit for his first myocardial infarction, a 45-year-old businessman refuses to be examined by the house officers and demands to see the most senior cardiologist in the hospital. He tells this individual that his secretary must be permitted unrestricted visiting privileges because he has many important business deals that require prompt attention. He adopts a condescending attitude toward the physicians and nurses. A reasonable management plan while the patient is acutely ill would include which of the following?
   - [A] Tell the patient that he must do what the doctors say or risk serious consequences.
   - [B] Restrict visits by the secretary until the patient is well.
   - [C] Discuss fears of dependency, loss of control, and damage to self-esteem.
   - [D] Agree that the patient is an important person.
   - [E] Refer the patient to a psychiatrist.

5. A 30-year-old man complains of panic attacks and anticipatory anxiety. Which of the following drugs would be an effective treatment?
   - [A] Carbamazepine
   - [B] Fluoxetine
   - [C] Haloperidol
   - [D] Meprobamate
   - [E] Pentobarbital

6. A 30-year-old woman cannot stop worrying about whether she might have accidentally run over a person when she last drove her car. She is temporarily reassured when she calls the local police station to see if anyone was killed by a hit-and-run driver while she was on the road, but the next time she drives, her fear returns with even greater intensity. What is the most likely diagnosis?
   - [A] Panic disorder
   - [B] Generalized anxiety disorder

C Obsessive-compulsive disorder (OCD)
D Posttraumatic stress disorder (PTSD)
E Substance-induced anxiety disorder

Directions: Each of the numbered items or incomplete statements in this section is negatively phrased, as indicated by a capitalized word such as NOT, LEAST, or EXCEPT. Select the ONE lettered answer or completion that is BEST in each case.

7. Correct statements about diazepam include all of the following EXCEPT:
   A Addiction is rare in medical practice.
   B Doses for generalized anxiety are effective for panic disorder.
   C Use should not exceed 8 weeks.
   D It can be used as a hypnotic.
   E Antipsychotic properties do not accompany the anxiolytic effect.

8. Treatment modalities that are usually helpful for posttraumatic stress disorder (PTSD) include all of the following EXCEPT:
   A Discussion of the precipitating event
   B Relaxation techniques
   C Biofeedback
   D Systematic desensitization
   E Administration of selective serotonin reuptake inhibitors (SSRIs)

9. Symptoms that predict a good response to a monoamine oxidase (MAO) inhibitor include all of the following EXCEPT:
   A Anxiety
   B Hypersomnia
   C Increased appetite
   D Psychosis
   E Rejection sensitivity

Directions: Each set of matching questions in this section consists of a list of lettered options followed by several numbered items. For each numbered item, select the ONE lettered option that is most closely associated with it. Each lettered option may be selected once, more than once, or not at all.

QUESTIONS 10–14

Match the subtype of phobia with its defining fear.
   A Agoraphobia
   B Social phobia
   C Blood–injection–injury phobia
   D Natural environmental phobia
   E Space phobia

10. Humiliation

11. Elevators

12. Venipuncture

13. Falling down

14. Thunderstorms

Answers and Explanations

1. The answer is B [*I A 1 e*]. Patients with panic anxiety become progressively more phobic of situations in which they have experienced spontaneous anxiety attacks. Although biologic factors are implicated in panic disorder and agoraphobia, these conditions do not seem to be inherited together. Phobias that develop after exposure to a frightening situation are called specific phobias, and they are only associated with panic when the patient is actually in the phobic situation. Patients may become phobic of benign situations that stimulate unconscious conflicts; however, the symbolism of the phobia is usually apparent, and spontaneous panic attacks do not occur. Antidepressants often initially increase anxiety, but they do not cause phobias.

2. The answer is C [*I B 7*]. Posttraumatic stress disorder (PTSD) may persist for years after the stress has abated. This condition may develop after any traumatic event involving a threat to life or physical integrity that evokes intense fear, helplessness, or horror. A soldier or anyone under stress may develop the more acute adjustment disorder, which resolves when the stressful situation ceases. Preoccupation with a stressful event is characteristic of many kinds of anxiety as an attempt to master the stress retroactively. Both disorders impair social or other aspects of functioning. Patients with acute stress disorder and PTSD frequently have depressive symptoms.

3. The answer is C [*II K 1*]. Projection is attributing to others one's own unacceptable feelings, thoughts, or impulses. Whereas denial involves ignoring elements of external reality, repression involves forgetting memories, thoughts, and feelings that cause internal conflict. Reaction formation—which involves adopting attitudes or interests that are the opposite of the underlying mental state—and isolation—which involves repressing the affect associated with the mental state—are defenses that help to support repression.

4. The answer is D [*II D*]. Supporting the patient's self-esteem and allowing him some control will decrease his need to keep demonstrating his importance. Attempts to assert the physician's control over the situation are likely to make the patient feel more threatened and increase the patient's attempts to reassure himself by becoming more demanding. Although a few acutely ill patients may benefit at some point from discussions of fears of dependency, loss of control, or damage to their self-esteem, confronting this issue during the acute phase of the illness tends to increase anxiety. A psychiatric referral at this point will make the patient feel rejected or insulted.

5. The answer is B [*I B 7 b; III C 1, 2*]. Antidepressants, including the selective serotonin reuptake inhibitors (SSRIs) such as fluoxetine but not bupropion, are effective treatments for panic disorder. Neuroleptics should be reserved for psychotic anxiety. The dangers of addiction and withdrawal preclude the use of meprobamate as an anxiolytic. Carbamazepine is not effective against panic attacks unless they are a symptom of partial seizures.

6. The answer is C [*I B 4 a*]. Obsessions are intrusive unrealistic ideas that may be recognized as absurd but cannot be resisted. Compulsions are irrational, repetitive behaviors that arise in response to an obsession, to reduce anxiety, or both. Panic disorder is characterized by sudden unprovoked episodes of intense anxiety without specific content. The worries about everyday events that occur in generalized anxiety disorder are more realistic and more responsive to reassurance than the obsessions of obsessive-compulsive disorder (OCD). Posttraumatic stress disorder (PTSD) is associated with intrusive recollection of actual rather than imagined traumatic experiences. Substance-induced anxiety usually is diffuse or episodic and is not centered around specific worries.

7. The answer is B [*III C 1*]. High doses of diazepam are often necessary to treat panic attacks. Diazepam, similar to any other benzodiazepine, can be used as a hypnotic, although daytime sedation may occur. Benzodiazepines should usually be prescribed for limited periods, although recurrent treatment is often necessary for generalized anxiety disorder. Diazepam does not have antipsychotic properties.

8. The answer is D [*I B 7 b*]. Discussion of the patient's feelings about the traumatic event is a cornerstone of treatment of posttraumatic states. Biofeedback, meditation, and related relaxation techniques are useful adjuncts in the treatment of any anxiety disorder. However, systematic desensitization is a treatment for agoraphobia and specific phobias. Selective serotonin reuptake inhibitors (SSRIs) may reduce arousal, depression, and intrusive recall.

9. The answer is D [*III C 3 a*]. Monoamine oxidase (MAO) inhibitors may be more effective in patients with atypical depression or depression accompanied by anxiety, rejection sensitivity, mood reactivity; and reverse vegetative symptoms. MAO inhibitors are no more effective than other antidepressants for psychotic depression (about 25% of patients respond to an antidepressant without an antipsychotic drug).

10–14. The answers are: 10-B, 11-A, 12-C, 13-E, and 14-D [*I B 2, 5, 6*]. Agoraphobia, which may occur with or without panic disorder, is characterized by fear of being trapped in situations from which escape would be difficult or embarrassing (e.g., elevators, crowded theaters). Social phobia involves fear of humiliating oneself in social or performance situations. Blood–injection–injury phobia is a familial form of specific phobia that produces fainting at the sight of blood. Natural environmental phobia is a type of specific phobia involving fears of natural events (e.g., thunderstorms). Space phobia is the fear of falling down if a source of physical support (e.g., a wall) is unavailable.

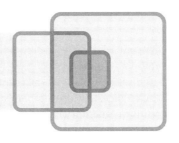

chapter 6

Cognitive and Mental Disorders Due to General Medical Conditions

ROBERT BREEN

I | INTRODUCTION

In the *Diagnostic and Statistical Manual of Mental Disorders*, 4th edition (*DSM-IV*), psychopathology that is caused by general medical conditions or by substances (e.g., abused drugs, medications, and toxins) is classified in three distinct groups. This classification replaced such terms as "organic mental disorders" that erroneously implied that other (primary) mental disorders are nonorganic.

A **Delirium, dementia, amnestic, and other cognitive disorders** are characterized by cognitive disturbances. They are caused by general medical conditions or are substance induced.

B **Mental disorders due to general medical conditions,** excluding cognitive disorders, are specific mental disorders due to general medical conditions. Examples include mood disorder due to a general medical condition, psychosis due to a general medical condition, sleep disorder due to a general medical condition, and sexual disorder due to a general medical condition. The description for each of these disorders is found in the *DSM-IV* chapter that describes the primary psychiatric disorders with similar syndromes. For example, the description of mood disorder due to a general medical condition is found in the *DSM-IV* chapter that concerns mood disorders.

1. **Diagnosis.** A mental disturbance is due to a general medical condition when evidence suggests that the disturbance results from the direct physiologic effect of the medical condition.

2. **Etiology.** The proposed general medical etiology should be known to cause the particular mental disturbance, and a temporal relationship should exist between the course of the general medical condition and the mental disturbance.

3. **Differentiation.** The disturbance should not be better explained by a primary mental disorder or one that is substance induced.

C **Substance-induced mental disorders** Specific substance-induced mental disorders are described in the *DSM-IV* with other disorders that have similar presenting syndromes. For example, cocaine-induced psychotic disorder is described in the *DSM-IV* chapter concerning schizophrenia and related psychotic disorders.

1. **Diagnosis.** A mental disturbance is substance induced if evidence suggests that the disturbance developed in association with substance use.

2. **Etiology.** The proposed substance should be known to cause the particular mental disturbance.

3. **Differentiation.** The disturbance should not be better explained by a primary mental disorder or one that is due to a general medical condition.

131

II COGNITIVE DISORDERS

Cognitive disorders are characterized by the syndromes of delirium, dementia, and amnesia. All are caused by general medical conditions, substances, or a combination of these factors. Disturbances of cognition involve symptoms such as confusion, memory impairment, speech and language difficulties, and impairment of the ability to plan or engage in complex tasks.

A **Delirium (Table 6–1)**

1. **Diagnostic features**
   a. **Disturbance of consciousness.** Individuals have reduced clarity of awareness of the environment. Their ability to focus, sustain, or shift attention is impaired. Affected individuals may appear confused, perplexed, or alarmed. They may have difficulty in responding to reassurance or in following directions.
   b. **Impaired cognition.** Individuals with delirium often have a marked disturbance of recent memory and may be unable to give a meaningful history. They may be disoriented to time and place. Speech may be rambling, incoherent, or sparse. Patients may have trouble finding words or identifying objects or people. Perceptual disturbances may include illusions and hallucinations. Often, actual perceptions are misinterpreted, and ordinary noises or objects are perceived as dangerous or disturbing. Hallucinations are often visual, but other senses can also be involved. Persecutory delusions based on sensory misperceptions are common.
   c. **Short and fluctuating course.** Delirium develops over a course of hours or days and fluctuates in severity. Individuals may have relatively lucid intervals of minutes or hours. Often, delirium worsens at night or during isolation.
   d. **Caused by a general medical condition or by a substance.** A comprehensive medical assessment should be undertaken to establish the relationship of the delirium to a general medical condition or to a substance. The disturbance should not be better explained by a primary mental disorder such as a manic episode occurring during the course of bipolar disorder.

TABLE 6–1 *DSM-IV* Classifications for Cognitive Disorders

Delirium

Delirium due to a general medical condition
Substance intoxication delirium
Substance withdrawal delirium
Delirium due to multiple etiologies
Delirium not otherwise specified

Dementia

Dementia of the Alzheimer's type
Vascular dementia
Dementia due to human immunodeficiency virus (HIV) disease
Dementia due to head trauma
Dementia due to Parkinson's disease
Dementia due to Huntington's disease
Dementia due to Pick's disease
Dementia due to Creutzfeldt-Jakob disease
Dementia due to other general medical conditions
Substance-induced persisting dementia
Dementia due to multiple etiologies
Dementia not otherwise specified

Amnesia

Amnestic disorder due to a general medical condition
Substance-induced persisting amnestic disorder
Amnestic disorder not otherwise specified
Cognitive disorder not otherwise specified

A general medical condition is more likely to be responsible for a delirium if its onset or exacerbation corresponds in time period to the course of the delirium and if it has previously been reported to cause delirium. Similarly, it is more likely that a substance is responsible for a delirium if history or laboratory results indicate that use of or withdrawal from the substance corresponds in time period to the delirium and if the substance is known to cause delirium.

    e. **Not explained by dementia.** When delirium is superimposed on a preexisting dementia, it is considered an associated feature of the dementia, not a separate diagnosis and is coded as the specific type of dementia **with delirium.**

2. **Associated features and diagnoses**
   a. **Disturbance in the sleep–wake cycle.** Individuals with delirium are often somnolent during the daytime or awake and agitated at night. They may have difficulty falling asleep and marked confusion on arousal.
   b. **Disturbance in psychomotor behavior.** Psychomotor behavior may be disorganized, with purposeless movements, psychomotor agitation, or decreased psychomotor activity.
   c. **Emotional disturbances.** Individuals with delirium are often emotionally labile. They may be extremely agitated and frightened or withdrawn and apathetic. Periods of irritability, belligerence, or euphoria can occur. Symptoms of delirium can cause affected individuals to strike out, struggle, or attempt to flee, sometimes resulting in patient injuries.
   d. **Abnormal electroencephalogram (EEG) findings.** EEG abnormalities are common in patients with delirium, usually showing either generalized slowing or fast wave activity. But delirium may occur without EEG changes.
   e. **Evidence of general medical conditions or substance use**
      (1) Individuals with delirium often have signs and symptoms of the underlying general medical condition. Metabolic disturbances and hypoxia due to perfusion or ventilation abnormalities are especially common.
      (2) Individuals with substance-induced delirium may have toxic levels of the responsible substance and other physical problems associated with the substance. Substance withdrawal delirium may occur while patients still test positive for significant amounts of a substance to which they have become tolerant. In many cases, delirium results from multiple concurrent etiologies.

3. **Epidemiology.** Older adults are most susceptible to delirium. Studies indicate that up to 25% of older patients have delirium at some point during hospitalization. Delirium also may occur in 30% to 40% of hospitalized patients with acquired immunodeficiency syndrome (AIDS).

4. **Etiology.** Delirium most often results from a variety of general medical conditions and from substances that interfere with brain function. Disturbance of the balance between cholinergic and dopaminergic neurotransmission is common in dementia. Some research findings suggest that the reticular-activating system may be specifically affected in individuals with delirium.
   a. **General medical conditions** most often associated with delirium include systemic infections, metabolic disturbances, hepatic and renal diseases, seizures, and head trauma.
   b. **Substance-induced delirium** is associated with either intoxication or withdrawal from drugs. Elderly and severely ill individuals are at highest risk of developing substance-induced delirium.

5. **Differential diagnosis.** Delirium must be distinguished from psychosis. The diagnosis of substance-induced delirium should not be made unless the symptoms exceed those that would be expected during typical intoxication or withdrawal.

6. **Treatment.** Delirium is treated by diagnosis and correction of the underlying physiologic problems. Environmental measures can reduce overstimulation and aid in orientation. Reassurance of the patient and family is important. Antipsychotic medications may aid in control of agitation. Judicious use of benzodiazepines is critical in sedative withdrawal delirium. Appropriate control of pain should be maintained. Restraints may be necessary but may also increase the risk of patient injury.

B **Dementia (see Table 6–1)**

1. The essential feature of dementia is progressive deterioration of memory and cognition that is due to general medical conditions or is substance induced. In dementia, cognitive deficits should

be apparent even with clarity of consciousness. A disturbance of both memory and at least one of the following aspects of cognition is necessary for diagnosis of dementia.

    a. Memory impairment, the hallmark of dementia, often develops insidiously as the condition progresses. Early on, individuals may appear more absentminded and distracted, misplacing personal objects and becoming disoriented in unfamiliar surroundings. As dementia progresses, recent memories are difficult to recall, learning deficits become more prominent, and individuals may become lost in what were familiar surroundings. Older memories are the most resistant to loss, but individuals with progressive dementia eventually forget even their own names. In addition to social and occupational compromise, memory impairment can lead to physical dangers such as fires from untended cooking, traffic accidents due to inattention, or exposure from wandering away while in a disoriented state.

    b. Possible cognitive deficits of dementia

        (1) Aphasia is an impairment or loss of language function. Affected individuals may have difficulty constructing sentences, finding words, naming objects, maintaining fluency, or comprehending instructions. Speech may become halting or characterized by circumlocution as aphasic individuals become frustrated and attempt to substitute more general words such as "it," "that," or "thing," rather than the correct noun. Communication deteriorates over time, sometimes resulting in mutism.

        (2) Apraxia is an inability to execute previously learned complex motor behaviors such as bathing, dressing, driving, or drawing. The difficulty is not due to impaired sensory or motor function.

        (3) Agnosia is a failure to recognize or identify previously known objects. This problem is not due to impaired sensory function. Affected individuals may be unable to recognize common objects or utensils and may not recognize familiar persons.

        (4) Disturbance in executive function refers to impaired ability to think abstractly and plan, initiate, sequence, monitor, and stop complex behavior. Individuals with dementia may have difficulty conceptualizing or solving problems such as creating a report, making a grocery list, or adjusting the thermostat in a house.

    c. Insidious and progressive course. Dementia usually develops over a course of months or years and progresses in severity. Traumatic or infectious dementias may develop more rapidly. Individuals may have brief periods of improvement only to lose some cognitive skills forever as the illness runs its course.

    d. Caused by a general medical condition or by a substance. A comprehensive medical assessment should be undertaken to determine the type of dementia and possible treatment. The disturbance should not be better explained by a primary mental disorder such as schizophrenia or a developmental disorder. Some of the medical conditions responsible for dementia are reversible. When a substance is responsible for dementia, abstinence may interrupt progression, but reversibility is limited. Some clinicians distinguish between cortical and subcortical dementias.

        (1) Cortical dementia is characterized by the early appearance of aphasia, difficulties with calculation, and memory loss. Disturbances of speech and psychomotor behavior are less predominant.

        (2) Subcortical dementia is characterized by the early appearance of problems with executive functioning and recall, dysarthria, motor skill impairment, and personality changes. These symptoms occur in the absence of significant aphasia.

    e. Not explained by dementia. When delirium is superimposed on a preexisting dementia, it is considered an associated feature of the dementia, not a separate diagnosis, and is coded as the specific type of dementia **with delirium.**

2. Associated features and diagnoses

    a. Disturbance in the sleep–wake cycle. Individuals with dementia lose orientation to time and may develop a dysfunctional sleep–wake cycle with agitation at night.

    b. Disturbance in psychomotor behavior. Psychomotor behavior may be disorganized, with restlessness, agitation, or decreased psychomotor activity. Specific psychomotor changes are seen in different types of dementia

    c. Emotional disturbances. Individuals with dementia may become emotionally disinhibited and labile. They may have outbursts of anger, anxiety, or despair. Depressive symptoms are common and may exacerbate cognitive deficits.

  d. **Personality disturbances.** Individuals with even relatively mild dementia may undergo marked changes in personality, becoming disinhibited, socially inappropriate, or moody. Irritability and argumentativeness may increase. Expansiveness and euphoria are sometimes present.

  e. **Psychotic symptoms.** Misperceptions are common because some individuals mistake old memories for current events. Delusions of a persecutory nature may be present. Hallucinations can also occur.

  f. **Neuroimaging.** Abnormal findings on computed tomography (CT) and magnetic resonance imaging (MRI) are common and reflect the pathophysiology of the underlying general medical condition. Neurodegenerative diseases often cause generalized or focal cerebral atrophy, with enlarged cerebral ventricles and deepened cortical sulci. Vascular disease, neoplasms, and traumatic injuries may cause focal lesions. Functional MRI (fMRI), positron emission tomography (PET), or single-photon emission computed tomography (SPECT) may reveal evidence of focal hypometabolic activity before structural changes are visible.

  g. **Evidence of general medical conditions or substance use.** Individuals may demonstrate diagnostic signs of the dementia subtype. Neurodegenerative diseases are frequently associated with motor and sensory deficits. Cerebrovascular lesions may be associated with focal motor and sensory deficits and with evidence of systemic vascular disease. Other dementing generalized medical conditions have characteristic physical findings such as evidence of infection, endocrine disturbance, or head trauma. Laboratory findings may reveal evidence of vitamin deficiencies, organ dysfunctions, and tumors. Substance-induced persisting dementia may be associated with physical signs of prolonged substance abuse such as alcohol-related liver disease.

3. **Epidemiology.** The prevalence of dementia increases with age; it affects 5% of the population older than age 65 years and 50% of the population older than age 85 years.

4. **Familial pattern.** Some types of neurodegenerative dementias are heritable such as dementia of the Alzheimer's type and Huntington's dementia.

5. **Etiology.** Many medical conditions that involve diffuse or focal cerebral damage can cause dementia. **Neurodegenerative diseases** account for more than 75% of dementias. **Cerebrovascular disease** is the other major cause of dementia. **Traumatic** causes of dementia will become more common as more people survive serious accidents with head injuries. **Infectious** causes of dementia had been on the decline until human immunodeficiency virus (HIV) disease began to spread. **Metabolic, nutritional, endocrine and substance-induced persisting dementias** also occur.

6. **Differential diagnosis.** Dementia must be distinguished from other psychiatric conditions. Cognitive functioning often deteriorates in patients with schizophrenia but when delusions develop in the course of a dementia, the diagnosis is **dementia with delusions.** Delirium may occur superimposed on dementia and should be diagnosed as **dementia with delirium.** Major depressive disorder may occur with cognitive dysfunction equal to dementia, but this should be reversible with effective treatment for depression. When depressive symptoms develop during the course of a dementia, the diagnosis is **dementia with depressed mood.**

7. **Treatment of dementia depends on proper diagnosis of the cause.**
  a. **Behavioral interventions** involve providing a low-demand environment. Familiar surroundings are reassuring for individuals with memory and cognitive impairment. Predictable routines and orientation with clocks and calendars may keep the day structured. The physical environment should be managed to reduce the risk of injury from falls, and appropriate lighting should correspond with times for activity and rest. Wandering can also be controlled with environmental management, and identification bracelets may aid in recovery of an individual who wanders away.

  b. **Family counseling** about managing the risks associated with dementia is important. Caring for a person with dementia is challenging, and **respite** is important for caregivers.

  c. **Somatic treatments** are under development for neurodegenerative dementias. Vascular dementia can be prevented with early control of cerebrovascular disease. Surgery may reverse progressive dementia from an intracranial process. Infectious metabolic, nutritional, endocrine, and substance-induced persisting dementias may also be reversible.

  d. **Agitation** occurs in at least half of all cases of dementia. When behavioral measures fail to ameliorate agitation, antidepressants, mood stabilizers, and antipsychotic medications have all been used to manage agitation. The use of substances such as alcohol, anxiolytics, hypnotics, and opioid analgesics often further impairs cognition and should be avoided.

C **Amnestic disorders (see Table 6–1)**

1. **Diagnostic features.** Memory impairment, which does not occur solely during the course of delirium or dementia, is the essential characteristic.
   a. **Memory impairment.** As with delirium and dementia, the memory impairment is manifested by difficulty in learning new information and, less often, by an inability to recall previously learned information. Immediate memory is usually relatively intact, but recent memory is severely affected. Individuals may not be able to recount recent events and may be disoriented. Long-term memory is usually preserved.
   b. The memory impairment **does not occur exclusively during the course of delirium or dementia.** In amnestic disorders, other aspects of cognition are relatively intact. Clarity of awareness is preserved.

2. **Associated features and diagnoses**
   a. **Confusion.** Individuals are often confused and disoriented as a result of recent memory impairment, and they may appear to be suffering from delirium.
   b. **Confabulation.** Individuals with memory impairment may imagine events to account for periods of time that they are unable to recall. They may adamantly defend their ideas.
   c. **Emotional changes.** Other subtle emotional changes often occur. Individuals sometimes appear inappropriately unconcerned and amotivated. Emotional lability is sometimes present.

3. **Epidemiology.** Amnestic disorders are more common in populations with a higher prevalence of alcohol abuse and head trauma. Young adult men and individuals with antisocial personality disorder are at greater risk.

4. **Course.** The **onset** of amnesia may be rapid when it results from trauma or acute biochemical injury (e.g., anoxia). More insidious onset is seen with neurodegenerative conditions and with chronic exposure to toxic substances. The **clinical course** depends on the underlying cause, and the symptoms may be transient or chronic.

5. **Etiology.** Bilateral damage (transient or chronic) to diencephalic and mediotemporal structures (e.g., mamillary bodies, fornix, hippocampus) may produce memory dysfunction in the absence of other cognitive symptoms. Such damage can be caused by thiamine deficiency associated with alcohol dependence, head trauma, cerebrovascular disease, hypoxia, severe hypoglycemia, local infection (herpes encephalitis), ablative surgical procedures, and seizures. Acute and chronic use of alcohol, anxiolytics, sedatives, and hypnotics can produce amnesia.

6. **Differential diagnosis**
   a. **Delirium and dementia** are both characterized by prominent memory disturbances but are accompanied by other cognitive deficits.
   b. **Dissociative disorders** also involve disturbances of memory but are often associated with emotional stress and unusual patterns of memory impairment.
   c. **Substance intoxication and withdrawal** often cause memory impairment, which does not persist.
   d. **Age-related cognitive decline** is associated with a decreased acuity of memory but not to a degree that causes significant functional impairment.

7. **Treatment.** As with delirium and dementia, stabilization or correction of the underlying general medical condition is the definitive treatment. Further physical or biochemical cerebral insults should be avoided. Familiar surroundings as well as reassurance and support are helpful as gradual reorientation occurs.

D **Cognitive disorder not otherwise specified** A variety of cerebral insults can lead to patterns of cognitive deficits, which are not better explained by delirium, dementia, or amnesia.

1. **Mild neurocognitive impairment.** Early in the course of neurodegenerative illness or after mild cerebral damage from various causes, symptoms of cognitive impairment are sometimes evident in the absence of dementia. In addition, subtle changes in personality are often present in individuals with such conditions.

2. **Postconcussion syndrome.** Chronic physical discomfort and disturbances in cognition some-times occur after significant closed-head trauma with transient loss of consciousness and amnesia. In such cases, sleep disturbances, headaches, and dizziness are often present. Automobile accidents are a common cause of concussion injury.

III MENTAL DISORDERS DUE TO GENERAL MEDICAL CONDITIONS

A Catatonic disorder due to a general medical condition

1. **Diagnostic features.** Catatonia is a syndrome characterized by **abnormalities of psychomotor activity,** which include any of the following:
   a. **Motoric immobility** (e.g., catatonic rigidity, waxy flexibility)
   b. **Excessive motor activity** (e.g., catatonic excitement)
   c. Extreme **negativism or mutism** (e.g., passive resistance to instructions, failure to speak)
   d. **Peculiarities of voluntary movement** (e.g., purposeless repeated movements, bizarre posturing)
   e. **Echolalia** (e.g., immediate purposeless repetition of words)
   f. **Echopraxia** (e.g., purposeless imitation of movements)

2. **Etiology.** General medical conditions that cause catatonia include both generalized and focal cerebral insults and systemic illnesses. It is not known whether specific central nervous system (CNS) structures must be affected to produce catatonia.
   a. Neurologic conditions that can produce catatonia include **neoplasms, head trauma, cerebro-vascular disease,** and **encephalitis.**
   b. Other general medical conditions associated with catatonia include **hypercalcemia, hepatic encephalopathy, homocystinuria,** thiamine **deficiency,** and **diabetic ketoacidosis.**

3. **Differential diagnosis.** Individuals with catatonia often appear bizarre and disturbed; this combination makes comprehensive medical assessment particularly difficult. The onset and course of catatonia depend entirely on the underlying general medical condition. Conditions that should be ruled out include the following:
   a. **Delirium** may occur, but when catatonic behavior occurs exclusively during the course of delirium, it is not diagnosed separately.
   b. **Movement disorders,** especially dystonias, can mimic catatonia.
   c. **Schizophrenia, catatonic type,** may be present with catatonia but is accompanied by other signs of schizophrenia. This syndrome is not due to a general medical condition.
   d. **Mood disorders** may occur with catatonia but are accompanied by a mood disturbance such as depression or mania.

4. **Treatment.** Stabilization or correction of the underlying general medical condition is the definitive treatment. Antipsychotic medications or restraints are sometimes indicated to prevent patient injury from disorganized behavior.

B **Personality change due to a general medical condition** The alteration of personality may include emotional lability, poor impulse control, aggressive or angry outbursts, apathy, or suspiciousness. *DSM-IV* subtypes of personality change due to a general medical condition are designated as labile, disinhibited, aggressive, apathetic, paranoid, and combined and unspecified types.

1. **Diagnostic features.** Affected individuals may become reclusive, querulous, or combative.

2. **Etiology.** The **pattern of personality changes** depends in part on the locus of the responsible lesion. Frontal lobe damage is characterized by disinhibition, shallow emotions, and occasionally euphoria (so-called "frontal lobe syndrome"). Many of the same general medical conditions that cause dementia can cause personality change when the lesion is relatively less severe or the clinical course is in its early stages. Head trauma is a major cause of personality change that does not progress to dementia.

3. **Differential diagnosis**
   a. Personality change due to a general medical condition must be distinguished from other mental disorders due to general medical conditions and from those due to substance use or abuse. Dementia and other cognitive disorders are characterized by memory impairment or other cognitive problems.

b. Other mental disorders, whether they are primary or due to a general medical condition, can secondarily result in personality change such as those that result form depressed mood, delusional beliefs, or immersion in a substance-abusing subculture.

4. **Treatment.** Stabilization or correction of the underlying general medical condition is the definitive treatment for personality disorder due to a general medical condition. Unfortunately, full recovery after traumatic damage does not always occur. Social and occupational rehabilitation plays an important role in treatment, as do counseling and support for patients' families.

IV   GENERAL MEDICAL CONDITIONS THAT CAUSE MENTAL DISTURBANCES

A Overview

1. **Examination of patients with mental disturbances.** The general availability of sensitive and specific diagnostic examinations makes it reasonable to screen for general medical conditions in almost all patients who have cognitive or behavioral changes.

2. **Pathophysiology.** General medical conditions and substances can adversely affect cerebral functioning through a number of mechanisms. Effects may be reversible or irreversible, depending on the nature of the lesion.
   a. **Disruption of metabolic homeostasis.** Levels of electrolytes, pH, hydration, and osmolarity can be altered by many metabolic and endocrine disorders and neoplasms.
   b. **Disruption of molecular synthesis.** Synthesis of neurotransmitters, neuroreceptors, cellular structures, and supporting elements can be disrupted by neurodegenerative disease, endocrine diseases, and nutritional deficiencies.
   c. **Deficiency of substrates.** Oxygen or metabolic substrates for oxidative metabolism may be deficient in patients with pulmonary disease, cerebrovascular disease, nutritional disease, and metabolic diseases.
   d. **Electrophysiologic disruption.** Synaptic transmission can be altered biochemically or by seizures.
   e. **Tissue damage.** Brain tissue can be damaged or destroyed by trauma, infection, or neoplasms.

B Neurodegenerative diseases

1. **Dementia of the Alzheimer's type (DAT).** This progressive neurodegenerative illness produces characteristic brain lesions and dementia.
   a. **Histopathology.** Classic histopathologic findings are neuronal loss, neurofibrillary tangles, neuritic (i.e., amyloid, senile) plaques, and amyloid angiopathy. Mediotemporal lobes are most severely affected.
      (1) **Neuronal loss.** Cholinergic neurons in the basal forebrain (including the nucleus basalis of Meynert) are affected early, but general neuronal loss ultimately occurs.
      (2) **Neurofibrillary tangles.** Intraneuronal deposits of abnormal microtubular elements and phosphorylated tau protein are common.
      (3) **Neuritic plaques.** Extraneuronal deposits of amyloid, dystrophic neuronal elements, and microglia are most prominent in the hippocampus and neocortex. They are also present in vascular tissue (amyloid angiopathy) throughout the body.
   b. **Gross pathology.** Diffuse frontotemporal cerebral atrophy, widened cortical sulci, and enlarged cerebral ventricles are characteristic.
   c. **Epidemiology.** DAT, which by itself accounts for more than 50% of cases of dementia, is seldom evident before age 50 years and is slightly more common in women. It affects 10% of the population older than age 65 years and 50% of the population older than age 85 years. Incidence of Alzheimer's disease is three to four times higher in relatives of patients, and the concordance rate is greater than 50% in monozygotic twins. Early-onset DAT is extremely common in individuals with Down syndrome.
   d. **Etiology.** No definite single cause for Alzheimer's disease has been identified, and a multifactorial etiology is plausible. Most postulated causes involve abnormal production of insoluble beta amyloid.
      (1) **Genetic lesions.** Several genetic lesions may produce the disease. Chromosome 21, the most commonly implicated locus, is the site of the genes for amyloid precursor protein.

Alzheimer's disease is very common in patients with Down syndrome (trisomy 21). Chromosomes 1 and 14 have also been implicated.

(2) **Abnormal amyloid precursor protein metabolism.** A product of amyloid precursor protein, beta A4 (amyloid), is a major component of neuritic plaques. Neuronal damage has been attributed to the immunologic response to insoluble beta amyloid.

(3) **Tau protein.** This substance, which stabilizes cellular microtubules, is found in neurofibrillary tangles.

(4) **Cholinergic neuronal dysfunction.** Cholinergic neurons in the hippocampus are affected early in the course of disease.

(5) **Other abnormalities. Increased oxidative changes** due to cerebrovascular disease may cause neuronal damage. **Aluminum,** a component of neuritic plaques, has been implicated. **Abnormal neuronal membrane phospholipid metabolism** has also been suggested.

(6) The presence of **apolipoprotein E** places individuals at 80% risk for development of Alzheimer's disease. Although a test for the presence of the protein does exist, lack of sensitivity and specificity precludes the recommendation of routine testing of family members of affected individuals.

e. **Symptoms and course**

(1) The **onset** is usually insidious, and the disease usually progresses slowly. The duration from the onset of dementia to death is usually 8 to 10 years.

(2) **Functional neuroimaging** (e.g., SPECT, PET) may show decreased parietal lobe metabolism bilaterally.

(3) **Early deficits** commonly involve recent memory disturbances, mood disturbances, emotional lability, and impulsivity.

(4) **DAT** becomes clinically evident as the disease progresses. *DSM-IV* subtypes include DAT with delirium, delusions, depressed mood, and behavioral disturbances.

(5) **Late in the disease,** motor disturbances supervene, especially gait disturbances, pathologic reflexes, and incontinence.

f. **Differential diagnosis.** Dementias due to other causes are the major differential diagnoses for DAT. The clinical diagnosis of DAT is one of exclusion and is usually histopathologically confirmed at autopsy. Major depressive disorder can be manifested by difficulties in mental concentration and apathy that can mimic dementia.

g. **Treatment.** The goals of treatment are to delay progressive loss of function, reduce behavioral disturbances, and help caregivers cope with the burden of illness.

(1) **Available somatic treatments involve reversible inhibition of acetylcholinesterase or modulation of glutaminergic neurotransmission. Tacrine, donepezil, rivastigmine,** and **galantamine** are reversible acetylcholinesterase (AChE) inhibitors, which may be effective in transiently reversing or slowing cognitive decline through enhancing cholinergic neurotransmission. Tacrine has fallen into disuse because of hepatotoxicity. **Memantine** is a modulator of N-methyl d-aspartate (NMDA) receptor function that may improve cognitive function through enhancing glutaminergic neurotransmission (Table 6–2.)

(2) **Antidepressants, mood stabilizers,** and **antipsychotic agents** may be used to stabilize mood and reduce agitation.

TABLE 6–2   Approved Alzheimer's Treatments

Generic Name	Trade Name(s)	Usual Oral Dosage Range (mg/day)
CHOLINESTERASE INHIBITORS		
Tacrine	Cognex	*No longer in widespread use*
Donepezil	Aricept	5–10
Rivastigmine	Exelon	3–6 bid
Galantamine	Razadyne ER	16–24
NMDA MODULATORS		
Memantine	Namenda	5–10 bid

(3) The role of **neuroprotective agents** in the prevention or slowing of the progression of DAT remains controversial. Trials of antiinflammatory medications (e.g., ibuprofen, steroids), antioxidants (e.g., α-tocopherol), and other drugs (e.g., selegiline, estrogen) have all failed to establish efficacy. Environmental factors that may have neuroprotective effects include avoidance of head trauma and maintenance of intellectually challenging activities.

(4) Caregivers should try to maintain **adequate food intake** and **good hygiene.** They should also encourage exercise as much as possible.

2. **Parkinson's disease.** This common, progressive neurodegenerative disease involves loss of dopaminergic neurons in the substantia nigra. It is manifested by resting tremor, rigidity, bradykinesia, and gait disturbances.

a. **Histopathology.** A progressive loss of dopaminergic neurons occurs in the substantia nigra. Lewy bodies are found in the neuronal cytoplasm of the remaining dopaminergic neurons.

b. **Epidemiology.** The prevalence of the disease is three per 1,000. Dementia occurs in at least 20% to 30% of cases.

c. **Etiology.** The precise cause of the disease is unknown. Mitochondrial dysfunction in dopaminergic neurons appears to be a key pathogenic component. The condition may be induced by several factors, including environmental toxins, infection, genetic predisposition, and aging.

d. **Symptoms and course**

(1) The **onset** of disease is usually between age 50 and 65 years. The course is progressive, but the rate is extremely variable.

(2) **Motor symptoms** include progressive tremor, rigidity, bradykinesia, and postural instability.

(3) **Dementia** is usually more evident in advanced disease, and it must be distinguished from the depressive symptoms that are also commonly present. The dementia is characterized by "subcortical" features such as psychomotor slowing and disturbances of executive function.

(4) **Cognitive problems** may be compounded by coexisting depression and by DAT and other age-associated cognitive impairments.

e. **Differential diagnosis.** Other diseases that cause movement disorders and dementia must be considered, including vascular dementia, progressive supranuclear palsy, diffuse Lewy body disease, Shy-Drager syndrome, amyotrophic lateral sclerosis (ALS)–dementia–Parkinson's disease complex, and olivopontocerebellar degeneration. Antipsychotic medications can also produce parkinsonian symptoms. A diagnosis of Parkinson's disease is usually confirmed at autopsy by the presence of Lewy bodies.

f. **Treatment.** Dopamine precursors (e.g., levodopa, carbidopa); dopamine agonists (e.g., bromocriptine; pergolide; ropinirole; pramipexole); anticholinergic medications (e.g., benztropine, trihexyphenidyl); amantadine; and selegiline, a selective monoamine oxidase (MAO)-B inhibitor, may be used. Antiparkinsonian medications can produce personality changes, cognitive changes, and psychotic symptoms. Pallidotomy may ameliorate dyskinesias in advanced disease that are unresponsive to medication.

3. **Huntington's disease.** This progressive neurodegenerative disease involves loss of γ-aminobutyric acid (GABA)-ergic neurons of the basal ganglia. It is manifested by choreoathetosis and dementia.

a. **Histopathology.** A loss of GABA-ergic neurons occurs in the striatum. Other neurons may also be involved.

b. **Gross morphology.** Functional neuroimaging reveals caudate hypometabolism at an early stage. Atrophy of the caudate nucleus, with resultant ventricular enlargement, is common.

c. **Epidemiology.** The prevalence is about one in 100,000. Fifty percent of offspring of patients with Huntington's disease develop the illness.

d. **Etiology.** Huntington's disease is caused by a defect in an autosomal dominant gene (*D4S10*) located on chromosome 4 that consists of unstable expanded cytosine–adenosine–guanine (CAG) repeats. The precise mechanism by which this defect produces the disease is unknown, but it may involve Huntington protein, an abnormal gene product.

e. **Symptoms and course**
   (1) The **onset** of clinically evident disease usually occurs at approximately age 40 years, but the variation is wide. Death usually occurs approximately 15 years after onset.
   (2) **Early symptoms** include personality changes and subtle movement disturbances.
   (3) **Later symptoms** include choreoathetosis and dementia. The dementia is characterized by subcortical features, with cognitive slowing and disturbances of executive function. Behavioral disorganization, severe mood instability, and psychotic features are fairly common.

f. **Differential diagnosis.** Other causes of dementia should be considered. Schizophrenia (especially with catatonic symptoms), schizoaffective disorders, mood disorders with psychotic and catatonic symptoms, and other psychotic disorders can resemble Huntington's disease. Other causes of choreoathetosis, including tardive dyskinesia from antipsychotic medications, are also in the differential diagnosis.

g. **Treatment.** There is no proven somatic treatment to reverse or prevent degeneration in Huntington's disease. Antipsychotic medications can ameliorate both choreoathetosis and psychotic symptoms. Antidepressant and mood-stabilizing medications may also provide symptomatic treatment. Family counseling, including genetic counseling, is essential.

4. **Pick's disease,** the most common neurodegenerative disease of the frontal and temporal lobes, is manifested by personality and language changes followed by other symptoms of dementia.
   a. **Histopathology.** Pick bodies (intraneuronal argentophilic inclusions) and Pick cells (swollen neurons) are found in affected areas of the brain.
   b. **Gross morphology.** Functional neuroimaging (PET or SPECT) reveals frontal and temporal hypometabolism before frontal and temporal atrophy become apparent by MRI.
   c. **Epidemiology.** The prevalence is unknown, but the condition may be relatively more common than previously believed.
   d. **Etiology.** The cause is unknown, but a chromosomal location has been identified in some families.
   e. **Symptoms and course**
      (1) The **age of onset** of clinical symptoms is usually between age 50 and 60 years.
      (2) **Early behavioral signs** often include personality changes suggestive of frontal lobe disturbance, including disinhibition and emotional lability or apathy.
      (3) **Dementia** caused by Pick's disease usually follows several years later, with "subcortical" features, including impairment in language and executive functioning.
   f. **Differential diagnosis.** Pick's disease must be distinguished from other causes of dementia. Pick's bodies are found only in patients with Pick's disease.
   g. **Treatment.** There is no specific treatment.

C Cerebrovascular disease

1. **Gross morphology.** Cerebral angiography may reveal flow abnormalities or abnormal vasculature (e.g., aneurysms). Neuroimaging by CT or MRI reveals lesions in brain structures, including hyperintensities and focal atrophy suggestive of old infarctions. Functional neuroimaging may reveal both global and focal reductions in cerebral metabolism, with asymmetric distribution.

2. **Epidemiology.** Cardiovascular disease accounts for perhaps 20% of cases of dementia and is more common in men than women.

3. **Etiology.** The most common etiologies for cerebrovascular disease are systemic arterial hypertensive disease, valvular heart disease, and extracranial vascular disease.

4. **Symptoms and course**
   a. The **onset** may be preceded by evidence of systemic hypertensive illness or other vascular pathology. In addition, patients may have a history of transient ischemic attacks. Depending on etiology, the onset of cerebrovascular disease may be sudden or insidious.
      (1) Large thrombotic or embolic strokes are associated with the sudden onset or exacerbation of symptoms.
      (2) Symptoms from smaller serial infarcts or damage from cerebral insufficiency may be more gradual, with personality changes and increasing disturbance of cognitive function.
      (3) Single strokes may be associated with specific motor, sensory, and cognitive deficits, but they rarely result in dementia.

     b. Neurologic findings include abnormal reflexes, focal motor weakness, and gait disturbances.

     c. With extensive cerebrovascular disease, **vascular dementia** becomes apparent. Symptoms depend on the location of the lesions. Some common patterns include:

          (1) Binswanger disease. Multiple small infarctions of deep hemispheric structures produce subcortical dementia, pseudobulbar palsy, spasticity, and weakness.

          (2) Left hemispheric disease involves cortical dementia, with prominent aphasia and apraxia. Depressive symptoms are more common with left than with right hemispheric disease.

          (3) Right hemispheric disease is characterized by cortical dementia, with prominent agnosia and visuospatial deficits.

     d. The illness is often characterized by **stepwise exacerbations,** which correspond to progressive cerebrovascular compromise. The developing patterns of cognitive and motor deficits are highly variable, depending on the location of lesions. Symptoms may fluctuate as brain tissue surrounding new lesions recovers from embolic or thrombotic insults. The overall course reflects the nature of the underlying vascular pathology, the location of lesions, and the effectiveness of treatment.

5. Differential diagnosis. Dementia due to neurodegenerative disease usually has a more insidious onset and gradual progression, with less scattered motor findings. Dementia due to other general medical conditions is usually accompanied by other suggestive physical findings.

6. Treatment. Therapy is directed both at the underlying cause and at lessening cell damage. Successful treatment may arrest or slow the course of dementia.

     a. Control of risk factors such as hypertension, smoking, diabetes, hypercholesterolemia, and hyperlipidemia is useful.

     b. Depending on the vascular pathology, endarterectomy, correction of sources of emboli, and anticoagulant therapy may be indicated.

     c. Thrombolytic agents (e.g., tissue plasminogen activator [TPA]) are often given in hopes of decreasing cellular ischemia during the first hours of an acute ischemic stroke. Various neuroprotective agents that reduce cell damage from ischemia are being investigated.

D Infectious diseases

1. Mechanisms. Infectious agents can cause mental disorders in a variety of ways.

     a. Physical destruction of brain tissue

     b. Inflammation of brain tissue, meninges, or cerebral vasculature

     c. Mass effects from infectious lesions

     d. Toxins

     e. Systemic metabolic alterations such as fever, renal failure, hepatic failure, or electrolyte disturbance

2. Viral encephalitis. This disorder can lead to delirium, sometimes accompanied by headache, fever, and photophobia. Focal CNS herpesvirus lesions, usually in the frontal or temporal lobes, can produce anosmia, personality changes, bizarre behavior, and complex partial seizures. Rabies encephalitis rapidly produces delirium. Subacute sclerosing panencephalitis (SSPE) can occur after measles infection in children and progresses from delirium with myoclonus, ataxia, and seizures to chronic dementia.

3. Chronic viral infections. These disorders can produce progressive destruction of CNS tissue resulting in dementia.

     a. Dementia due to HIV disease. HIV directly destroys brain parenchyma, and the course of the dementia is progressive. It becomes clinically apparent in at least 30% of individuals with AIDS. Diffuse multifocal destruction of brain structures occurs, and cognitive impairment may be accompanied by signs of delirium. Motor findings include gait disturbance, hypertonia and hyperreflexia, pathologic reflexes (e.g., frontal release signs), and oculomotor deficits. The differential diagnosis for dementia due to HIV disease includes other HIV-associated general medical conditions that cause dementia, including CNS tumors and opportunistic CNS infections. Mood disturbances in individuals with HIV infection may mimic cognitive impairment.

     b. Dementia due to Creutzfeldt-Jakob disease. This rare spongiform encephalopathy is believed to be caused by a slow virus (prion). Affected individuals present with dementia, myoclonus, and EEG abnormalities (e.g., sharp, triphasic, synchronous discharges and, later, periodic discharges). Over a course of several months, symptoms progress from vague malaise and personality changes to dementia. Other findings include visual and gait disturbances, choreoathetosis or other abnormal movements, and myoclonus. Atypical presentations and slower courses have been described in some patients. So called "new variant" Creutzfeldt-Jakob disease may be related to bovine spongiform encephalopathy. Kuru, a slow virus found in New Guinea, causes dementia and motor disturbances.

   c. **Progressive multifocal leukoencephalopathy (PML).** This demyelinating condition, which is usually caused by papovavirus JC (JCV) infection, occurs predominantly in immuno-compromised hosts. Over several months, increasing multiple motor deficits and cognitive deficits lead to death. HIV infection has increased the incidence of PML.

4. **Neurosyphilis** (general paresis). This parenchymal form of CNS tertiary syphilis typically occurs 5 to 30 years after incompletely treated primary syphilis. Personality changes are usually noted before the onset of dementia. Prominent psychotic symptoms are sometimes present. Physical findings include papilledema, optic atrophy, Argyll Robertson pupils (i.e., constriction reaction to near objects [accommodation reflexes present] but not to light [pupillary reflexes absent]), gait disturbances, and spasticity.

5. **Acute bacterial meningitis.** This disease usually has a rapid onset. Affected individuals present with systemic signs of infection (e.g., high fever) that are accompanied by headache, stiff neck, and delirium. In most cases, the causal bacteria are *Streptococcus pneumoniae, Neisseria meningitides,* and *Listeria monocytogenes.*

6. **Chronic meningitis.** This form of meningitis is characterized by a more gradual onset of cognitive impairment, progressing in some cases to delirium. The most common infections are tuberculosis and cryptococcal and coccidioidal mycoses. **Syphilitic meningitis** is a form of tertiary syphilis that usually occurs 1 to 3 years after incompletely treated primary syphilis, and patients present with delirium. Chronic basilar meningitis is accompanied by pupillary abnormalities, ptosis, hearing impairment, and facial paralysis. Chronic hemispheric meningitis is accompanied by marked cognitive impairments and seizures.

7. **Mass lesions.** Depending on their location, lesions resulting from granulomatous infections or abscesses can cause a variety of cognitive disturbances. Infections that most commonly produce mass lesions include tuberculosis, parasitic disease (cysticercosis, schistosomiasis), and mycoses.

E **Myelin diseases** Several diseases involve myelin, the white matter that sheaths neuronal axons, and are associated with motor and sensory disturbances. Depending on the nature of the disorder and sites affected, cognitive symptoms, personality changes, and mood disturbances can occur.

1. **Acute disseminated encephalomyelitis.** This demyelinating illness of abrupt onset presents with delirium followed by sensory and motor deficits, seizures, and coma. The mortality rate is 50%, and marked residual neurologic and cognitive impairments are present. It sometimes occurs after viral illnesses or vaccinations and may have an immune origin. MRI is diagnostic.

2. **Multiple sclerosis (MS).** A multifocal demyelinating disease of unclear viral or immune origin, MS has a waxing and waning clinical course. Episodes of focal disturbances occur and remit, sometimes with increasing residual motor and sensory deficits. It has an overall prevalence of about 50 in 100,000 and is slightly more common in women, with a peak incidence between age 20 and 40 years. It is more common in temperate climates.

   a. **Sensory symptoms** include transient visual impairment (initial presentation in 40% of patients) and impaired vibratory and position sense.

   b. **Transient motor symptoms** include nystagmus, dysarthria, tremor, ataxia, bladder dysfunction, and focal motor weakness.

   c. **Personality changes** depend on the loci of lesions but may include emotional lability, shallow emotions, depression, suspiciousness, apathy, and impulsiveness.

   d. **Cognitive symptoms** occur, and persisting dementia occasionally develops late in the course of the illness. The transient and patchy distribution of lesions often leads to somatic preoccupation in affected individuals, suggesting a somatoform disorder.

3. **Other diseases of myelin.** A number of other leukodystrophies caused by genetic lesions of myelin metabolism cause progressive neurologic impairment and dementia in children and adults. These

diseases include metachromatic leukodystrophy (cerebroside sulfatase deficiency), globoid cell (Krabbe) leukodystrophy (galactocerebrosidase deficiency), and adrenoleukodystrophy.

F **Epilepsy** This disorder is characterized by recurrent seizures and is associated with a variety of mental disturbances that occur both intra- and interictally.

1. **Definition.** Seizures, also referred to as convulsions or ictal episodes, are characterized by transient bursts of abnormal CNS electrical activity that cause disturbances of movement, autonomic activity, and consciousness. Seizure manifestations depend on the location of the seizure focus and the electrophysiologic state of the CNS.

2. **Pathophysiology.** Seizures result from disturbances of the electrophysiologic activity of brain cells, leading to paroxysmal discharges, which spread to large groups of neurons and produce characteristic EEG findings.

3. **Types of seizures**
   a. **Generalized seizures** involve the entire brain.
      (1) **Tonic–clonic (grand mal) seizures** are manifested by loss of consciousness and postural control, followed by generalized muscular rigidity (tonic phase). This is followed by rhythmic contractions (clonic phase) of the upper and lower extremities. Incontinence may occur. EEG tracings show a wide range of abnormalities.
      (2) **Absence (petit mal) seizures** are characterized by brief disruptions of consciousness during which affected individuals may seem inattentive or unresponsive. There may be subtle motor findings such as loss of muscle tone, chewing, or lip-smacking movements. EEG tracings show characteristic bilaterally synchronous 3-Hz spikes and slow wave activity. Absence epilepsy is more common in children.
      (3) **Atonic seizures** (drop attacks) are characterized by brief losses of consciousness and postural tone. Episodes can resemble the cataplexy symptom of narcolepsy.
      (4) **Myoclonic seizures** involve muscle contractions without loss of consciousness. They are seen in individuals with a variety of neurodegenerative diseases.
   b. **Partial seizures** involve specific brain foci.
      (1) **Simple partial seizures** are manifested by motor, sensory, or autonomic disturbances, depending on the location of the seizure focus.
      (2) **Complex partial seizures** cause disturbances of consciousness, including decreased awareness and alterations of cognition, emotion, and sensory experience. Recurrent complex partial seizure is the most common form of adult epilepsy, sometimes called psychomotor epilepsy or temporal lobe epilepsy. During seizure episodes, affected individuals may have dream-like sensations and may exhibit poorly organized behavior that can appear inappropriate, bizarre, or violent. Complex partial seizures may resemble symptoms seen with dissociative fugue and depersonalization disorder. Interictal personality changes may occur.

4. **Etiology.** Focal brain lesions resulting from trauma, infections, and neoplasms may cause seizures. Metabolic disturbances, neurodegenerative diseases, and various substances may also precipitate seizures. Autism and mental retardation are associated with a higher incidence of seizures.

5. **Symptoms**
   a. **Preictal symptoms** are often referred to as an **aura** and can include motor, sensory, emotional, and cognitive experiences. Motor twitching, olfactory hallucinations (e.g., burning rubber), autonomic sensations (e.g., a feeling of epigastric discomfort), peculiar emotion states or reveries, and intrusive thoughts or memories have been described as components of auras.
   b. **Postictal mental symptoms** due to generalized seizures and complex partial seizures are characteristic of resolving delirium. The duration of confusion varies from minutes to hours. Amnesia is usually complete for intraictal events during generalized seizures. Varying degrees of amnesia for events occur during complex partial seizures. After tonic–clonic seizures, focal motor paralysis may be present for minutes, hours, or days (Todd paralysis).
   c. **Interictal symptoms** are absent in many patients with epilepsy. Some affected individuals, especially those with complex partial seizure disorders, may develop a variety of personality changes or cognitive deficits. Psychotic symptoms may also occur. Some of these symptoms may be caused by subclinical seizure episodes. With long-standing and poorly controlled seizure disorders, cognitive deficits become more common.

6. **Other psychopathology associated with epilepsy.** Individuals with epilepsy have a higher incidence of mental disorders.
    a. Some mental disorders such as mental retardation and autism may stem from the same cause as the comorbid seizure disorder.
    b. In cognitive disorders and other mental disorders due to general medical conditions, seizures may be the physiologic cause of the comorbid mental disturbance.
    c. Individuals with epilepsy may develop mood, anxiety, or somatoform disorders as a result of the psychological stress associated with the illness. The incidence of suicide is relatively high in individuals with epilepsy.
7. **Differential diagnosis**
    a. Seizure-like episodes can occur in **conversion disorder** and **factitious disorder,** but there is rarely incontinence or physical harm (e.g., tongue biting) from tonic–clonic motor activity. Patients with factitious seizures are more likely to suffer from actual seizures as well.
    b. **Dissociative disorders** can be manifested by alterations of consciousness and cognition that are suggestive of complex partial seizures. It is sometimes difficult to distinguish between these conditions. Repeated EEGs or 24-hour EEG recordings may be required. Nasopharyngeal EEG leads are sometimes used.
8. **Treatment.** Definitive treatment requires amelioration of the underlying cause through management of systemic illness or surgical removal of seizure foci in the brain. Control of epilepsy can often be accompanied with anticonvulsant medications. However, these medications themselves may cause cognitive impairment and mental disturbances.

G Neoplasms   Neoplastic disease can cause mental disturbances through a variety of physiologic mechanisms, including intracranial mass effects, destruction of brain tissue, seizures, metabolic alterations, production of neuropeptides and toxins, and autoimmune reactions.

1. The **type of mental disturbance produced** by neoplasia depends on the nature of the neoplasm, the location of the tumor, the size of the tumor, and the rate of tumor growth.
2. **Rapidly growing intracranial neoplasms** in any location can produce **delirium** accompanied by other signs of increased intracranial pressure, including headache, papilledema, and vomiting. Slowly growing intracranial neoplasms can produce more insidious changes in cognition and personality.
3. The **location of intracranial neoplasms** influences the nature of the mental disturbances and physical findings.
    a. **Frontal lobe tumors** may be associated with personality changes, including disinhibition, emotional lability, and apathy.
    b. **Parietal lobe tumors** may be associated with sensory deficits, agnosia, and visual neglect.
    c. **Temporal lobe tumors** may be associated with complex motor, perceptual, and behavioral symptoms that resemble complex partial seizures.
    d. **Occipital lobe tumors** may be associated with visual hallucinations.
    e. **Brain stem tumors** may lead to an alert yet immobile and mute state (akinetic mutism or vigilant coma).
4. **Neuropeptide- and hormone-secreting tumors** in any location can produce mental changes through direct effects on CNS activity or by alteration of systemic metabolism.
5. **Paraneoplastic syndromes** are distant effects of neoplasms mediated by tumor-induced autoimmune reactions, tumor-produced neurotoxic substances, and perhaps other mechanisms. Paraneoplastic syndromes can produce mental disturbances. Small-cell lung carcinoma can produce encephalitis and delirium. When limited to limbic structures (limbic encephalitis), the condition can produce memory impairment and personality changes.
6. **Adjustment disorders** arising from the psychosocial effects of neoplastic disease must be considered in the differential diagnosis of mental disorders due to neoplasms.

H Head trauma   Injury to the head that leads to traumatic brain injury can produce subtle or profound cognitive symptoms and personality changes that may be transient or chronic. Head trauma can cause **brain injury** by direct destruction of brain tissue, by shearing of neuronal axons, by increased intracranial pressure, and by resultant vascular hemorrhage. The symptoms and course of resultant mental disturbances depend on the nature, location, and extent of damage.

1. **Acute head trauma** may result in immediate delirium or delirium that occurs after recovery of consciousness. The delirium is of variable duration, from a few seconds to days or weeks of confusion. The duration may reflect the extent of overall damage. Recovery is often gradual over several weeks and frequently involves amnesia for events surrounding the trauma.

2. **Subdural hematomas** arising from head injury (occurring in 10% of individuals with serious head injury) may manifest as headache, cognitive or personality changes, and focal neurologic deficits reflecting the location of the lesion. Individuals with alcoholism are predisposed to development of posttraumatic subdural hematomas.

3. **Postconcussion syndrome** (diagnosed in the *DSM-IV* as cognitive disorder not otherwise specified) is a disturbance of at least 3 months' duration that sometimes occurs after significant head trauma. It is characterized by cognitive, somatic, and behavioral symptoms that include headaches, fatigue, sleep disturbances, dizziness, and personality changes.

4. **Personality change** sometimes results from head trauma, even in the absence of obvious cognitive changes.

5. **Chronic amnestic disorder** can result from damage to diencephalic and mediotemporal lobe structures (e.g., mamillary bodies, hippocampus, fornix).

6. **Dementia due to head trauma** is usually nonprogressive. This condition may persist indefinitely or may gradually ameliorate over many months or years. It is often accompanied by emotional lability and impulsivity. A history of head trauma is a risk factor for development of dementias caused by neurodegenerative disorders.

7. In **children,** head trauma may lead to either loss of developmental competencies or a slowing of mental development. When either occurs, diagnoses of both mental retardation and dementia may be appropriate.

I **Nutritional deficiencies**   Mental disturbances resulting from nutritional deficiencies are characterized by development of cognitive deficits and personality changes with occasional psychotic symptoms. Without treatment, such disorders may progress to dementia.

1. **Etiology.** Several nutritional substances are essential for the structural integrity of the CNS. Deficiencies can be caused by inadequate intake, impaired absorption, and abnormal metabolism. Deficiency diseases are more common in areas of severe food shortage and in individuals with limited or unusual diets or alcoholism. Often, multiple deficiencies and general malnutrition are present in a single individual.

2. **Thiamine (vitamin B$_1$)** is required as a coenzyme for oxidative decarboxylation and for neural conduction.
   a. **Beriberi** results from thiamine deficiency caused by malnutrition. Individuals can present with high-output cardiac failure (wet beriberi), peripheral neuropathy with bilateral distal impairment of motor and sensory skills and reflexes (dry beriberi), and CNS damage with motor and cognitive impairments (cerebral beriberi).
   b. **Wernicke's encephalopathy** and **Korsakoff psychosis** describe forms of cerebral beriberi most commonly found in alcohol-dependent individuals.
      (1) **Wernicke's encephalopathy** is characterized by the rapid onset of ataxia, oculomotor abnormalities (ophthalmoplegia and nystagmus), and delirium. Histopathologic changes occur in the mamillary bodies and walls of the third ventricle. Symptoms usually quickly resolve if thiamine is administered early.
      (2) Repeated or incompletely treated encephalopathy may result in alcohol-induced persisting amnestic disorder (**Korsakoff psychosis**), which is not responsive to treatment with thiamine. Associated symptoms include confabulation, personality changes, and motor deficits. Dementia may supervene.

3. **Nicotinic acid (niacin)** deficiency (pellagra) usually results from a dietary deficiency of tryptophan as a consequence of alcohol dependence, from some vegetarian diets, or from starvation. Symptoms include dermatitis, diarrhea, peripheral neuropathies, cognitive deficits, and personality changes that progress to delirium. Irreversible dementia can result if the deficiency is not treated.

4. **Pyridoxine (vitamin B$_6$)** deficiency leads to dermatitis, neuropathies, and cognitive changes. It is usually found only in association with use of medications (e.g., isoniazid) that act as pyridoxine antagonists.

5. **Cobalamin (vitamin B$_{12}$)** deficiency usually occurs when gastric mucosal cells fail to produce intrinsic factor necessary for ileal absorption of vitamin B$_{12}$. Symptoms include megaloblastic anemia (**pernicious anemia**), paresthesias and other sensory and motor peripheral neuropathies, gait disturbance, and cognitive disturbances. Delirium may occur. If treatment is inadequate, irreversible dementia may supervene.

J **Metabolic disorders** These conditions can cause mental disturbances through systemic metabolic alterations or by direct toxic effects on the CNS.

1. **Genetic metabolic diseases of childhood** (i.e., disorders of lipid, carbohydrate, and protein metabolism) can produce progressive mental retardation and other neurologic conditions in childhood. Some childhood disorders can be ameliorated by dietary control.

2. **Wilson's disease (hepatolenticular degeneration)** is an autosomal recessive genetic illness characterized by abnormal copper metabolism that results in copper deposition. As a result, copper deposition occurs, with damage to the liver, renal tubules, and brain structures (e.g., corpus callosum, putamen). Personality changes may become apparent in early adulthood and progress to dementia if untreated. Gait disturbances, incoordination, and chorea also develop. Treatment often includes a copper-restricted diet and administration of chelating agents (e.g., D-penicillamine, zinc).

3. **Acute intermittent porphyria (AIP),** an autosomal dominant genetic disorder, is characterized by abnormal heme biosynthesis and excessive accumulation of porphyrins. AIP leads to episodes of abdominal pain, motor neuropathies, and mental disturbances that range from personality changes to psychotic symptoms and delirium. This disease is more common in women and is often first apparent in young adulthood. Episodes are sometimes precipitated by use of barbiturates, estrogens, and sulfonamides. Treatment is symptomatic, involving analgesic and antipsychotic medications. Two other porphyrias, hereditary coproporphyria and variegated porphyria, have similar psychiatric symptoms.

4. **Hepatic encephalopathy** results from acute or chronic liver failure. Patients present with delirium accompanied by a characteristic flapping tremor (asterixis). Other symptoms include jaundice, hyperventilation, and EEG abnormalities. Treatment requires a nitrogen-restricted diet.

5. **Uremic encephalopathy** results from acute or chronic renal failure. Patients present with delirium accompanied by diffuse polyneuropathy, twitching, and hiccups. Untreated uremic encephalopathy may result in irreversible dementia. Treatment involves renal dialysis, which can also produce delirium.

6. **Disorders of glucose metabolism**
   a. **Hypoglycemic encephalopathy** results from the presence of excessive endogenous or exogenous insulin or the unavailability of glucose. Such episodes are most common after nighttime fasting, after vigorous exercise, or several hours after a heavy meal. Early symptoms include hunger, sweating, tremulousness, and anxiety. When untreated by administration of sugar, symptoms progress to delirium, coma, and seizures. Repeated severe hypoglycemic episodes can result in irreversible cognitive deficits.
   b. **Diabetic ketoacidosis** results from inadequately treated diabetes mellitus and presents with weakness, polyuria, polydipsia, nausea, vomiting, headache, and fatigue. Delirium may supervene. Dementia may result from repeated episodes.

7. **Fluid and electrolyte disturbances** cause mental disturbances that range from personality change to delirium.

8. **Hypoxia** can result from pulmonary, cardiovascular, and hematologic diseases and from toxins (e.g., carbon monoxide). Acute cognitive changes and delirium can occur. Chronic amnestic disorder or dementia are possible sequelae.

K **Endocrine disorders** These conditions often cause changes in personality, mood, and cognitive function.

1. **Pituitary disorders.** Pituitary tumors may impair cognitive functions by causing pressure to hypothalamic and temporal lobe structures. Compression of the optic chiasm can cause bitemporal

hemianopia. Endocrine disturbances reflect the area of the pituitary that is affected. Postpartum infarction and hemorrhage into the pituitary result in Sheehan syndrome, which is characterized by thyroid and adrenal failure with associated mental disturbances.

2. **Hypothalamic disorders.** Tumors of the hypothalamus may cause appetite and sleep disturbances accompanied by personality changes. Resultant metabolic disturbances from dysregulation of antidiuretic hormone can result in delirium from fluid and electrolyte disturbances.

3. **Thyroid disorders.** Disorders of thyroid metabolism can be caused by genetic lesions; neoplasms of the thyroid gland, pituitary gland, or hypothalamus; autoimmune diseases of the thyroid gland; surgical or radiochemical ablation of the thyroid gland; exogenous thyroxin; and iodine deficiencies.

   a. **Hyperthyroid disorders.** Presenting symptoms include weakness and fatigue, insomnia, weight loss, tremulousness, palpitations, and sweating. Exophthalmos and eyelid lag sometimes occur. Anxiety and restlessness are early mental symptoms, and cognitive impairment and personality changes may emerge. In severe cases, manic and psychotic symptoms can develop. Cognitive deficits in the absence of anxiety can occur in elderly individuals. Treatment results in resolution of the associated mental disturbances.

   b. **Hypothyroid disorders.** Individuals with hypothyroidism (myxedema) present with fatigue, somnolence, weakness, dry skin, brittle hair, cold intolerance, and hoarse speech. Depression and irritability are common. Cognitive slowing may progress to dementia. Occasionally, persecutory delusions and hallucinosis develop. Without timely treatment (i.e., exogenous thyroxin, iodine), residual dementia occurs. Untreated hypothyroidism in children results in mental retardation.

4. **Parathyroid disorders.** Disorders of parathyroid metabolism can be caused by genetic lesions, neoplasms of the parathyroid gland and other tissues, and surgical or radiochemical ablation of the parathyroid gland. In addition to parathyroid pathology, abnormal calcium metabolism can also result from diseases with bone lesions such as Paget disease, multiple myeloma, and metastatic disease.

   a. **Hyperparathyroidism** with resultant hypercalcemia can cause muscular weakness, anxiety, and personality changes. Delirium, seizures, and death can occur in parathyroid storm.

   b. **Hypoparathyroidism** with resultant hypocalcemia leads to neuromuscular signs and symptoms, including increased excitability, transient paresthesias, cramping, twitching, tetany, and seizures. Delirium may occur even in the absence of tetany.

5. **Abnormalities of adrenal cortical functioning.** These disorders can be caused by adrenal and pituitary neoplasms, excessive use of exogenous corticosteroids, or sudden cessation of corticosteroid use.

   a. **Adrenocortical hyperactivity (Cushing syndrome)** or excessive levels of exogenous corticosteroids produce a variety of mental disturbances. Restlessness, sleep disturbances, and mood symptoms are common. Mood changes can include agitated depression or manic symptoms. Psychotic symptoms are sometimes seen, and suicide can occur. Treatment of the underlying pathology or gradual tapering of exogenous corticosteroids causes resolution of associated mental disturbances.

   b. **Chronic adrenal insufficiency (Addison disease)** produces apathy, fatigability, irritability, and depression. Occasionally, psychotic symptoms or delirium occurs. Treatment with corticosteroids eliminates the mental disturbances.

6. **Pheochromocytoma.** This catecholamine-secreting neoplasm of the adrenal medulla can produce panic attacks, hypertension, excessive perspiration, palpitations, tremulousness, lightheadedness, headaches, and pallor.

L **Autoimmune disorders** These conditions can produce cognitive deficits and personality changes resulting from direct damage to brain tissue, damage to cerebral vasculature, and metabolic disturbances due to damage to other organ systems. Treatment of autoimmune disorders with steroids and other immunosuppressants can also produce mental disturbances.

1. **Systemic lupus erythematosus (SLE).** Characteristic damage to multiple organ systems results from deposition of antinuclear antibody–antigen complexes in renal glomeruli and systemic vascular beds. Arthralgias, cutaneous rashes, adenopathy, pericarditis, pleurisy, and renal failure are

common manifestations. Mental disturbances, the initial presentation, eventually occur in at least 50% of SLE patients. Mental symptoms commonly involve personality changes. Mood symptoms and psychotic symptoms are sometimes present, and occasionally, delirium and dementia occur. Treatment with corticosteroids often produces mental disturbances, including psychosis and mood symptoms. SLE is much more common in women.

2. **Vasculitides.** Individuals with other autoimmune vasculitides may present with psychiatric symptoms when cerebral vasculature is involved. Such vasculitides may be associated with infection, transplant rejection, or other systemic autoimmune disease. Isolated vasculitis of the CNS sometimes occurs without identified associated illness, and affected individuals present with headache, focal neurologic deficits, and altered mental status.

Study Questions

Directions: *Each of the numbered items or incomplete statements in this section is followed by answers or by completions of the statement. Select the ONE lettered answer or completion that is BEST in each case.*

1. On examination in the emergency department, a 32-year-old man has an unsteady gait, mild bilateral oculoparesis, and spider angiomas. He is confused and agitated. Which of the following agents is the best immediate pharmacologic treatment?

   (A) Anticoagulants
   (B) Acetylcholinesterase (AChE) inhibitors
   (C) Pentobarbital
   (D) Salicylates
   (E) Thiamine

2. Which of the following medications for dementia of the Alzheimer's type affects glutaminergic neurotransmission?

   (A) Donepezil
   (B) Memantine
   (C) Rivastigmine
   (D) Tacrine
   (E) Galantamine

3. A 46-year-old woman has been found unconscious in her garage. Her car was running, and all the doors to the garage were closed. On examination, the woman is confused. Which of the following is the most likely cause of her confusion?

   (A) Dissociative fugue
   (B) Gasoline inhalation
   (C) Hypoglycemia
   (D) Hypoxia
   (E) Lead poisoning

4. A 58-year-old man has gradually become more apathetic and moody. At times, he is confused and forgetful. His gait is unsteady, his deep tendon reflexes are diminished, and he complains of tingling in his legs. Which of the following disorders is the most likely diagnosis?

   (A) Cerebellar neoplasm
   (B) Cobalamin (vitamin B_{12}) deficiency
   (C) Hyperthyroidism
   (D) Manganese intoxication
   (E) Multiple sclerosis (MS)

5. A 26-year-old woman presents with a history of episodic anxiety, emotional lability, confusion, and abdominal pain. She takes birth control pills but uses no other substances. Which of the following disorders is the most likely diagnosis?

   (A) Absence (petit mal) seizures
   (B) Acute intermittent porphyria (AIP)
   (C) Exposure to organophosphates
   (D) Premenstrual syndrome
   (E) Wilson disease (hepatolenticular degeneration)

6. A 29-year-old man presents with a history of three distinct episodes of emotional lability. Five years ago, when the first episode occurred, he experienced a right visual field deficit that resolved after 3 months. Two years ago, during another episode, he experienced transient mild ataxia. He now has a 2-month history of chronic fatigue, nonrestorative sleep, anxiety attacks, and irritability. Which of the following disorders is the most likely diagnosis?

   A Cobalamin (vitamin B_{12}) deficiency
   B Herpes encephalitis
   C Multiple sclerosis (MS)
   D Neurosyphilis
   E Systemic lupus erythematosus (SLE)

7. A 39-year-old man with Down syndrome has exhibited increasing forgetfulness and angry outbursts over the past several months. He has become neglectful of personal hygiene and has trouble finding items in his room. Which of the following conditions is the most likely cause of these problems?

   A Alzheimer's disease
   B Cerebrovascular disease
   C Intracranial neoplasm
   D Human immunodeficiency virus (HIV)
   E Thiamine deficiency

8. A 23-year-old woman with no history of alcohol abuse reports that she has been troubled by morning episodes of tremulousness, anxiety, tachycardia, and sweating. Which one of the following test results is most likely to be abnormal?

   A Serum ammonia measurement
   B Serum glucose measurement
   C Serum sodium measurement
   D Thyroid function test
   E Toxicologic screen

9. A 28-year-old woman presents with complaints of irritability and moodiness. She gives a history of brief episodes of auditory hallucinosis and suspiciousness. Her speech is slightly slurred. Which one of the following conditions is the most likely diagnosis?

   A Folate deficiency
   B Hyperparathyroidism
   C Pick's disease
   D Sydenham chorea
   E Wilson disease

Directions: *Each set of matching questions in this section consists of a list of four to 26 lettered options (some of which may be in figures) followed by several items. For each numbered item, select the ONE lettered option that is most closely associated with it. To avoid spending too much time on matching sets with large numbers of options, it is generally advisable to begin each set by reading the list of options. Then, for each item in the set, try to generate the correct answer and locate it in the option list, rather than evaluating each option individually. Each lettered option may be selected once, more than once, or not at all.*

QUESTIONS 10–13

For each of the following symptoms, select the most commonly associated neoplasm.

   A Frontal lobe neoplasm
   B Parietal lobe neoplasm
   C Pituitary neoplasm
   D Occipital lobe neoplasm
   E Temporal lobe neoplasm

10. Trance-like states

11. Apathy

12. Uninhibited behavior

13. Visual hallucinations

QUESTIONS 14–17

For each of the following conditions, select the associated symptom.

- A Anxiety attacks
- B Depressive episodes
- C Insidious personality changes
- D Psychotic symptoms
- E Reduced clarity of awareness

14. Pheochromocytoma

15. Adrenocortical hyperactivity (Cushing syndrome)

16. Pick's disease

17. Delirium due to hyponatremia

Answers and Explanations

1. The answer is E [*IV 1 2 b*]. This case is most suggestive of Wernicke encephalopathy, which is a delirium characterized by gait disturbance, oculomotor abnormalities, and cognitive impairment. This delirium is caused by acute thiamine deficiency, usually resulting from alcohol abuse. Treatment involves rapid administration of thiamine. Pentobarbital is likely to worsen the symptoms. Salicylates, anticoagulants, and acetylcholinesterase (AChE) inhibitors would have no effect.

2. The answer is B [*IV B 1 g*]. Memantine is a modulator of N-methyl d-aspartate (NMDA) receptor function that may improve cognitive function through enhancing glutaminergic neurotransmission. Tacrine, donepezil, rivastigmine, and galantamine are reversible acetylcholinesterase (AChE) inhibitors that may be effective in transiently reversing or slowing cognitive decline through enhancing cholinergic neurotransmission.

3. The answer is D [*IV J 8*]. The particular circumstances strongly suggest that the woman has been exposed to levels of carbon monoxide sufficient to interfere with the oxygen-carrying capacity of her hemoglobin. Thus, cerebral anoxia and delirium have resulted. Although the other choices can cause cognitive disturbances, they are less likely causes in this case.

4. The answer is B [*IV I 5*]. The evidence of gradual cognitive, motor, and sensory impairments is most suggestive of cobalamin deficiency. Megaloblastic anemia is likely to be present. Although multiple sclerosis (MS) might also cause such impairments, the course would most likely wax and wane. A patient with a neoplasm is more likely to present with seizures. Hyperthyroidism causes increased reflexes and palpations.

5. The answer is B [*IV J 3*]. The woman's history is characterized by episodes of cognitive impairment, personality changes, mood disturbance, and abdominal pain. The episodes started when she began using estrogen. This pattern is most suggestive of acute intermittent porphyria (AIP), a disorder of heme synthesis that includes wine-colored urine. AIP is most common in women; often, it is first evident in the third decade of life and can be precipitated by use of estrogens and barbiturates.

6. The answer is C [*IV E 2*]. The man has experienced relapsing and remitting symptoms involving a variety of CNS sites, a course that is characteristic of multiple sclerosis (MS). The visual deficit is suggestive of optic nerve involvement, which is often an early symptom of this illness and is uncommon in any of the other choices. The peak incidence of diagnosis of MS is approximately age 30 years. Cobalamin deficiency causes megaloblastic anemia. Herpes encephalitis produces bizarre behavior and seizures. Psychosis is prominent in patients with neurosyphilis. Mood disturbance is seen in individuals with systemic lupus erythematosus.

7. The answer is A [*IV B 1 c*]. The symptoms are very suggestive of dementia, with impairment in memory and other cognitive processes. Alzheimer's disease causes 55% of cases of dementia. It is usually seen in older individuals, but individuals with Down syndrome are very likely to develop this disease by age 40 years.

8. The answer is B [*IV J 6 a*]. The patient describes an episodic disturbance that occurs in the morning. This episode is most suggestive of hypoglycemia, which most often occurs after nighttime fasting or after vigorous exercise. Symptoms are strongly reminiscent of anxiety attacks. Hyperthyroidism might also manifest as anxiety and tremulousness, but it would not be limited to the morning. Ammonia levels are associated with liver disease secondary to alcohol abuse. Sodium is likely to be normal without gastrointestinal disturbance. Thyroid symptoms would occur at other times. Toxicology screen is less productive, unless ingestion occurred within a few hours.

9. The answer is E [*IV J 2*]. Wilson disease (hepatolenticular degeneration) usually becomes symptomatic in the second or third decade of life. The initial signs often include personality and mood changes.

Transient episodes of psychosis may occur. The disease process involves the putamen and the corpus callosum, resulting in movement or muscular signs such as the dysarthria manifested here. Hyperparathyroidism is associated with anxiety and personality change, and folate deficiency is associated with birth defects. Pick's disease causes dementia. Sydenham chorea is noted for movements.

10–13. The answers are 10-E *[IV G 3 c]*, **11-A** *[IV G 3 a]*, **12-A** *[IV G 3 a]*, and **13-D** *[IV G 3 d]*. Temporal lobe neoplasms are most commonly associated with trance-like states and disturbances of complex behavior. Mood symptoms can be prominent.

Frontal lobe neoplasms are most associated with insidious personality changes. These changes can include apathy as well as loss of inhibitions.

Occipital lobe neoplasms are most often associated with visual symptoms, which can include misperceptions and hallucinations.

14–17. The answers are 14-A *[IV K 6]*, **15-B** *[IV K 5 a]*, **16-C** *[IV B 4]*, and **17-E** *[II A 1 a]*. Pheochromocytoma is a catecholamine-secreting neoplasm of the adrenal medulla, which can produce attacks of severe anxiety as well as hypertension and headaches.

Adrenocortical hyperactivity (Cushing syndrome) produces excessive levels of corticosteroids that lead to restlessness, sleep disturbances, and mood symptoms. Psychotic symptoms occasionally occur but are less likely.

Pick's disease is a neurodegenerative condition that results in personality disturbances and supervening dementia.

Delirium caused by hyponatremia or any other cause is distinguished by a reduced clarity of consciousness.

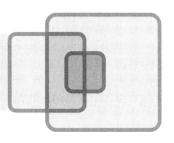

chapter **7**

Substance-Related Disorders

ANGELA D. HARPER

I   **INTRODUCTION**

The *Diagnostic and Statistical Manual of Mental Disorders,* 4th edition (*DSM-IV*) recognizes two broad categories of disorders related to the use of psychoactive substances. Substance use disorders are syndromes of pathologic use of a substance, and substance-induced disorders are disturbances of thinking, emotion, or behavior caused by intoxication with or withdrawal from a psychoactive substance.

A   **Substance use disorders** are subdivided into two categories: substance dependence and substance abuse.

1. **Substance dependence** is a pathologic pattern of substance use that results in impairment or distress. Substance dependence is diagnosed when three or more of the following consequences of substance use occur together at any time in the same year:
   a. **Tolerance,** which is defined as:
      (1) A requirement for increased amounts of the substance to achieve the same effect
      (2) Decreased effect with continued use of the same amount of the substance
   b. **Withdrawal,** which is defined as:
      (1) Typical withdrawal syndrome for the substance (see I B 2)
      (2) The substance or a related compound is taken to relieve or avoid withdrawal symptoms
   c. Use of the substance in greater amounts or for a longer time than was originally intended
   d. Unsuccessful attempts or wishes to cut down on or control substance use
   e. Significant amounts of time spent in activities necessary to obtain or use the substance or recover from its effects
   f. Giving up important social, occupational, or recreational activities because of substance use
   g. Continued use of the substance despite knowledge that it is causing or aggravating physical or mental problems

2. **Physiologic dependence** is defined in the *DSM-IV* as the presence of either tolerance or withdrawal (I A 1 a, b).

3. **Substance abuse,** according to the *DSM-IV,* is a maladaptive pattern of abuse with fewer and different consequences than substance dependence. Substance abuse is diagnosed if one of the following four problems has occurred over a 12-month period and if the patient does not meet criteria for substance dependence:
   a. Failure to fulfill major role obligations
   b. Recurrent use of a substance in situations in which it is hazardous (e.g., while driving)
   c. Recurrent legal problems resulting from substance use
   d. Continued use of a substance despite social or interpersonal problems caused by the substance (e.g., arguments with a spouse about substance use, getting into fights when drunk)

B   **Substance-induced disorders** include a diverse group of physical and mental syndromes caused by psychoactive substances or their withdrawal:

1. **Substance intoxication** is a reversible, substance-specific syndrome (see II).

2. **Substance withdrawal** is a substance-specific syndrome that appears when a substance is withdrawn (see III).

3. **Substance-induced delirium** is an acute disturbance of cognition and awareness caused by taking a psychoactive substance. Of the substances in the *DSM-IV* considered to be psychoactive, only nicotine is not thought to cause delirium.

4. **Substance-withdrawal delirium** is caused by withdrawal of alcohol, sedative-hypnotics, anxiolytics, and related substances.

5. **Substance-induced persisting dementia,** which is caused by intoxication with or withdrawal from substances (e.g., alcohol, inhalants, sedatives), is characterized by memory impairment plus one or more of four signs of cognitive dysfunction. These signs include **aphasia, apraxia, agnosia,** and **disrupted executive function.** Signs of dementia persist after intoxication or withdrawal has cleared.

6. **Substance-induced, persisting amnestic disorder** consists of impairment of recall of previously learned material or of the ability to learn new information. It is associated with the use of alcohol, sedative-hypnotics, anxiolytics, and related substances. The memory disorder persists after intoxication or withdrawal has resolved.

7. **Substance-induced psychotic disorder** is characterized by prominent hallucinations or delusions caused by substances such as alcohol, amphetamines, cannabis, cocaine, hallucinogens, inhalants, opioids, phencyclidine, and sedatives. According to the *DSM-IV,* this diagnosis cannot be based on hallucinations if the patient realizes that the hallucinations are caused by the substance, although the significance of this distinction is not established scientifically. If transient psychotic symptoms are associated only with delirium caused by substance intoxication or withdrawal, the diagnosis is substance-induced delirium or substance-induced withdrawal delirium.

8. **Substance-induced mood disorder** is depressed or manic mood that either is clearly caused by substances such as alcohol, amphetamines, cocaine, hallucinogens, inhalants, opioids, phencyclidine, sedatives, and anxiolytics or develops within 1 month of using these substances.

9. **Substance-induced anxiety disorder** (see Chapter 4) consists of generalized anxiety, panic attacks, obsessions, or compulsions that either are clearly caused by a substance or develop within 1 month of substance use or withdrawal.

10. **Substance-induced sexual dysfunction** either develops within 1 month of substance intoxication or is clearly caused by substances such as alcohol, amphetamines, cocaine, opioids, and a number of medications (e.g., reserpine, serotonin reuptake inhibitors, monoamine oxidase [MAO] inhibitors).

11. **Substance-induced sleep disorder** either is obviously caused by a psychoactive substance or appears within 1 month of substance use or withdrawal. Typical offending agents include alcohol, amphetamines, caffeine, cocaine, opioids, sedatives, hypnotics, and anxiolytics.

12. **Hallucinogen-persisting perception disorder (flashbacks)** are the reexperiencing of perceptual symptoms that were caused by intoxication with a hallucinogen but occur after the drug is no longer being taken. Because hallucinogens act on the serotonin 5HT2 receptor, medications that increase synaptic serotonin availability (e.g., selective serotonin reuptake inhibitors [SSRIs]) may overstimulate receptors previously sensitized by hallucinogens to produce flashbacks years after substance discontinuation.

C **Addiction** is a term used by some clinicians to refer to overwhelming involvement with seeking and using drugs or alcohol and a high tendency toward relapse after substance withdrawal. It is, therefore, a quantitative description of the degree to which drug use pervades an individual's life. Addiction may be described as a form of substance dependence, as defined in I A.

1. It is possible for an individual to develop tolerance and undergo withdrawal without being addicted; that is, the individual's life is not organized around finding and using the drug. This is common in patients who become physically dependent on narcotics, tranquilizers, or sedatives during treatment of prolonged illness or insomnia but who do not experience intrusion of drug use into many aspects of their lives.

2. It may be possible to be addicted in the sense that drug-seeking behavior is paramount in an individual's life without being physically dependent.

D **Substances subject to dependence and abuse** The *DSM-IV* categorizes substance-related disorders according to which of 13 types of substances is used. All of these substances are believed to be associated with dependence and abuse, except caffeine (which in the *DSM-IV* is said to produce neither syndrome but recently has been shown to produce physical dependence) and nicotine (which causes dependence only). Any of these substances may produce the other syndromes listed in I B. The specific substance categories include:

1. Alcohol
2. Amphetamines
3. Caffeine
4. Cannabis
5. Cocaine
6. Hallucinogens
7. Inhalants
8. Nicotine
9. Opioids
10. Phencyclidine
11. Sedatives, hypnotics, and anxiolytics
12. Polysubstance
13. Other (e.g., digitalis, amyl nitrite)

II INTOXICATION SYNDROMES

Because the manifestations and treatment of intoxication with different drugs can vary drastically and may require different treatments, it is crucial to be able to differentiate between common intoxication syndromes.

A **Alcohol** often is combined with other substances. The odor on the patient's breath that is characteristically associated with alcohol intoxication is caused by impurities in the preparation and is unreliable in diagnosing intoxication. In addition, head injuries and metabolic encephalopathies (e.g., ketoacidosis) often are mistaken for alcohol intoxication. Blood and urine screens may help to make the diagnosis. The central nervous system (CNS) concentration of alcohol parallels the concentration in the blood.

1. **Alcohol intoxication** is diagnosed in the *DSM-IV* when the following signs appear in association with drinking:
   a. Slurred speech
   b. Loss of coordination
   c. Unsteady gait
   d. Nystagmus
   e. Impaired attention or memory
   f. Stupor or coma
2. **Mild intoxication** is characterized by disorganization of cognitive and motor processes. The first functions to be disrupted are those that depend on training and previous experience. As intoxication becomes more noticeable, the following changes occur:
   a. **Overconfidence.** If performance is initially impaired by psychological inhibitions, an individual may transiently function better after ingestion of small amounts of alcohol. However, although the intoxicated individual tends to feel more efficient, all aspects of physical and mental performance are impaired by alcohol.
   b. **Mood swings, emotional outbursts,** and **euphoria** may occur.
   c. **Initial enhancement of spinal reflexes** may develop as they are released from higher inhibiting circuits, followed by progressive general anesthesia of CNS functions.
   d. **An increased pain threshold** may be evident, but other sensory modalities are unaffected.
   e. **Nausea, vomiting, restlessness,** and **hyperactivity** may be present.

3. **Severe intoxication** is characterized by:
   a. Stupor or coma
   b. Hypothermia
   c. Slow, noisy respiration
   d. Tachycardia
   e. Dilated pupils (may be normal in some intoxicated individuals)
   f. Increased intracranial pressure
   g. Death (rare in the absence of ingestion of additional substances, trauma, infection, or unconsciousness lasting longer than 12 hours)

4. **Treatment** depends on whether or not the patient is conscious.
   a. **Conscious patients** need little treatment beyond waiting for the alcohol to be metabolized.
      (1) Stimulants and caffeine do not hasten sobriety.
      (2) Restraint for severe agitation is safer than administration of tranquilizers or sedatives, which may potentiate the CNS depressant effects of alcohol.
      (3) In low doses, antipsychotic drugs (e.g., ziprasidone or haloperidol given intravenously or risperidone or olanzapine given orally) may decrease hyperactivity without increasing sedation.
   b. **Stuporous or unconscious patients** should be kept warm with legs elevated. It also may be necessary to:
      (1) Prevent aspiration, especially if gastric lavage is performed.
      (2) Treat increased intracranial pressure with mannitol or by other measures (e.g., corticosteroids) in addition to the normal management of overdoses of CNS depressants.
      (3) Remove alcohol by hemodialysis in extreme situations.

B Sedatives, hypnotics, and anxiolytics

1. **Specific substances**
   a. Benzodiazepine tranquilizers (e.g., diazepam, oxazepam, chlordiazepoxide, lorazepam, prazepam, clorazepate, alprazolam, clonazepam)
   b. Benzodiazepine hypnotics or sleeping pills (e.g., flurazepam, temazepam, triazolam, estazolam)
   c. Barbiturates (e.g., phenobarbital, amobarbital, pentobarbital, secobarbital)
   d. Drugs related to barbiturates: ethchlorvynol, glutethimide, propanediols (e.g., meprobamate), methyprylon, paraldehyde, and others
   e. Chloral compounds (e.g., chloral hydrate)

2. **Mild to moderate intoxication** with benzodiazepines, barbiturates, and related compounds causes:
   a. Euphoria
   b. Hypalgesia (increased pain threshold)
   c. Increased seizure threshold
   d. Sedation
   e. Paradoxical excitement in:
      (1) Susceptible individuals
      (2) Elderly persons
      (3) Children
      (4) People with preexisting neurologic impairment
   f. Nystagmus, dysarthria, ataxia, impaired attention and memory
   g. Psychomotor impairment
   h. Postural hypotension

3. **Severe intoxication** usually is caused by purposeful overdoses in suicide attempts and accidental overdoses by addicts. A few patients, especially those with preexisting brain disease, may take too much medication because of drug automatism (the patient forgets that the drug has already been taken and continues to take more pills, usually in an effort to get to sleep). Severe intoxication can cause:
   a. Stupor and coma
   b. Respiratory depression
   c. Depressed reflexes

    d. Hypotension

    e. Decreased cardiac output

    f. Hypoxemia

    g. Bullous skin lesions and necrosis of sweat glands

    h. Hypothermia

    i. Coma

    j. Death

       (1) Death from barbiturate intoxication usually is caused by pneumonia or renal failure.

       (2) Short-acting preparations (e.g., amobarbital) are more lethal at lower doses than are long-acting compounds (e.g., phenobarbital).

       (3) Death from an overdose of benzodiazepines alone is rare. However, combinations of benzodiazepines and other CNS depressants, especially combinations with alcohol, can be fatal.

4. Treatment of CNS depressant intoxication involves emesis if the ingestion has occurred within 30 minutes of initiation of treatment and the gag reflex is intact. Gastric lavage should be performed for less recent ingestions of substances that have not been fully absorbed. A cathartic agent should be given to decrease intestinal absorption of the drug. For severe poisoning, the following steps are taken:

    a. Protection of the airway

    b. Oxygen administration

    c. Ventilation when necessary

    d. Prevention of further loss of body heat

    e. Correction of hypovolemia and maintenance of blood pressure with dopamine

    f. Forced diuresis with maximal alkalinization of the urine

    g. Hemodialysis

C CNS stimulants

1. Specific substances

    a. Amphetamines and related compounds include the prescription drugs dextroamphetamine, methylphenidate, and pemoline sodium and the illicit drugs methamphetamine (speed), cocaine, and smokable cocaine (crack). Medical indications for amphetamines include:

       (1) Attention deficit disorder

       (2) Depression in elderly patients

       (3) Depression in medically ill patients who cannot tolerate antidepressants

       (4) Augmentation of antidepressants in patients with treatment-resistant depression

       (5) Narcolepsy

    b. Cocaine is used to treat nosebleeds and is sometimes used as a local anesthetic in the ears, nose, and throat.

    c. Phenmetrazine

    d. Phenylpropanolamine

    e. Antiobesity drugs. Long-term treatment of obesity with stimulants is almost always unsuccessful because of tolerance.

2. Mild to moderate intoxication produces:

    a. Elevated mood

    b. Increased energy and alertness

    c. Increased ability to perform repetitive tasks when the individual is tired or bored

    d. Decreased appetite

    e. Talkativeness

    f. Anxiety and irritability

    g. Insomnia

    h. Hypertension or hypotension

    i. Increased or decreased heart rate

    j. Hyperthermia

   k. Nausea or vomiting
   l. Loss of appetite and weight
3. Severe intoxication may produce agitation, anger, and psychosis. Although tolerance develops to many of the effects of stimulants, there is no tolerance to the tendency to develop psychotic symptoms, which may be indistinguishable from those of functional paranoid psychoses. **Signs and symptoms** include:
   a. Visual, auditory, and tactile hallucinations
   b. Delusions, especially of being infested with parasites
   c. Paranoia and loose associations in a clear sensorium
   d. Mania
   e. Fighting
   f. Hypervigilance
   g. Dilated pupils
   h. Elevated blood pressure and pulse (may be normal in some chronic abusers)
   i. Arrhythmias
   j. Seizures
   k. Exhaustion
   l. Coma
   m. Intracranial hemorrhage
   n. Multiple cerebral infarcts
4. Treatment
   a. Hypertension and hyperthermia can be treated with **phentolamine.**
   b. Psychotic symptoms can be treated with **haloperidol,** which antagonizes the dopaminergic properties of stimulants.

D **Hallucinogens and phencyclidine**
1. Specific substances
   a. Lysergic acid diethylamide (LSD)
   b. Psilocybin
   c. Mescaline
   d. 2,5-Dimethoxy-4-methylamphetamine (STP)
   e. Phencyclidine (PCP)
2. Intoxication depends on the substance.
   a. Most hallucinogen intoxications produce:
      (1) Dilated pupils
      (2) Increased heart rate and blood pressure
      (3) Fever
      (4) Paranoia in a clear sensorium
      (5) Illusions
      (6) Hallucinations
      (7) Depersonalization
      (8) Anxiety
      (9) Distortion of time sense
      (10) Inappropriate affect
   b. PCP intoxication also can cause:
      (1) Violent behavior
      (2) Hyperactivity
      (3) Hyperacusis
      (4) Mutism
      (5) Echolalia
      (6) Analgesia
      (7) Nystagmus
      (8) Ataxia
      (9) Muscular rigidity
      (10) Focal neurological signs
      (11) Seizures

    (12) Coma

    (13) Intracranial hemorrhage

  3. Treatment of intoxication and "bad trips" depends on the substance.

    a. The psychological effects of most hallucinogens are usually decreased by reassurance in a quiet setting. Oral administration of diazepam is sometimes a useful adjunct.

    b. Patients intoxicated with PCP may react violently to any environmental stimulation, including attempts at reassurance. They should generally be left alone in a quiet area. If they become violent, they may be sedated with intravenously administered haloperidol or diazepam. Seizures should be treated with intravenous administration of diazepam.

E **Cannabis**   Specific substances include marijuana, hashish, and Δ-tetrahydrocannabinol (TCH).

  1. Intoxication by marijuana and related substances rarely produces hallucinations. More common effects include:

    a. Euphoria

    b. Anxiety

    c. Increased appetite

    d. Increased suggestibility

    e. Distortion of time and space

    f. Red conjunctivae

    g. No change in pupils

    h. Dry mouth

    i. Tachycardia

  2. Treatment. The psychological effects of the cannabis group of drugs, similar to those of most hallucinogens, are generally eased by reassurance in a quiet setting. Oral administration of diazepam is sometimes useful.

F **Opioids**   Many street preparations are adulterated with quinine, procaine, lidocaine, lactose, or mannitol and are contaminated with bacteria, viruses, or fungi.

  1. Specific substances

    a. Morphine

    b. Heroin

    c. Hydromorphone

    d. Oxymorphone

    e. Levorphanol

    f. Codeine

    g. Hydrocodone

    h. Oxycodone

    i. Methadone

    j. Meperidine

    k. Alphaprodine

    l. Propoxyphene

    m. Pentazocine, which has both narcotic antagonist and agonist properties

  2. Mild to moderate intoxication may produce:

    a. Analgesia without loss of consciousness

    b. Drowsiness and mental clouding

    c. Nausea and vomiting

    d. Apathy and lethargy

    e. Euphoria

    f. Itching

    g. Constricted pupils

    h. Constipation

    i. Flushed, warm skin caused by cutaneous vasodilation

    j. Dysarthria

    k. Impaired attention and memory

    l. Illusions

3. Severe intoxication is associated with:
   a. Miosis
   b. Respiratory depression, which may recur up to 24 hours after apparent recovery from an overdose with most narcotics and up to 72 hours after apparent recovery from a methadone overdose
   c. Hypotension or shock
   d. Depressed reflexes
   e. Coma
   f. Pulmonary edema
   g. Seizures (with propoxyphene or meperidine)

4. Treatment
   a. Severe intoxication is treated primarily by **supportive care.**
   b. Naloxone, a narcotic antagonist, can:
      (1) Reverse coma and apnea (The effects of concomitantly self-administered drugs [e.g., barbiturates] are not altered, and detoxification from these drugs also should be undertaken.)
      (2) Precipitate a severe abstinence syndrome in narcotic-dependent patients
      (3) Cause vomiting

G **Inhalants**   Sniffing ("huffing") inhalants is becoming an increasingly severe problem among children and adolescents. Because brain damage may occur with repeated use, and no antidote or specific treatment of intoxication exists, it is important to identify the problem and institute remedial therapy.

1. Specific substances
   a. Gasoline
   b. Glue
   c. Paint thinner
   d. Solvents
   e. Spray paints

2. Intoxication may cause:
   a. Dizziness
   b. Euphoria
   c. Altered states of consciousness
   d. Confusion
   e. Nystagmus
   f. Ataxia
   g. Dysarthria
   h. Lethargy
   i. Depressed reflexes
   j. Psychomotor retardation
   k. Tremor
   l. Muscular weakness
   m. Blurred vision
   n. Delirium

3. Chronic use may result in dementia.

4. There is no specific treatment for inhalant dependence and abuse other than prevention of further access to the substance.

H **Anticholinergic drugs**   A number of psychiatric medications have anticholinergic side effects. Some anticholinergic substances grow wild, and some are included in various herbal medications.

1. Specific substances
   a. Most over-the-counter cold and sleeping preparations
   b. Atropine
   c. Belladonna
   d. Henbane
   e. Scopolamine

    f. Antiparkinsonian drugs (e.g., trihexyphenidyl, benztropine)
    g. Tricyclic and tetracyclic antidepressants and paroxetine
    h. Low-potency neuroleptics (e.g., thioridazine)
    i. Jimson weed
    j. Mandrake
    k. Propantheline

2. **Intoxication** with anticholinergic substances is coded as "other intoxication" in the *DSM-IV* and may produce:
    a. Confusion
    b. Memory loss
    c. Delirium
    d. Hallucinations
    e. Amnesia
    f. Body image distortions
    g. Drowsiness
    h. Psychosis
    i. Tachycardia
    j. Decreased peristalsis
    k. Fever
    l. Warm, dry skin
    m. Fixed, dilated pupils
    n. Coma

3. **Treatment** is primarily directed toward protecting the patient and waiting for the drug to be metabolized. Intravenous administration of physostigmine can temporarily reverse coma or severe hyperpyrexia but should be used cautiously. Relief is transient because of the short half-life of the drug; gastrointestinal and cardiac side effects may be significant. Persistent signs of intoxication can be treated with longer-acting cholinesterase inhibitors such as donepezil (Aricept).

I **Club drugs** are the newest category of drugs that hit the scene in nightclubs and "raves" or all-night dance parties during the 1990s. These so called "designer drugs" are most popular in young adults.

1. **Specific substance**
    a. GHB (GABA-hydroxybutyrate)
    b. MDMA (3,4–methylenedioxymethamphetamine) or Ecstasy or "X"
    c. Ketamine or "Special K"

2. **Intoxication**
    a. Euphoria and disorientation
    b. Relaxation and emotional warmth
    c. Increased sexuality
    d. Amnesia
    e. Disinhibition
    f. Hypertension and hyperthermia
    g. Dehydration and tachycardia
    h. Jaw clenching and bruxism
    i. Liver or renal failure in extreme cases

3. **Treatment** is similar to that of other stimulants. Supportive care such as adequate rehydration is crucial. Occasionally, the use of alprazolam for extreme agitation is needed.

III   SUBSTANCE WITHDRAWAL

Substance withdrawal produces substance-specific, physiologically determined syndromes that appear after abrupt withdrawal or decrease in dosage of the drug. Withdrawal from some compounds produces mild syndromes. Withdrawal from others produces phenomena that are uncomfortable but not dangerous. Life-threatening abstinence syndromes result from abrupt discontinuation of a few substances. Blood levels are often zero in abstinence syndromes.

A Alcohol abstinence syndromes

1. **Alcohol withdrawal ("the shakes")** usually appears within a few hours of stopping or decreasing alcohol consumption. Generally, this lasts for 3 to 4 days; occasionally, it may last as long as 1 week.
   a. **Signs and symptoms** include:
      (1) Tachycardia
      (2) Tremulousness
      (3) Diaphoresis
      (4) Nausea
      (5) Orthostatic hypotension
      (6) Malaise or weakness
      (7) Anxiety
      (8) Irritability
   b. **Treatment**
      (1) The standard practice has been to administer a mid- to long-acting benzodiazepine, such as diazepam or chlordiazepoxide, in a tapering dose over 4 to 5 days.
      (2) Thiamine can be given parenterally at 100 mg/day for 3 days if one is extremely concerned about the patient's nutritional status, but this is usually not necessary.

2. **Major motor seizures ("rum fits")**
   a. **Symptoms.** Major motor seizures occur during the first 48 hours of alcohol withdrawal in a small percentage of patients.
   b. **Treatment** is via intravenous administration of diazepam. Phenytoin is not administered unless the patient has epilepsy.

3. **Alcohol withdrawal delirium (delirium tremens)** begins on the second or third day (rarely later than 1 week) after withdrawal or decrease of alcohol intake. It occurs in fewer than 5% of alcohol-dependent patients, usually after they have been drinking heavily for at least 5 to 15 years. If seizures also occur, they always precede the development of delirium. If a patient decompensates to the point of delirium tremens, the mortality rate is approximately 10%.
   a. **Symptoms** of delirium tremens include:
      (1) Delirium
      (2) Autonomic hyperactivity (e.g., increased pulse rate, increased blood pressure, and sweating)
      (3) Agitation
      (4) Vivid hallucinations
      (5) Gross tremulousness
   b. **Treatment**
      (1) Hydration
      (2) Vital signs every hour
      (3) A benzodiazepine (e.g., diazepam) administered in divided doses. The maximum dosage depends on the amount that it takes to keep the patient calm, comfortable, and seizure free.
      (4) An antipsychotic drug such as haloperidol or risperidone in severe cases of agitation or psychosis
      (5) Consider if parenteral administration of thiamine is necessary
      (6) Consider the addition of valproic acid as a seizure prophylaxis, augmentation to the benzodiazepine, and to assist in keeping the patient calm and comfortable if the patient is not responding well to the benzodiazepine alone.

4. **Alcohol hallucinosis** (alcohol-induced psychotic disorder with hallucinations in the *DSM-IV*) is a rare condition that develops within 48 hours of cessation of drinking or at the end of a long binge with gradual decreases in blood alcohol levels.
   a. **The principal symptom** is vivid auditory hallucinations without gross confusion. Usually, the patient hears threatening or derogatory voices that discuss the patient in the third person or speak directly to the patient. Command hallucinations are absent. Symptoms usually last a few hours or days, but in approximately 10% of patients, they may persist for weeks or months. Occasionally, the syndrome may become chronic, in which case it may be indistinguishable from schizophrenia.
   b. **Treatment.** Antipsychotic drugs may relieve hallucinations in patients who do not improve spontaneously. Although they are not well studied for alcohol hallucinations, the atypical

antipsychotic drugs (e.g., risperidone, ziprasidone) are good initial choices because they are better tolerated than neuroleptics such as haloperidol.

B **Withdrawal from sedatives, hypnotics, and anxiolytics** produce syndromes that vary in time of onset, duration, and severity. Withdrawal syndromes are likely to occur after chronic use of 400 to 600 mg/day of pentobarbital, 3200 to 6400 mg/day of meprobamate, and 40 to 60 mg/day of diazepam or their equivalents. Milder withdrawal syndromes may develop in individuals taking lower doses for longer periods of time. It is difficult to predict whether an individual will develop a withdrawal syndrome and how severe it may be.

1. **Symptoms** usually begin within 12 to 24 hours, peak at 4 to 7 days, and last about 1 week after withdrawal from short-acting compounds such as pentobarbital and alprazolam. Withdrawal from long-acting compounds such as diazepam or phenobarbital begins later (4 to 10 days after drug discontinuation) and reaches its peak more slowly (around the seventh day). Signs and symptoms include:
   a. Anxiety and agitation
   b. Orthostatic hypotension
   c. Weakness and tremulousness
   d. Hyperreflexia and clonic blink reflex
   e. Fever
   f. Diaphoresis
   g. Delirium
   h. Seizures
   i. Cardiovascular collapse

2. **Treatment.** Withdrawal from CNS depressants can be life threatening, so treatment is mandatory when the syndrome is diagnosed. Although some patients with uncomplicated withdrawal may be managed as outpatients, hospitalization is required for the management of more severe and complicated withdrawal to ensure compliance with the treatment protocol and adequate coverage if the condition worsens. Treatment is not as effective if it is initiated after the appearance of delirium.
   a. Because all CNS depressants produce cross-tolerance, a known compound (pentobarbital or phenobarbital) is substituted for the offending substance to suppress the abstinence syndrome and is then gradually withdrawn. The amount of phenobarbital or pentobarbital that the patient is likely to tolerate—and that therefore will suppress withdrawal—can be calculated by observing the results of administering 200 mg of pentobarbital or 60 to 100 mg of phenobarbital when the patient no longer appears to be intoxicated (usually within 12 to 16 hours after discontinuation of the offending substance).
      (1) If the patient becomes severely intoxicated or falls asleep with the test dose, tolerance does not exist, and the patient does not need further treatment.
      (2) If the patient develops moderate symptoms after the test dose (e.g., dysarthria, nystagmus, ataxia without sleepiness), moderate tolerance exists, suggesting that the patient requires 200 to 300 mg/day of pentobarbital or 60 to 90 mg/day of phenobarbital.
      (3) Absence of symptoms or nystagmus without other signs of intoxication in response to the test dose indicates significant tolerance. The patient should then be administered a total daily (divided) dose of 600 to 1000 mg of pentobarbital or 180 to 300 mg of phenobarbital every 6 hours to suppress withdrawal.
      (4) Tolerance also may be assessed by giving successive 60- to 100-mg doses of phenobarbital every 1 to 4 hours until the patient is intoxicated. The amount necessary to produce definite signs of intoxication (to a maximum of 500 mg/day) is then administered in divided doses every 6 hours to suppress the abstinence syndrome.
   b. As soon as the patient is stabilized, the dose of pentobarbital is decreased by 10% every 1 to 2 days. Phenobarbital, which is longer acting, may be withdrawn more rapidly. Reappearance of abstinence phenomena indicates that the dose needs to be reduced more gradually. Unexpected intoxication during the phenobarbital protocol indicates accumulation of the barbiturate and a need for faster dosage reduction.
   c. Because cross-tolerance exists between barbiturates and alcohol, phenobarbital or pentobarbital can also be used to suppress alcohol abstinence syndromes, as well as withdrawal from more than one CNS depressant.

    d. Benzodiazepines can also be used to suppress withdrawal from any cross-reacting CNS depressant. With the exception of alcohol withdrawal, standardized protocols using benzodiazepines have not been established, however.

C **Stimulant withdrawal**   There is no observable physiologic disruption with stimulant withdrawal; psychological and behavioral manifestations may be severe, however.

1. **Symptoms**
   a. Increased sleep
   b. Nightmares caused by rapid eye movement (REM) rebound
   c. Fatigue
   d. Lassitude
   e. Increased appetite
   f. Depression ("cocaine blues")
   g. Suicide attempts
   h. Craving for the drug

2. **Treatment**
   a. Antidepressants (e.g., bupropion, venlafaxine, desipramine) are helpful for withdrawal depression.
   b. Hospitalization may be necessary if the patient is suicidal.

D **Cessation of hallucinogens** does not produce a significant abstinence syndrome.

1. **Symptoms.** Flashbacks (brief reexperiences of the hallucinogenic state) may be precipitated by marijuana, antihistamines, and SSRIs.

2. **Treatment.** Reassurance that symptoms will subside and administration of a benzodiazepine are usually sufficient therapy.

E **Opioid withdrawal** is not life threatening; however, it may be extremely uncomfortable.

1. **Symptoms** usually appear 8 to 10 hours after cessation of morphine. The onset is slower when long-acting drugs, such as methadone, have been withdrawn. Symptoms peak at 48 to 72 hours and disappear in 7 to 10 days. Disturbances include:
   a. Lacrimation and rhinorrhea
   b. Sweating
   c. Restlessness and sleepiness
   d. Gooseflesh
   e. Dilated pupils
   f. Irritability
   g. Violent yawning
   h. Insomnia
   i. Coryza
   j. Craving for the drug

2. **Treatment**
   a. **Buprenorphine** was introduced in the late 1990s. Administered intramuscularly up to four times a day with a daily taper, it is highly effective for acute opiate withdrawal. Buprenorphine is a partial agonist/antagonist to the mu receptor. If given too soon after the patient's last use of opiates, acute and painful withdrawal will occur because of buprenorphine's antagonistic properties. The patient must show clear evidence of opiate withdrawal before receiving the first dose. **Subutex** is a sublingual form of buprenorphine that is absorbed in the mucosal lining of the oral membranes. It is given in divided doses of 2 to 6 mg up to four times a day and tapered until detox is complete.
   b. The effects of narcotic withdrawal are lessened by **methadone** substitution. When the patient demonstrates objective signs of withdrawal, a sufficient dose of methadone to suppress abstinence, or a maximum dose of 20 to 50 mg/day (never more than 100 mg), is administered. The dose of methadone is then decreased by 10% to 20% at each reduction, every few days. Although any licensed physician may prescribe methadone for pain, the use of methadone to detoxify a narcotic addict (as well as methadone maintenance to prevent relapse of addiction)

violates federal law in any setting other than a federally approved site for the treatment of narcotic addiction.

    c. **Clonidine** administered at 0.1 to 0.3 mg three times per day for 2 weeks may help to suppress withdrawal symptoms, although it can cause hypotension. Clonidine should be tapered rather than abruptly discontinued because rapid withdrawal causes rebound hypertension.

F **Anticholinergic drug withdrawal** occasionally produces influenza-like syndromes, depression, mania, or seizures. Discontinuation of clinically significant doses taken for more than 1 month should, therefore, be gradual. Treatment is with **atropine** or reintroduction of the offending agent with more gradual discontinuation.

G **Nicotine withdrawal** has been found to be a significant impediment to smoking cessation. Symptoms include malaise, irritability, anxiety, and craving for tobacco. Treatment with nicotine patches containing gradually decreasing doses of nicotine is effective only when it is combined with a behavioral program. Clonidine administered as described in III E 2 c or by means of a patch may be a useful adjunct.

H **Caffeine withdrawal** produces insomnia, depression, and headaches. Gradual reduction of intake may prevent withdrawal symptoms.

IV   PRINCIPLES OF TREATMENT OF SUBSTANCE-RELATED DISORDERS

Certain approaches are useful for treatment of abuse and dependence with all substances.

A **Detoxification**   It is impossible to address the causes of substance abuse and dependence while the patient continues to use the substance. The first goal of treatment, therefore, is to withdraw the substance.

B **Insistence on abstinence**   A few individuals may be able to use addicting substances in moderation after successful treatment of dependence or abuse, but it is impossible to identify them. Complete abstinence is safest.

C **Avoidance of other substances associated with dependence or abuse**   Frequently, people who have been dependent on alcohol or another substance ask to be treated with benzodiazepines or related compounds for anxiety or insomnia. Acceding to this request is dangerous for several reasons:

1. It introduces another substance that can be associated with dependence.

2. Taking a pill for rapid relief of dysphoria reinforces the association between taking the drug and feeling better, thereby increasing the tendency to go back to the drug of choice for the same result.

3. There is no evidence that tranquilizers decrease the use of alcohol as a self-treatment for anxiety, and some reports suggest that using benzodiazepines increases the risk of relapse of alcoholism.

4. Controversy surrounds the use of stimulants such as methylphenidate and dextroamphetamine to treat attention deficit hyperactivity disorder (ADHD) in individuals who are presumed to have used cocaine and other illicit stimulants as self-treatments for ADHD. It is usually safer to use treatments for ADHD with a lower risk of dependence and abuse (e.g., bupropion, venlafaxine, desipramine).

D **Involvement of the family**   Family members may encourage use of the substance in the patient, especially if there is family strife that everyone is able to ignore because all attention is focused on the identified patient. For example, a family may ignore or overlook sexual abuse of one child by focusing attention on another child's problem with drugs or alcohol. A spouse may also be drug dependent. The family can be important allies in insisting that the patient deal with the problem. Similarly, it is very difficult to prevent use of a substance by a patient whose spouse continues to use that substance or is not willing to reduce its availability in the home. Encouragement of families to enlist the help of **Al-Anon** is often helpful when treating a patient with addiction issues.

E **Unscheduled toxicology screens**   Despite technical problems that may reduce reliability, periodic urine screens often are essential in identifying relapse and noncompliance.

F **Self-help groups**   Peer support groups provide credibility and encouragement from individuals who have had similar problems and who are adept at dealing with common resistances to treatment. Twelve-step programs have been developed for most substances.

G **Sanctioned treatment**   When a patient is forced to remain in therapy by a legal sanction (e.g., threatened loss of driver's license or professional license for relapse), the outcome is better than when the patient is free to withdraw from therapy at any time.

H **Contingency contracting**   Contingency contracting provides a powerful negative contingency for leaving treatment or relapsing and a positive contingency for remaining drug free. In the most widely used form of contingency contracting, the patient agrees in advance that the therapist will notify an employer or licensing body if relapse occurs. The patient may leave a letter with the therapist outlining the problem, which is to be mailed if a urine screen result is positive or the patient does not keep an appointment. Some patients deposit a sum of money with the therapist; a certain amount is then paid back to the patient for each week of abstinence. When the contingency for relapse is a report to the appropriate medical licensing authority, the relapse rate of substance-dependent physicians is less than 25%.

I **Change of peer group**   For many patients, especially adolescents, substance use is encouraged by peers. Such individuals must be helped to find a different peer group in which substance use is not a prerequisite to social support.

V   ALCOHOLISM

Alcoholism affects approximately 12% of the population at some point during their lifetimes. Alcohol abuse or dependence usually develops during the first 5 years of regular use of alcohol.

A **Three patterns of chronic alcohol abuse** have been described:

1. Regular daily excessive drinking

2. Regular heavy drinking on weekends only

3. Long periods of sobriety interspersed with binges that last days, weeks, or months

B **Familial influences** seem to play a role in the development of alcoholism. Individuals are at an increased risk of being alcoholic if they have:

1. A family history of alcoholism, especially if the individual is the son of an alcoholic father

2. A family history of teetotalism (i.e., avoidance of alcohol under any circumstance)

3. An alcoholic spouse

C **Diagnostic clues** to alcoholism include:

1. Inability to decrease or discontinue drinking

2. Binges lasting at least 2 days

3. Occasional consumption of a fifth of spirits or the equivalent in wine or beer in a single day

4. Blackouts (transient amnesia for events that occur while the patient is intoxicated)

5. Continued drinking despite a physical illness that is exacerbated or caused by drinking

6. Drinking nonbeverage alcohol (e.g., shaving lotion)

7. Drinking in the morning

8. Withdrawal syndromes

9. Apparent sobriety in the presence of an elevated alcohol level in the blood, indicating tolerance to the sedative effects of alcohol

10. Arrest for driving under the influence (DUI)

11. Frequent trips to the emergency room for falls or other "accidents"
12. Absenteeism from work

[D] **Physical, psychiatric, and social complications**

1. **Physical complications,** which may be caused by associated nutritional deficiencies or by a direct toxic effect of alcohol, are not uncommon in patients who drink more than 3 to 6 oz of whiskey a day or the equivalent. More familiar syndromes include:
   a. Cerebral atrophy
   b. Wernicke encephalopathy
   c. Korsakoff psychosis
   d. Nicotinic acid deficiency encephalopathy
   e. Polyneuropathy
   f. Cardiomyopathy
   g. Hypertension
   h. Skeletal muscle damage of uncertain clinical significance
   i. Gastritis
   j. Peptic ulcer
   k. Constipation
   l. Pancreatitis
   m. Cirrhosis
   n. Impotence
   o. Various anemias
   p. Teratogenicity
      (1) **Fetal alcohol syndrome,** characterized by mental retardation, microcephaly, slowed growth, and facial abnormalities, may be a risk even if moderate amounts of alcohol are consumed during pregnancy.
      (2) Because safe quantities have not been established, complete abstinence from alcohol during pregnancy is recommended. If a patient does drink, she should be advised to do so on a full stomach to minimize rapid increases in blood alcohol levels. Folate supplementation may have the potential to ameliorate the risk of fetal malformations, but it has not been shown to make it possible to drink safely during pregnancy.
   q. **Accidents**
      (1) Almost half of all traffic fatalities involve alcohol.
      (2) Drunk drivers who are killed in motor vehicle accidents are four to 12 times more likely than drivers who are not killed to have had a previous arrest for driving under the influence, indicating that drinking and driving is a recurrent problem. Many people continue to drink and drive after their licenses are revoked.

2. **Psychiatric complications.** The major psychiatric complication of alcoholism is **suicide.** More than 80% of individuals who kill themselves are depressed, alcoholic, or both. Alcohol is a frequent component of many suicides, even in patients who are not alcoholic.
   a. Seventy-five percent of alcoholics have no other primary psychiatric diagnoses, although depression is a common complication of the direct effects of alcohol on the brain and the consequences of drinking on the patient's life.
   b. Alcoholism may be an attempt at self-treatment of another psychiatric disorder, such as depression, anxiety, mania, psychosis, or posttraumatic stress disorder. This possibility should be considered when psychiatric symptoms clearly preceded heavy drinking. However, the history often is unreliable, and only a trial period of abstinence reliably distinguishes between primary alcoholism and alcohol abuse that is secondary to another condition. If psychological distress resolves after a period of abstinence, alcoholism is likely to have been a cause rather than a result of the psychiatric disorder.
   c. Alcoholism is a common comorbid condition with mood disorders, anxiety disorders, and personality disorders. In such situations, both conditions must be treated.

3. **Social complications** occur with the use of all psychoactive substances. The on-the-job accident rate is increased three to four times in workers who use psychoactive substances. Alcohol and other drugs cause sexual, marital, and legal problems.

E **Specific treatment approaches** result in approximately one-third of patients remaining sober, one-third enjoying a period of sobriety followed by relapse, and one-third continuing to drink. Useful interventions include the following:

1. **Confrontation of denial.** The major obstacles to therapeutic success are the patient's denial of the severity of the problem and his or her wish to continue drinking. Repeated statements that the patient is not in control of the drinking and repeated confrontation with the complications of the alcoholism may be necessary before the patient agrees to treatment.

2. **Insistence on abstinence.** Because it is not possible to identify in advance the very few patients who may be able to succeed with controlled drinking, total abstinence is the only realistic goal.

3. **Assessment of motivation.** The patient who is willing to consider abstaining completely for 1 month has at least some motivation to give up alcohol completely. If the patient insists on some continued alcohol intake (usually while assuring the doctor that it will be easy to keep from drinking excessively), treatment is less likely to be successful. Further therapeutic efforts may be unsuccessful until the patient is willing to give up alcohol completely for at least a brief period of time.

4. **Disulfiram (Antabuse).** Many alcoholics' efforts at abstinence are supported by disulfiram, which causes severe nausea and vomiting when it interacts with alcohol. Even if the patient does not need the drug, willingness to take it is a favorable prognostic sign. The only contraindications to the use of disulfiram are organic brain syndromes, severely impaired liver function, or other conditions that might interfere significantly with compliance. The usual dose is 250 to 500 mg/day. Vitamin C and antihistamines may abort the alcohol–disulfiram reaction. Disulfiram may, in rare instances, increase liver enzymes; therefore, yearly monitoring of liver functioning is recommended. Patients must be warned about not using metronidazole, alcohol containing mouthwash, and certain cough syrups because these substances will produce the disulfiram reaction.

5. **Naltrexone** is approved for reduction of craving for alcohol, although its effectiveness has been limited.

6. **Acamprosate (Campral)** is approved and designed to reduce the craving for alcohol while still allowing the patient to consume alcohol and not get sick. It works on GABA and glutamate neurotransmission. The patient must abstain from alcohol for 5 days before taking the medication for it to be effective.

7. **Involvement of the family.** The patient's family can be an important source of support, or the family may openly or covertly encourage the patient to go on drinking.
   a. A family "intervention," in which all family members confront the patient's drinking, helps the patient to deal with denial.
   b. Refusal by the spouse to remain with the patient unless he or she stops drinking may be the only force strong enough to convince the patient to agree to a trial of abstinence. Such threats should be mobilized only when they are a true expression of the spouse's feelings, or they will not be credible.
   c. Contingency contracting that involves remaining in the hospital may be very effective.
   d. Employers and other important individuals in the patient's life should also be involved in treatment whenever possible.

8. **Alcoholics Anonymous (AA).** AA is a highly useful treatment group and has actually been found to be the most effective treatment model in maintaining sobriety in multiple studies. Other peer counseling programs also provide peer support and encouragement for patients to stop drinking.

9. **Behavior therapy.** Punishing drinking (e.g., with disulfiram) and rewarding sobriety (e.g., by paying the patient for abstinence through contingency contracting) are useful for patients who consider their drinking a bad habit. Expressive psychotherapy is appropriate for patients who believe that their drinking is motivated by unresolved emotional conflicts.

10. **Ongoing emotional support by the primary physician.** Primary care physicians provide an important source of encouragement for patients to confront the problem and to maintain sobriety. The physician should accept periodic relapses in a nonjudgmental manner. If the patient refuses specific therapy for alcoholism, the physician should continue to be available to the drinking patient in case a psychosocial crisis precipitates the patient's wishing to become involved in treatment.

VI OPIOIDS

Opioid dependence and abuse is a major public health problem. The incidence of heroin use increased during the 1960s, and use of this drug is now a problem in smaller communities in the United States as well as in large cities. After a period of decreased use, narcotic use is undergoing a resurgence in middle-class groups.

A The epidemiology of narcotic use, particularly heroin, deserves consideration. Between 2% and 3% of adults age 18 to 25 years have tried heroin at some time in their lives. Abuse of narcotics usually occurs in the context of abuse of other drugs. Using "soft" drugs such as marijuana seems to break down a psychological barrier to using "hard" drugs. Approximately 50% of individuals who abuse narcotics become physically dependent. Most addicts tend to become abstinent over time. Often they finally discontinue drug dependence approximately 9 years after its onset.

1. **Patterns of narcotic abuse vary widely.** Some addicts, particularly those who are maintained on methadone, lead productive lives and enjoy good health. For others, the need to obtain illicit drugs and money to buy them leads to prostitution and other crimes. However, to a significant extent, personality and behavior before drug use predict behavior while using opioids. Many narcotic abusers lead an antisocial lifestyle that persists until the drug is withdrawn. These individuals differ from those with antisocial personality disorder who are also narcotic abusers in that the antisocial behavior in persons with the personality disorder antedated substance abuse. Because of physical complications of abuse and a lifestyle associated with violence, the death rate is two to 20 times higher (10 in 1000) in opioid addicts than it is in the general population. Patterns of narcotic use and dependence are as follows:

   a. **Acquired during medical treatment.** A small but definite percentage of narcotic users become dependent in the course of medical treatment. This can often provide a gateway into obtaining greater quantities off the streets when their physicians finally cut off their supply or may lead them into harder drugs, such as heroin.

   b. **Recreational use.** More commonly, narcotic abuse develops when an adolescent or young adult who is engaged in experimental or recreational drug use progresses to use of more dangerous substances. Although between 60% and 90% of adolescents experiment to some extent with drugs (experimentation with drugs has been reported in children as young as age 5 years), the number who go on to opioid dependence is not great. Progression to dependence on CNS stimulants and depressants is more common.

   c. **Methadone maintenance.** A significant number of individuals who have become dependent on opioids receive methadone from organized treatment programs.

   d. **Health care personnel.** The incidence of narcotic addiction is higher in physicians, nurses, and other health care personnel than in any other group of individuals with comparable education and socioeconomic class. Most physician–addicts initially use a narcotic to relieve depression, fatigue, or a physical ailment rather than for pleasure. The pattern and consequences of the addiction are no different than they are for other addicts, except that health care personnel are more likely to make drugs available to themselves through prescriptions written for real and imaginary patients. Health care professionals are often caught diverting narcotics from the floor medication dispensers, partially used vials of medication, or even from patients.

2. **Epidemic transmission.** Heroin abuse tends to be transmitted in an epidemic fashion among individuals who know each other. These epidemics begin slowly, peak rapidly, and then decline quickly. They tend to abate completely after 5 to 6 years.

   a. **Susceptibility** to heroin addiction varies in different populations. Young African American men are at highest risk, and women seem to be at lower risk.

   b. **Dependence** is initiated in a susceptible individual by someone known to the individual who is already addicted. The risk of such initiators exposing their acquaintances to heroin use continues for about 1 year. Drug "pushers" actually cause few new cases of dependence, although they obviously are a major source of the drug.

   c. **Heroin abuse** tends to spread until all susceptible individuals within a given group have been exposed. New addicts then tend to expose their friends in other circles, who produce a third generation of abusers.

3. **Drug cultures.** When cultural norms support heroin use and relatively pure preparations are available, a large percentage of users become dependent.

   a. More than 40% of the U.S. Army enlisted men stationed in Vietnam reported trying narcotics at least once, and approximately 50% of those who tried it became physically dependent at some time during their stay in Vietnam. However, very few individuals who became dependent on narcotics in Vietnam continued drug use when they returned to the United States. This suggests that removal of peer group support for drug abuse, removal of the easy availability of drugs, and, possibly, removal of major environmental stresses ended the reasons for drug abuse.

   b. Most individuals in the United States who become dependent on narcotics have a psychological predisposition to abuse and tend to remain in peer groups that encourage substance use. Relapse is likely when they return to an environment in which drugs are available and friends and colleagues condone abuse.

4. **Psychiatric illness.** Approximately 50% to 87% of people with opioid dependence suffer from another psychiatric illness, especially depression, anxiety states, and borderline and antisocial personality disorders. Individuals from disorganized social backgrounds are also more susceptible to narcotic dependence. A combination of a susceptible psychosocial constellation, availability of narcotics, an environment that encourages abuse, and friends or colleagues who already are users may be necessary for the development of addiction.

B Medical complications of narcotic abuse may result from contaminants of illicit preparations and the patient's lifestyle.

1. **Sexually transmitted diseases** are common in female drug abusers as a result of engaging in prostitution to obtain the narcotic.

2. **Fatal overdose** caused by fluctuations in the purity of available compounds is common.

3. **Anaphylactic reactions** may be caused by the intravenous injection of impurities.

4. **Hypersensitivity reactions** to impurities may also cause the formation of granulomata and neurologic, musculoskeletal, and cutaneous lesions.

5. **Infections** commonly caused by contaminated products and shared needles include hepatitis, endocarditis, septicemia, tetanus, and formation of pulmonary, cerebral, and subcutaneous abscesses. Up to two-thirds of individuals in narcotic treatment centers test positive for human immunodeficiency virus (HIV).

6. **Suicide and death** at the hands of associates are more common in narcotic abusers than in the general population.

C Treatment of opioid dependence requires a multidisciplinary approach.

1. **Methadone maintenance** for the treatment of addiction can only be carried out by a federally approved program.

   a. If the patient has strong psychosocial supports available and is highly motivated to discontinue drug use, the patient can be withdrawn from opioids immediately using methadone (see III E 2 b).

   b. If supports are weak or motivation to undergo withdrawal is uncertain, a period of methadone maintenance is instituted while motivation, social supports, and the relationship with the treatment team are strengthened. The usual dosage of methadone in this setting is 40 to 150 mg/day. The role of methadone is to take away craving and prevent a "high" from self-administered opiates because of the blockage of the mu receptor by the methadone. Patients must come to the clinic 6 out of 7 days a week for the first 90 days. If their urine is clean, they "phase up" to the next level, which allows them less restrictions every 3 months.

      (1) The patient must have clear-cut signs of addiction (e.g., intoxication, needle tracks, and medical or psychosocial consequences of abuse) to qualify for methadone maintenance.

      (2) Periodic unscheduled urine and blood screens are performed to assess compliance with the program. Persistent noncompliance (i.e., continued self-administration of narcotics, cocaine, benzodiazepines) results in dismissal.

(3) Very gradual withdrawal from methadone is attempted when the patient seems ready. Most addicts note some abstinence symptoms when the dosage is reduced below 20 mg/day, and reduction in dosage by as little as 1 mg/wk below this level may be necessary for the detoxification of long-term methadone users.

2. **L-α-Acetylmethadol (LAAM),** also known as methadyl acetate, a long-acting preparation, suppresses narcotic withdrawal for 72 hours. When it is used instead of methadone for maintenance, less frequent administration of the drug is necessary. However, more patients drop out of LAAM maintenance than methadone maintenance.

3. **Naltrexone,** a long-acting narcotic antagonist, has been used in a manner analogous to disulfiram to precipitate withdrawal when narcotics are used.

4. **Suboxone,** a combination of Subutex and naloxone, can be prescribed on an outpatient basis by physicians who have completed a training course on the use of this medication. Naloxone was added so that if anyone tried to inject the drug, the addict would experience the antagonist effect of the drug. Suboxone is given in pill form and instead of being used for detoxification, it is used for opiate replacement and maintenance. Patients usually take 8 to 24 mg/day in divided doses. Similar to methadone, it reduces craving and prevents a high if opiates are used while taking Suboxone. Benefits of Suboxone over methadone are that a 30-day prescription of Suboxone can be given instead of going to a methadone clinic every day. Patients must be very motivated and reliable for this treatment to work. Each doctor may provide treatment for only 30 patients in his or her practice.

5. **Therapeutic communities** play an important role in the treatment of narcotic addiction. Confrontation by fellow addicts of lying and rationalization of drug use has more credibility to an addict than therapies that are administered by professionals. Most of the time, this occurs during 12-step meetings.

6. **Residential treatment.** If outpatient therapy is unsuccessful, residential treatment is necessary to remove the patient from easy access to the drug and from associates who encourage continued narcotic use. Group confrontation and support are used extensively in these settings. Compliance with treatment is higher when it is mandated by the courts than when it is voluntary and the patient is free to withdraw at any time.

7. **Licensure restrictions.** Physicians and nurses who abuse narcotics are increasingly being identified by state licensing bodies and professional societies. Treatment programs have been very successful when the problem is identified early and when continued licensure for medical practice is made contingent on documentation of ongoing abstinence (i.e., contingency contracting).

8. **Prevention of addiction in a medical setting.** Health care providers should not permit fears of addiction from interfering with the administration of appropriate doses of narcotics to patients in pain. The following guidelines apply to the administration of opioids to patients at risk of dependence:
   a. Adequate doses of narcotics should be administered to patients with bona fide acute pain syndromes. As a result of tolerance, addicts generally require higher doses than other patients.
   b. Narcotics should be administered on a set schedule rather than as needed. This approach prevents patients from becoming preoccupied with pain and its relief and provides a constant blood level that results in lower individual doses being necessary.
   c. An addict should not be detoxified during an acute physical illness.
   d. Prescriptions should not be written for outpatients with suspicious complaints or those with a high abuse potential, as indicated by:
      (1) Losing prescriptions or running out of medication early
      (2) Requests for a specific drug
      (3) History of abuse of alcohol or other drugs
      (4) Physician shopping
      (5) Claims that a physician who originally wrote a prescription is unavailable
      (6) Threats when narcotics are not prescribed
      (7) Dishonesty with the physician
      (8) When a narcotic is not the standard of care for that particular complaint (e.g., migraine headaches, fibromyalgia, general back pain)

VII TRANQUILIZERS AND SLEEPING PILLS

Abuse of and dependence on tranquilizers and sleeping pills are created or encouraged in everyday medical practice more often than opioid dependence and abuse.

A **Manifestations of dependence and abuse** Barbiturates and related compounds are particularly prone to pathologic use. Whereas benzodiazepines with short half-lives are more prone to dosage escalation to reduce interdose withdrawal, highly lipid-soluble benzodiazepines produce a more rapid effect that may be experienced as a high. Diazepam, which is very lipid soluble; lorazepam, which has a short half-life; and alprazolam, which has both properties, are the most commonly abused benzodiazepines. Dependence may first be suspected only when an abstinence syndrome that responds to phenobarbital or pentobarbital appears in a patient who is admitted to the hospital and is denied access to the abused substance.

1. Because they suppress REM sleep, barbiturates and related sedatives (e.g., secobarbital, glutethimide, ethchlorvynol) subject the patient who uses them to a **rebound of REM sleep,** usually in the form of **nightmares,** when the drug is discontinued. Although it seems to the patient that he or she cannot sleep without the drug, continued drug use serves only to prevent withdrawal and suppress REM rebound, and escalating doses often are needed to accomplish this result.

2. When barbiturates and related compounds are used as tranquilizers, drug withdrawal tends to be mistaken for a return of anxiety, which leads to an increase in dosage to suppress the symptoms. Fear of withdrawal symptoms then leads to continued drug use and an inability to function without the drug, as well as other manifestations of dependence.

3. Symptoms of benzodiazepine withdrawal may persist for months after drug discontinuation, leading to prolonged use of the benzodiazepine to suppress withdrawal.

B **Identification and management of abuse** Misuse of sedatives and tranquilizers can be minimized if the physician does not prescribe barbiturates for insomnia and anxiety or benzodiazepines for patients with a history of substance dependence. Identification and management of problems with CNS depressants involve the following steps:

1. A **detailed history** of amounts and kinds of all prescription and nonprescription drugs that have ever been taken should be obtained. Often, the patient continues to take drugs that were prescribed by a physician that he or she is no longer seeing.

2. **Prescriptions** for a patient who has terminated treatment should be **discontinued.**

3. **Toxicology screening** in patients who abuse any drug should be performed to identify mixed abuse. Drugs are not present in the blood of a patient who is experiencing a withdrawal syndrome.

4. **Regular appointments** should be scheduled for patients who have been taking barbiturates for years and who are reluctant to discontinue them. Assurance of an ongoing relationship with a physician the patient trusts may make the patient more willing to consider tapering drug intake. Insistence on discontinuation of barbiturates and related medications is mandatory for patients who escalate the dose, have withdrawal symptoms, or experience psychomotor impairment.

5. **Hospitalization** should be considered for detoxification of patients with severe or mixed dependence. This permits adequate treatment of what may be life-threatening withdrawal and ensures compliance with the withdrawal protocol.

VIII COCAINE

Cocaine abuse and dependence have become extremely serious public health problems. One-fourth of young adults have used cocaine, and adverse consequences are common.

A **Routes of administration** Cocaine may be self-administered by three routes.

1. **Nasal** administration is associated with the onset, over a period of about 20 minutes, of euphoria that lasts approximately 1 hour.

2. **Intravenous** administration produces immediate euphoria.

3. Crack, an easily synthesized compound that is not inactivated by high temperature, is **smoked,** producing immediate euphoria.

B **Addictive potential**   Contrary to the popular wisdom of a few years ago, cocaine is highly addictive. The advent of crack and the flooding of the market with cheap cocaine have made cocaine a drug of abuse at all socioeconomic levels.

1. Animals will choose self-administration of cocaine over food and water until they die.

2. Some patients report feeling addicted from the very first dose of cocaine.

3. Crack is the cheapest and most addictive form of cocaine.

4. Cocaine often is used in conjunction with other substances, especially alcohol and tranquilizers.

C **Psychomotor impairment**   In one report, more than 50% of a group of drivers who were stopped by the police for reckless driving and who were not intoxicated with alcohol were intoxicated with cocaine, marijuana, or both.

D **Psychiatric disorders**   Cocaine use may be a means of self-treatment for certain psychiatric disorders, especially depression and attention deficit disorder. Some individuals who suffer from bipolar disorder abuse cocaine to achieve a sense of control over excitement and mood swings that occur spontaneously without the drug. In any of these situations, cocaine is so inherently rewarding that attempts to treat the comorbid condition without treating cocaine abuse are invariably unsuccessful. In addition, as a potent kindling stimulus, cocaine exacerbates mood instability in bipolar disorder.

E **Treatment**   The same approaches that have been applied to abuse of opioids and alcohol have been found helpful in the treatment of cocaine abuse and dependence

1. **Bupropion and possibly venlafaxine** are thought to potentially reduce craving because of their action on dopamine.

2. **Amantadine** decreases cocaine craving in the first few weeks after withdrawal. It may also be useful in long-term treatment.

3. **Cognitive therapy** has been found to have a delayed onset of action in promoting abstinence from cocaine. The benefits of medications tend to dissipate after the medication is discontinued.

4. **Topiramate and Antabuse** are being considered as potential treatments for cocaine craving.

IX   CANNABIS

Cannabis abuse and dependence is often not considered an important problem. However, in addition to producing medical and psychological complications, marijuana has been shown in adolescents to serve as a "gateway drug." That is, use of marijuana reduces the threshold for using more dangerous substances, with progression from use of alcohol and marijuana to use of hallucinogens, stimulants, and narcotics.

A **Manifestations of dependence and abuse**   Chronic marijuana use results in an amotivational syndrome that may persist after drug discontinuation. Intellectual function may also be impaired. Although marijuana traditionally has not been thought to cause physical dependence, recent reports indicate that people who use this substance regularly experience craving for the drug and prolonged dysphoria with drug withdrawal that is reduced by restarting the drug.

B **Treatment**

1. No medication is specifically useful in the treatment of marijuana use, although 5HT3 antagonists may turn out to reduce the craving and "highs" that reinforce marijuana use.

2. As with any substance, reducing access to the drug, learning other means of coping with stress, changing peer groups, toxicology screens, and involving the family are essential components of any treatment plan.

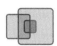 *Study Questions*

Directions: *Each of the numbered items or incomplete statements in this section is followed by answers or by completions of the statement. Select the ONE lettered answer or completion that is BEST in each case.*

1. What feature of addiction differentiates it from other forms of substance misuse?
   - A Overwhelming involvement in seeking and using a drug
   - B Physical dependence
   - C Use of narcotics
   - D Antisocial behavior
   - E Tolerance and withdrawal

2. The percentage of United States Army enlisted men who became dependent on narcotics while in Vietnam was roughly
   - A 5%
   - B 20%
   - C 40%
   - D 75%
   - E 90%

3. Which of the following abnormalities is a manifestation of barbiturate intoxication but not of barbiturate withdrawal?
   - A Agitation
   - B Confusion
   - C Disorientation
   - D Nystagmus
   - E Postural hypotension

4. A patient's blood alcohol level is 10 mg/100 ml, but there is no clinical evidence of intoxication. It is a reasonable assumption that the patient
   - A Is tolerant to opioids
   - B Is dependent on alcohol
   - C Has pancreatitis
   - D Is impotent
   - E Has cerebral atrophy

Directions: *Each of the numbered items or incomplete statements in this section is negatively phrased, as indicated by a capitalized word such as NOT, LEAST, or EXCEPT. Select the ONE lettered answer or completion that is BEST in each case.*

5. Opioid overdoses produce all of the following signs EXCEPT:
   - A Coma
   - B Depressed reflexes
   - C Decreased respiration
   - D Dilated pupils
   - E Hypotension

6. Amphetamine psychosis (stimulant-induced psychotic disorder) is characterized by all of the following EXCEPT:
   - A Clear sensorium
   - B Depression
   - C Loose associations
   - D Paranoia
   - E Tactile hallucinations

7. All of the following statements characterize marijuana EXCEPT:

- Ⓐ Physical dependence can develop.
- Ⓑ Its use increases the likelihood of narcotic use.
- Ⓒ Overdose causes seizures.
- Ⓓ Chronic use causes an amotivational state.
- Ⓔ It causes tachycardia.

8. A patient is in the hospital for heroin detoxification. He just received his first injection of buprenorphine. Thirty minutes later, he begins vomiting, sweating, and cramping. What happened?

- Ⓐ He is allergic to buprenorphine.
- Ⓑ He does not really use heroin.
- Ⓒ He lied about when he last used.
- Ⓓ He has the stomach flu.
- Ⓔ The nurse gave him Antabuse instead of buprenorphine.

Directions: *Each set of matching questions in this section consists of a list of four to 26 lettered options followed by several numbered items. For each numbered item, select the ONE lettered option that is most closely associated with it. Each lettered option may be selected once, more than once, or not at all.*

QUESTIONS 9–14

Match each of the following substances with the withdrawal syndrome it usually causes.

- Ⓐ Anxiety
- Ⓑ Flashbacks
- Ⓒ Hypersomnia
- Ⓓ Influenza-like symptoms
- Ⓔ Piloerection
- Ⓕ Tremors

9. Alcohol

10. Anticholinergics

11. Benzodiazepines

12. Hallucinogens

13. Opioids

14. Stimulants

Answers and Explanations

1. The answer is A [*I C*]. Although the definition of addiction varies, most definitions share the concept of overwhelming involvement in and preoccupation with obtaining and using any type of drug. Addictive behavior may occur with any substance; even addiction to placebo has been reported. Physical dependence is defined as the presence of tolerance, withdrawal, or both. Antisocial behavior may play a role in attempts to make enough money to obtain substances, but it is not a defining feature of addiction or any other form of misuse.

2. The answer is B [*VI A 3 a*]. Forty percent of enlisted men tried narcotics while they were in Vietnam, and approximately half of those who tried it became dependent. The finding that only a small minority of men continued to use narcotics on return to the United States suggests that the easy availability of drugs and the encouragement of a peer group allow opioid abuse to continue.

3. The answer is D [*II B 1 c, 2 e; III B 1*]. Both intoxication and withdrawal from barbiturates may cause confusion, delirium, anxiety, agitation, and postural hypotension. If caused by withdrawal, these signs improve with administration of a barbiturate. Nystagmus, which is a sign of intoxication but not of withdrawal, may appear.

4. The answer is B [*V C 9*]. Absence of intoxication in the presence of a high blood alcohol level indicates that the patient is tolerant to the central nervous system depressant effects of alcohol, which is a major criterion for alcohol dependence. Pancreatitis, impotence, and cerebral atrophy are complications of alcoholism that should be investigated, but these are not diagnosed by a blood alcohol level. Because opioids and alcohol are not cross-tolerant, tolerance to alcohol does not provide any information about tolerance to opioids.

5. The answer is D [*II F 2 g*]. Similar to alcohol, barbiturates, and benzodiazepines, narcotics can produce depression of consciousness, reflexes, blood pressure, and respiration. Narcotics cause constricted rather than dilated pupils. Opioid intoxication can be diagnosed with intravenous naloxone.

6. The answer is B [*II C 3*]. Stimulant psychosis often is associated with paranoia and loose associations in a clear sensorium, which may make it indistinguishable from schizophrenia. Tactile hallucinations and delusions of infestation with parasites also may occur. Depression is usually associated with stimulant withdrawal, not stimulant intoxication.

7. The answer is C [*II E 1, IX A*]. Contrary to popular wisdom, physical dependence on marijuana may occur, and withdrawal symptoms may appear with discontinuation. Marijuana has been found to be a "gateway drug" that lowers the threshold for use of "harder" drugs. Marijuana use can produce tachycardia and an amotivational state. Overdose can cause distortions in time sense and injected conjunctivae, but not seizures.

8. The answer is C [*III E 2 a*]. The patient is going into acute opiate withdrawal 30 minutes after receiving his first buprenorphine injection. He most likely told the nursing staff and physician that he had used his last dose of heroin several hours earlier from the time of his admission than he actually did. He probably feared going into withdrawal and did not wait long enough for withdrawal signs to appear before getting his first dose of buprenorphine. As a result, buprenorphine's antagonistic properties knocked off the remaining heroin still attached to the mu receptors and threw the patient into acute opiate withdrawal.

9–14. The answers are 9-F, 10-D, 11-A, 12-B, 13-E, and 14–C [*III B 1 a, C 1 f, D 1, E 1 d, and F 1 a-2*]. Withdrawal of stimulants causes increased sleep (hypersomnia). Abrupt withdrawal of anticholinergic substances leads to cholinergic rebound, with influenza-like symptoms and, occasionally, mania. Opioid withdrawal causes piloerection (gooseflesh). Withdrawal of benzodiazepines often causes anxiety, which may be difficult to distinguish from return of the original symptoms. Flashbacks on withdrawal of hallucinogens may be precipitated by marijuana. Alcohol causes elevation of blood pressure, pulse, and tremors as the first signs of withdrawal.

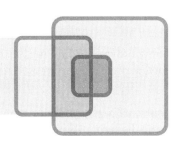

chapter 8

Somatoform and Associated Disorders

MARGARET A. SHUGART

I   **DEFINITIONS**

The somatoform disorders form a heterogeneous group of disorders that have common presenting features suggestive of physical illnesses, symptoms, or preoccupations. As a feature of this group, the physical symptoms are unexplained by a general medical condition or are disproportionate to symptoms that might be expected from a general medical condition. To establish one of these diagnoses, the clinician must rule out occult physical illnesses or conditions, other psychiatric disorders that might better explain the symptoms (e.g., a patient with major depressive illness who has a delusion of having a fatal cancer), and substance abuse. The condition must be of sufficient severity to impair social and occupational or other important areas of functioning. Disorders and conditions with a mixed picture of physical and psychiatric symptoms might be divided into the following groups.

A   **Disorders involving subjective symptoms unexplained by physical findings**   This group of disorders includes symptoms such as conversion symptoms (see II A 2 d) and may involve many body systems, including the joints, reproductive organs, gastrointestinal tract, nervous system, and special senses. This group does not include disorders that involve a conscious or intentional misrepresentation of symptoms (see I F).

B   **Disorders involving unusual attention to and preoccupation with symptoms, organs, and body parts**   This group of disorders includes either preoccupation with a body part or parts that patients consider defective, deformed, weak, or ugly in contrast with external evidence to the contrary (e.g., body dysmorphic disorder) or unusual degrees of attention to physical symptoms (e.g., a mole that the person incorrectly believes to be malignant) or organ systems (e.g., excessive preoccupation with examining feces for blood or deformity believed to be evidence of malignancy).

C   **Disorders in which psychological symptoms may exacerbate a general medical condition**   Conditions in this group include general medical conditions exacerbated by a psychological factor (e.g., stress), including some cardiovascular disorders, irritable bowel syndrome, psoriasis, and many other medical conditions. Included in this category may be disorders exacerbated or caused by immune and neuroendocrine dysfunctions (associated with affective and anxiety disorders) and mitral valve prolapse (common in individuals with panic disorder).

D   **Psychiatric disorders that present with primarily physical symptoms or present physical symptoms as an unusual or atypical form of the disorder**   Disorders in this category include unusual presentations of familiar psychiatric disorders (e.g., a patient with depression who presents with headaches or malaise; a patient with panic disorder who presents with symptoms of a myocardial infarction).

E   **Disorders in which psychiatric symptoms are caused or exacerbated by a general medical condition**   Medical conditions can cause psychiatric symptoms resembling almost any psychiatric disorder. Common examples are hypothyroidism mimicking depressive disorders, toxic delirium mimicking schizophreniform disorder, and paroxysmal atrial tachycardia resembling panic disorder.

(F) **Disorders in which physical symptoms are incorrectly reported or are created by patients for the purpose of gaining a specific benefit** Familiar disorders in this group include **factitious disorder** and **malingering**. The hallmark of these conditions is conscious fabrication of symptoms (e.g., a man putting blood from a finger stick into his urine sample and complaining of flank pain).

(G) **Disorders of a primarily medical nature that the practitioner mistakes for psychiatric conditions** The *Diagnostic and Statistical Manual of Mental Disorders,* 4th edition (*DSM-IV*), emphasizes that clinicians frequently dismiss unusual physical symptoms and physical disorders early in their course as having a psychiatric basis. This mistake may lead to unfortunate consequences for the clinicians as well as patients. Therefore, clinicians should note the formal diagnostic criteria for somatoform disorders to avoid this serious and costly mistake.

II   DIAGNOSIS

(A) **Somatization disorder**

1. **History.** Patients have **recurring multiple physical complaints** beginning before age 30 years, occurring over several years, and resulting in treatment for or significant impairment in social, occupational, or other important areas of functioning.

2. **Symptoms.** Each of the following criteria must be met, with individual symptoms occurring at any time during the course of the disturbance. The **symptoms are not intentionally produced or feigned** (e.g., as in factitious disorder or malingering).
   a. **Four pain symptoms.** History of pain related to at least four different sites (e.g., head, abdomen, back, joints, extremities, chest, rectum) or functions (e.g., menstruation, sexual intercourse, urination)
   b. **Two gastrointestinal symptoms.** History of at least two gastrointestinal symptoms other than pain (e.g., nausea, bloating, vomiting, diarrhea, intolerance of several different foods)
   c. **One sexual symptom.** History of at least one sexual or reproductive symptom other than pain (e.g., sexual indifference, erectile or ejaculatory dysfunction, irregular menses, excessive menstrual bleeding, vomiting throughout pregnancy)
   d. **One pseudoneurological symptom.** History of at least one symptom or deficit suggesting a neurologic condition not limited to pain such as conversion symptoms (e.g., impaired coordination or balance, paralysis or localized weakness, difficulty swallowing or lump in throat, aphonia, urinary retention, hallucinations, loss of touch or pain sensation, double vision, blindness, deafness, seizures) or dissociative symptoms (e.g., amnesia or loss of consciousness other than fainting)

3. **Other criteria.** Patients **have either of the following conditions:**
   a. After appropriate investigation, each of the symptoms described in II A 2 cannot be fully explained by a known general medical condition or the direct effects of a substance (e.g., a drug of abuse, a medication).
   b. If a related general medical condition is present, the physical complaints or resulting social or occupational impairment exceed what would be expected from the history, physical examination, or laboratory findings.

(B) **Undifferentiated somatoform disorder**

1. Occurrence of one or more physical complaints (e.g., fatigue, loss of appetite, gastrointestinal or urinary problems) for 6 months or more

2. **Occurrence of either of the following conditions:**
   a. After appropriate investigation, the **symptoms cannot be fully explained by a known general medical condition or the direct effects of a substance** (e.g., a drug of abuse, a medication).
   b. **If a related general medical condition is present,** the physical complaints or resulting social or occupational **impairment exceed what would be expected** from the history, physical examination, or laboratory findings.

3. The **symptoms cause clinically significant distress or impairment** in social, occupational, or other important areas of functioning.

4. The **duration of the disturbance is at least 6 months.**

5. The **disturbance is not better explained by another mental disorder** (e.g., another somatoform disorder, sexual dysfunction, mood disorder, anxiety disorder, sleep disorder, psychotic disorder).

6. The **symptom is not intentionally produced** or feigned (e.g., as in factitious disorder or malingering).

[C] Conversion disorder (*DSM-IV* criteria)

1. One or more symptoms or deficits affecting voluntary motor or sensory function suggest a neurologic or other general medical condition.

2. Psychological factors are judged to be associated with the symptom or deficit because the initiation or exacerbation of the symptom or deficit is preceded by conflicts or other stressors.

3. The symptom or deficit is not intentionally produced or feigned (e.g., factitious disorder and malingering).

4. The symptom or deficit cannot, after appropriate investigation, be fully explained by a general medical condition, by the direct effects of a substance, or as a culturally sanctioned behavior or experience.

5. The symptom or deficit causes clinically significant distress or impairment in social, occupational, or other important areas of functioning or warrants medical evaluation.

6. The symptom or deficit is not limited to pain or sexual dysfunction, does not occur exclusively during the course of somatization disorder, and is not better accounted for by another mental disorder.

7. The *DSM-IV* requires specification of the subtype of conversion disorder:
   a. **With motor symptoms or deficits** (e.g., impaired coordination or balance, paralysis or localized weakness, difficulty swallowing or "lump in throat," aphonia, urinary retention)
   b. **With sensory symptoms or deficits** (e.g., loss of touch or pain sensation, double vision, blindness, deafness, hallucinations)
   c. **With seizures or convulsions** (includes seizures or convulsions with voluntary motor or sensory components)
   d. **With mixed presentation** (if symptoms are evident in more than one category)

[D] Pain disorder

1. Pain in one or more anatomic sites is the predominant focus of the clinical presentation and is of sufficient severity to warrant clinical attention.

2. The pain causes clinically significant distress or impairment in social, occupational, or other important areas of functioning.

3. Psychological factors are judged to have an important role in the onset, severity, exacerbation, or maintenance of the pain.

4. The symptoms or deficit are not intentionally produced or feigned (e.g., as in factitious disorder and malingering).

5. The pain is not better explained by a mood, anxiety, or psychotic disorder and does not meet criteria for dyspareunia.

6. **Subtypes** are defined as follows:
   a. **Pain disorder associated with psychological factors.** Psychological factors are judged to play a major role in the onset, severity, exacerbation, or maintenance of the pain. If a general medical condition is present, it does not play a major role in the onset, severity, exacerbation, or maintenance of the pain. This disorder is not diagnosed if criteria for somatization disorder are met. **Acute** or **chronic** duration should be specified.
   b. **Pain disorder associated with both psychological factors and a general medical condition.** Both psychological factors and a general medical condition are judged to have important roles in the onset, severity, exacerbation, or maintenance of the pain.
   c. **Pain disorder associated with a general medical condition.** A general medical condition has a major role in the onset, severity, exacerbation, or maintenance of the pain. This category is

for medical conditions and for conditions in which the relationship between anatomic and psychological factors is not clearly established (e.g., low back pain). This subtype is not a mental disorder and is coded on Axis III.

E Hypochondriasis   This condition is a preoccupation with fears of having (or the idea that one has) a serious disease because a person has misinterpreted bodily symptoms.

1. The preoccupation persists despite appropriate medical evaluation and reassurance.

2. The belief in the preoccupation is not of delusional intensity (e.g., as in delusional disorder, somatic type) and is not restricted to a circumscribed concern about appearance (e.g., as in body dysmorphic disorder).

3. The preoccupation causes clinically significant distress or impairment in social, occupational, or other important areas of functioning.

4. The duration of the disturbance is at least 6 months.

5. The preoccupation is not better explained by generalized anxiety disorder, obsessive-compulsive disorder (OCD), panic disorder, a major depressive episode (MDE), separation anxiety, or another somatoform disorder.

F Body dysmorphic disorder is a preoccupation with an imagined defect in appearance. If a slight physical anomaly is present, the person's concern is markedly excessive. *Dysmorphophobia* is the historical term for this disorder.

1. The preoccupation causes clinically significant distress or impairment in social, occupational, or other important areas of functioning.

2. The preoccupation is not better explained by another mental disorder (e.g., dissatisfaction with body shape and size as in anorexia nervosa).

G Somatoform disorder not otherwise specified   This category includes disorders with somatoform symptoms that do not meet the criteria for any specific somatoform disorder. Examples include:

1. **Pseudocyesis.** This false belief of being pregnant is associated with objective signs of pregnancy, which may include abdominal enlargement (although the umbilicus does not become everted), reduced menstrual flow, amenorrhea, subjective sensation of fetal movement, nausea, breast engorgement and secretions, and labor pains at the expected date of delivery. This condition cannot be explained by a general medical condition such as a hormone-secreting tumor.

2. A disorder involving nonpsychotic hypochondriacal symptoms of less than 6 months' duration.

3. A disorder involving unexplained physical complaints that are of less than 6 months' duration and are not caused by another mental disorder.

H Factitious disorder   This condition involves the intentional production or feigning of physical or psychological signs or symptoms. The motivation for the behavior is assumption of the sick role. External incentives for the behavior (e.g., profiting economically, avoiding legal responsibility, improving physical well-being, as in malingering) are absent. **Subtypes** include the following:

1. With predominantly psychological signs and symptoms

2. With predominantly physical signs and symptoms (Münchausen syndrome)

3. With combined psychological and physical signs and symptoms

I Factitious disorder not otherwise specified   This disorder, also known as **Munchausen's by proxy**, includes production of intentional symptoms in another individual such as a child for the purpose of having the other person assume a sick role.

J Malingering   This intentional production of false or grossly exaggerated physical or psychological symptoms is motivated by external incentives (e.g., avoiding military duty, avoiding work, obtaining financial compensation, evading criminal prosecution, obtaining drugs). Malingering is listed in the

DSM-IV as a V code. (A V code describes a condition that may be the focus of clinical attention.) Malingering should be strongly suspected if a combination of the following is noted:

1. Medicolegal context of presentation (e.g., the person is referred by an attorney to the clinician for examination)
2. Marked discrepancy between the person's claimed stress or disability and the objective findings
3. Lack of cooperation during the diagnostic evaluation and in complying with the prescribed treatment regimen
4. The presence of antisocial personality disorder

III ETIOLOGIC THEORIES

A **Specificity theory** The theory of emotional specificity (i.e., the physiologic expression of blocked emotions) has led to personality studies of patients with peptic ulcers, coronary artery disease, and cancer. Although these studies have lent some support to the theory, it has generally lost favor as a comprehensive explanation.

1. **Sigmund Freud** and his followers studied somatic involvement in psychological conflict and were particularly interested in **conversion reactions,** in which a psychological problem is symbolically manifested physically, although physiologic tissue damage cannot be demonstrated.
2. **Flanders Dunbar** suggested that **specific conscious personality traits** cause specific psychosomatic diseases.
3. **Franz Alexander** theorized that **specific unconscious conflicts** cause specific illnesses in organs innervated by the autonomic nervous system. These illnesses occur because prolonged tension can produce physiologic disorders, leading to eventual pathology. Alexander also believed that constitutional predisposing factors are involved. His theory led to the concept of the **classic psychosomatic diseases,** including:
   a. Bronchial asthma
   b. Rheumatoid arthritis
   c. Ulcerative colitis
   d. Essential hypertension
   e. Neurodermatitis
   f. Thyrotoxicosis
   g. Peptic ulcers

B **Stress response theories** Whatever event is perceived by patients as stressful can produce stress, whether it is the death of a loved one, divorce, financial loss, or illness. In each culture, different events may carry different "weights" as stressors. Within a culture, however, stressful life events can be assessed quantitatively for their risk of producing psychophysiologic illnesses in a large group of people. Psychological reactions to stress can alter neuroendocrine, immune, cardiovascular, and other physiologic parameters that can lead to a **nonspecific cause of disease**.

1. **Neurophysiologic reactions to stress** activate the pituitary–adrenal axis and are known as the **general adaptation syndrome.** The nonspecific systemic reactions of the body to stress include:
   a. **Alarm reaction** (shock)
   b. **Resistance** (adaptation to stress)
   c. **Exhaustion** (resistance to prolonged stress, which cannot be maintained)
2. **Physiologic reactions to stress** include the following:
   a. **Fight-or-flight response.** Arousal of the sympathetic nervous system results in increased production of epinephrine and norepinephrine (NE), with an increase in pulse and muscle tension. When an affected individual can neither fight nor flee, this state of arousal can lead to organic dysfunction.
   b. **Withdrawal and conservation.** George Engel and coworkers have shown that when an individual is threatened with loss (real or imagined), the metabolism can slow down. The individual withdraws, and this action conserves energy.

(1) Pulse and body temperature decrease.

(2) The individual may become susceptible to illness, particularly infection. Studies on the psychophysiologic effects of bereavement support the following hypothesis: Morbidity and mortality rates are higher during the first year after death of a spouse in a bereaved group compared with those rates in an age-controlled, nonbereaved group. Elderly people removed from their homes and placed in nursing homes have an increased risk of death from cardiovascular causes.

C **Biopsychosocial model** This model, proposed by George Engel, offers the interaction of biologic, psychological, and social events as the means for understanding the etiology, pathologic process, and treatment for psychiatric disorders as well as psychophysiologic conditions. This model is reciprocal rather than linear. In other words, a biologic event can alter psychological perceptions and cognitive set. These changes, in turn, can alter social behaviors. The social environment responds by treating the individual differently, and the response to that different treatment is an alteration in physiology.

1. **Biologic factors** reflect the physiologic, neurophysiologic, and pathophysiologic functioning of the individual.
   a. **Hereditary and congenital factors** include inherited risks for psychiatric disorders (e.g., affective and anxiety disorders), physiologic vulnerabilities (e.g., risks for heart disease or some cancers), and defects (e.g., malformations, biochemical abnormalities, differences in pain threshold).
   b. **Physical disease processes** can affect the functioning of the brain and other physiologic processes.
   c. **Environmental factors** (e.g., exposure to toxic substances, medications being prescribed, substances of abuse, amount of daylight, alterations of circadian rhythms related to a job) can affect the physiology of the brain and body.
   d. **Normal physiologic responses** to environmental events may place the individual at risk for a variety of additional physical and psychological events.
      (1) **Immune system compromise,** which is reflected in the increased risks of death after significant losses from causes such as infectious illnesses and some neoplasms
      (2) **Cardiovascular responses to stress,** which include hypertension and increased heart rate (which may unmask some arrhythmias)
      (3) **Neuroendocrine systems,** which are altered by environmental stressors, major mental illnesses, and many of the medications used to treat mental illnesses. Many of these abnormalities may reflect changes in hypothalamic–pituitary functioning modulated in the brain. Major systems involved include the following:
         (a) **Cortisol** is altered in relation to stress, anxiety, and depression.
         (b) **Prolactin** is altered in a variety of psychiatric disorders as well as in normal stress responses. Interestingly, prolactin also may modulate T-lymphocyte function.
         (c) **Thyroid function** is variably altered in major mental illnesses, particularly depression. Thyrotropin-releasing hormone (TRH) has been the focus of recent study, as has depression in mildly hypothyroid people.
         (d) **Other hormones** such as growth hormone have been studied in relation to psychiatric disorders. Their role in stress response is less clear than the role of those factors just listed.
      (4) **Neurohumoral factors** are reported to be altered in major mental illness and stress response. β-Endorphin and dynorphin abnormalities are associated with anxiety-related disorders. Somatostatin, corticotropin-releasing hormone, and TRH also appear to be altered with stress, as do dopamine, γ-aminobutyric acid (GABA), NE, and serotonin. These neurohumoral factors may be an intermediary mechanism by which stressful events are translated into longer term alterations in brain function. However, any primary role for this function remains unclear.

2. **Psychological factors**
   a. **Perception of pain or physiologic events** is the conscious registering of a stimulus or event. Perception of physical events has been shown to be altered by a number of factors such as a state of arousal, individual differences in threshold, mood, other stimuli, and physiologic events.

    b. Attention to the pain or physiologic event is perhaps the best example of the conscious effect of the physical event on the person. For example, a patient with chronic pain notices the pain very frequently despite efforts to ignore it.

    c. The **meaning or context of the symptom** determines how much attention it gets. For example, the literature contains many reports of broken legs and war wounds that go unnoticed by the injured person. In contrast, a patient who believes that a change in a physical symptom is the sign of a worsening or fatal illness pays a great deal of attention to the symptom.

    d. Primary gain from a physical symptom is the abatement of a psychological symptom that results from the attention demanded by the physical symptom. For example, a broken leg takes attention away from worries about a relationship and may even be more "comfortable."

3. Social factors help determine the meaning of the physical symptom or pain and may serve to extinguish or perpetuate attention to the symptom. Some social factors that determine how a physical symptom is perceived are considered in the following discussion.

    a. The **sick role** is defined by the culture, the family group, and the beliefs of the individual. The sick role can be understood as the expected behavior of the person as a result of illness. In some cultures, the sick role is very limited; a person, when sick, is allowed only to lie down and stop eating. In other cultures, the sick role may be highly elaborated on the basis of the type of sickness, chronically, and the supposed role of the individual in bringing on the illness. Some positive and negative aspects of the sick role include the following:

        (1) Secondary gain results from the social benefits of the sick role. Individuals may be able to avoid work, gain financial rewards, avoid conflict, and gain sympathy.

        (2) The sick role of some **"socially stigmatized" illnesses** such as human immunodeficiency virus (HIV), mental illness, and epilepsy may preclude persons from working, finding housing, or enjoying social relationships, all of which are independent of concrete evidence contradicting the need for social isolation (e.g., actual contagiousness of HIV, low evidence of dangerousness).

        (3) Some sick roles may create disability independent of or disproportionate to the disability associated with the illness. For example, in mental hospitals and tuberculosis sanitariums, **institutionalism** produced adaptation to the hospital culture, which was often more socially disabling than the condition itself.

    b. Interpersonal relationships are often altered by illness.

        (1) A family member (often a child) may be placed in the sick role to help the family avoid other major issues (e.g., substance abuse by a parent).

        (2) Acutely, the sick role normally elicits caring responses from others. As the sick role becomes more chronic, it elicits increasing anger and rejection from others (including from unsophisticated physicians and caregivers).

        (3) Development of socially stigmatized illnesses may elicit acute rejection from the social network (e.g., HIV, mental illness).

        (4) Illness and the sick role may upset the power dynamics in a relationship. Individuals may seek to reestablish the power dynamics by precipitating another crisis.

        (5) Communication between ill persons and others may become increasingly centered on the illness, creating a cycle in which exacerbation of symptoms becomes the mechanism for eliciting a response from others.

        (6) Family communication style involving high levels of **expressed emotionality** is associated with many psychophysiologic disorders, as well as major mental illnesses (see Chapter 3: III C 2 c).

    c. Health-related behaviors

        (1) Social, educational, and psychological factors may contribute to the tendency of individuals to avoid or engage in behaviors that increase their risk of disease or injury (e.g., unprotected sex and HIV risk, smoking, substance abuse, motorcycle riding).

        (2) Little is known about psychiatric comorbidity of many of these high-risk behaviors.

        (3) Public health approaches to the reduction of high-risk behaviors have been largely educational and, in many cases, have been less effective than expected.

        (4) Relatively little work has been done on altering lifestyle to reduce health risk using means other than education and substance abuse treatment.

IV COMORBIDITY AND DIFFERENTIAL DIAGNOSIS

Although somatoform disorders are presented as discrete diagnostic entities, in reality, the phenomenologic overlap between these disorders and other physical and psychological disorders is great. Furthermore, in contrast to other groups of psychiatric disorders such as schizophrenia and major affective disorders, relatively little phenomenologic and diagnostic work has been done. However, the costs of these patients to the health care system in excessive disability, needless diagnostic tests, and poorly justified surgery are enormous. Patients in this group usually have mixed, complex diagnostic and treatment pictures. Some of the diagnostic blurring in the *DSM-IV* is intentional: it helps clinicians avoid dichotomous thinking about patients (e.g., "The patient has somatization disorder; now I can make a psychiatric referral and stop looking for physical disease.")

A **Major illnesses with psychological factors**

1. **Gastrointestinal disorders.** Emotional states have long been known to cause a reaction in the gastrointestinal tract. Vague complaints of nausea, indigestion, diarrhea, constipation, and abdominal pain are common in association with psychiatric disorders.

   a. **Peptic ulcers**

      (1) **Etiology.** Gastric, duodenal, and acute posttraumatic stress ulcers all have different etiologies. The Mirsky study of United States Army recruits showed that several factors are necessary for the development of ulcers, including high stress, high pepsinogen secretion, and psychological conflict (dependency). Although conflicts involving dependency are noticeable in some ulcer patients, not all individuals affected by these conflicts are prone to developing ulcers, nor are all ulcer patients psychologically distressed.

      (2) **Treatment.** Patients who comply with good medical management do not usually require psychotherapy. Physicians should help patients identify the areas of their lives that seem to cause stress. Also, it may be useful to teach patients relaxation techniques in which the patient tenses all muscles, relaxes them in groups (e.g., arms, hands, legs, feet), and then notes the resultant feeling. Hypnotic techniques may also offer good relaxation for some patients. Antianxiety agents are occasionally indicated, as are antispasmodics.

   b. **Ulcerative colitis**

      (1) **Etiology.** A large proportion of cases of ulcerative colitis have a familial occurrence, which suggests a genetic cause. However, the exact etiology is unknown. It has been demonstrated that exacerbation of ulcerative colitis is associated with psychological stress and remission is associated with psychological support. Stress such as unresolved grief on the anniversary of a death can precipitate episodes of the disorder. Associated psychological features include:

      (a) Immaturity

      (b) Indecisiveness

      (c) Conscientiousness

      (d) Covertly demanding behavior

      (e) Fear of loss of an important individual

      (2) **Treatment.** Although psychotherapy cannot guarantee that the condition will not recur, it is useful when it focuses on helping patients develop mature ways of expressing needs, as well as helping them deal with unresolved losses.

   c. **Irritable bowel syndrome** (also termed spastic colon and nervous diarrhea) is disordered bowel motility, including both hypermotility and hypomotility.

      (1) **Etiology.** Although the syndrome is usually associated with environmental stress, patients tend to have other psychological symptoms such as anxiety and depression.

      (2) **Treatment.** Brief psychotherapy to help patients identify environmental stress and effect changes usually aids in decreasing symptoms. Tricyclic antidepressants are also effective.

2. **Cardiovascular disorders.** Much evidence suggests that the cardiovascular system reacts to a patient's emotional state.

   a. **Coronary artery disease** is the most common cause of death in the United States.

      (1) **Etiology.** Multiple nonpsychiatric elements are implicated in the development of coronary artery disease, including genetics, diet, smoking, high blood pressure, obesity, and

amount of physical activity. A personality type has also been implicated, according to some studies. The **type A behavior pattern** is only one risk factor out of many, and its exact role in the development of coronary artery disease is unclear. However, men who fall into this type of behavior pattern are at twice the risk for coronary artery disease as those who do not. Characteristics of the type A personality include:

(**a**) Competitiveness
(**b**) Ambition
(**c**) Drive for success
(**d**) Impatience
(**e**) A sense of time urgency
(**f**) Abruptness of speech and gesture
(**g**) Hostility

    (**2**) **Treatment.** Behavioral methods designed to decrease environmental stress and modify lifestyle when mutable are increasingly common.

  b. **Essential hypertension**

    (**1**) **Etiology.** Causes are unknown, but psychological factors were initially thought to involve conflicts between passive-dependent and aggressive tendencies in patients who repressed their hostility. Unfortunately, no reliable evidence is available to support this theory. On the other hand, a common reaction to stress is elevation of blood pressure. Patients who have a biologic susceptibility to essential hypertension may react to stressful situations by exacerbating that hypertension rather than, for example, increasing gastrointestinal motility.

    (**2**) **Treatment.** Therapy for hypertension may involve biofeedback, in which a patient is attached to a machine that provides information about ordinarily unnoticed biologic parameters. For example, a tone sounds when the patient's blood pressure rises. The patient then learns to relax to decrease the tone as well as the blood pressure. Biofeedback therapy, however, tends not to be long lasting and must be repeated to maintain the effect. Many antihypertensive agents have psychiatric effects, particularly that of producing depression. When treating depressed patients, care should be taken to avoid administering antihypertensive agents that cause depression.

  c. **Arrhythmias**

    (**1**) **Etiology.** Even in the absence of heart disease, psychological factors can influence the normal rhythm of the heart beat. **Stress** may cause arrhythmias by arousing the sympathetic nervous system (as is evident in the fight-or-flight reaction). Sinus tachycardia, paroxysmal atrial tachycardia, and ventricular ectopic beats are the most common arrhythmias to arise in reaction to stress. These reactions may be more common in patients who are already fearful of heart disease.

    (**2**) **Treatment.** Therapy involves questioning patients about unreasonable fears of heart disease and helping patients identify environmental stresses that precipitate the reaction. The condition may be part of either an anxiety disorder or a depression, which should be treated. Benzodiazepines may be useful for a limited time, as may β-blocking agents (e.g., propranolol). Contrary to a common belief among some physicians, effective treatment of depression with careful use of antidepressant medications (some of which have specific antiarrhythmic properties) may be safer than avoiding treatment for depressed patients with cardiac disease.

3. **Respiratory disorders.** Changes in respiration in normal individuals may correspond to an emotional state (e.g., the sigh of boredom, the gasp of surprise). The strongest psychological reactions associated with respiratory disease, however, are those that develop secondary to the illness. The panic associated with shortness of breath can be quite disabling.

  a. **Hyperventilation syndrome**

    (**1**) **Etiology.** This disorder is often associated with **anxiety,** particularly panic disorder (see Chapter 5: I B 1 a), which may cause an increased depth or rate of breathing. In turn, this response leads to **respiratory alkalosis** and then to lightheadedness, paresthesias, and carpopedal spasms. These symptoms increase the patient's anxiety, resulting in a vicious circle of increased hyperventilation and respiratory alkalosis. Hyperventilation may occur with the typical symptoms of shortness of breath; numbness of the fingers, nose, and lips; and lightheadedness.

(2) **Treatment.** Educating patients about the syndrome after the acute event is past may be sufficient. However, if underlying anxieties continue to provoke the syndrome, psychotherapy is indicated. If patients satisfy the criteria for panic disorder, pharmacotherapy should be considered as well.

b. Bronchial asthma

(1) **Etiology.** Once thought to be caused by psychological factors, asthma attacks now are believed to be the result of a genetic vulnerability exacerbated by allergies and infections. Nevertheless, stress and an inconsistent relationship between an asthmatic child and an overly protective mother may be factors in the onset of specific episodes of illness. Overly dependent patients who react to any slight changes of symptoms and overly independent patients who deny symptoms are both at greater risk for hospitalization than are psychologically normal patients.

(2) **Treatment.** Psychotherapy is usually indicated when anxiety, which may precipitate an asthma attack, is not relieved by the supportive care of a physician. Family therapy may be helpful in separation issues, which may also exacerbate asthma symptoms.

4. Migraine headache

a. Etiology. More than 90% of chronic, recurrent headaches are migraine, tension, or mixed migraine–tension. Whereas muscle tension headaches (often with bilateral occipital or bitemporal distribution) represent muscle spasms, migraine headaches are usually unilateral and represent a period of vasoconstriction (aura) followed by vasodilatation (headache). Although anxiety and stress commonly precipitate all three types of headache, the theory that specific psychological dynamics (e.g., repressed hostility) lead to migraine headaches has not been proved. Many true migraine patients report development of headaches during a period of relaxation after a stressful period. Depression should be ruled out as a cause but treated if present.

b. Treatment

(1) **Drug therapy**

(a) Serotonin-receptor agonists (sumatriptan)

(b) Ergot derivatives and combinations (ergotamine)

(c) β-adrenergic blocking agents (propranolol)

(d) Tricyclic antidepressants

(e) Divalproex sodium

(f) Calcium channel blockers (e.g., verapamil)

(2) **Biofeedback**

(3) **Psychotherapy** in patients with chronic stress

(4) **Hypnosis** and **imagery** to increase peripheral blood flow (e.g., imagining that hand is in warm water) to abort progression from aura to headache

5. Immune disorders. Psychological states affect immune response in complex ways that are not yet fully understood. Stress may depress cell-mediated immune response (via T lymphocytes). Disorders of immune response may involve susceptibility to various conditions.

a. Autoimmune diseases

(1) Systemic lupus erythematosus (SLE)

(2) Rheumatoid arthritis

(3) Pernicious anemia

b. Allergic disorders

c. Cancer. Studies show that patients who react to stress with feelings of hopelessness or depression are at higher risk for cancer.

d. Immune system. Although a controversial subject, increasing evidence suggests **immune system dysfunction** in disorders such as depression.

(1) Evidence also suggests abnormal diurnal variation in circulating natural killer cell phenotypes and cytotoxic activity in patients with major depression.

(2) Interleukin-1β is produced in increased amounts in patients with depression, which in turn may contribute to hypothalamic–pituitary axis dysregulation.

(3) Mortality studies such as record linkage studies report increased mortality from physical illnesses that are at least indirectly associated with lack of full immunologic competence (e.g., deaths from infectious disease, neoplasms associated with major depression).

(4) Clinicians have long noted that stresses, loss, and mental illness are associated with flare-ups in disorders usually kept in some control by the immune system (e.g., melanoma, tuberculosis).

B **General medical conditions presenting as somatoform disorders**   In all of the somatoform disorders, patients may have an undiagnosed physical disorder with inconsistent, vague, or confusing symptoms. Several illnesses should be considered.

1. **SLE and several other autoimmune disorders.** These diseases, which are associated with multiple organ systems, are characterized by exacerbations and remissions. SLE typically begins in late adolescence or the early twenties, and women are nine times more likely to develop SLE than men. The onset may be vague, and psychiatric symptoms (e.g., mood disorders, schizophreniform disorder) may be present.

2. **Endocrine disorders**
   a. **Hyperthyroidism** (thyrotoxicosis) may be present, with complaints of fatigue, palpitations, dyspnea, and anxiety.
   b. **Hypothyroidism** may also manifest with fatigue and anxiety. Mood disorders, including depression, are possible. Menstrual problems are commonly seen and may be dismissed as a somatization problem.
   c. **Hyperparathyroidism** can manifest with severe anxiety, gastrointestinal symptoms, polyuria, and some pain.

3. **Neurologic disorders.** Any physical illness that begins early in life and is associated with an insidious or intermittent onset of symptoms should be considered in the differential diagnosis of somatoform disorder.
   a. **Multiple sclerosis** (MS) may have transient, remitting neurologic symptoms associated with dysphoric mood and anxiety. It often is misdiagnosed as a psychiatric illness early in its course.
   b. **Temporal lobe** or **complex partial seizures** may cause a distorted body image as well as mood disorders and changes in personality.
   c. **Acute intermittent porphyria** (AIP) is rare but may mimic somatization disorder with its gastrointestinal pain and neurologic complaints.
   d. **Other systemic diseases** and toxic or metabolic diseases can present physicians with confusing symptom pictures, particularly early in their course. They should not be dismissed as somatoform disorders, particularly if the symptoms do not fit the "classic" picture of the somatoform disorders.

4. **Psychiatric disorders**
   a. **Major depression** is perhaps the most common illness, with presenting complaints that are comorbid with or mistaken for somatoform disorders.
   b. **Acute adjustment reactions** can manifest as multiple somatic symptoms or preoccupation with symptoms.
   c. **Schizophrenia** occasionally manifests as multiple somatic complaints or delusions.
   d. **Panic disorders** can manifest as multiple somatic complaints and extreme preoccupation with symptoms.
   e. **Personality disorders** frequently coexist with somatoform disorder and should be differentiated from the somatoform disorder for purposes of treatment and diagnosis.

C **Substance abuse**

1. **Alcoholism** remains the major comorbid substance abuse disorder in various psychosomatic and psychophysiologic illnesses.

2. **Opiates** are probably underprescribed for acute pain (e.g., after surgery, acute physical trauma); however, when they are prescribed for chronic pain in patients with somatization disorder, pain disorder, factitious disorder, or conversion disorder represent a threat for addiction.

3. **Other substances** may be abused by vulnerable patients. Benzodiazepines, barbiturates, psychomotor stimulants, and others may be abused by substance-abusing, somaticizing patients.

4. After a particular patient has become **habituated to a prescription** medication and uses it for relief of psychological as well as physical symptoms, **secondary drug-seeking behaviors** may develop (e.g., using multiple doctors simultaneously, magnifying or creating symptoms, and using other people's medications).

D **Dissociative disorders** (see VI)

1. **Significant association** is present among somatization disorder, conversion symptoms, and dissociation symptoms.
   a. An association between somatization disorder and dissociative symptoms is so frequent that they were considered to be in the same diagnostic class in previous editions of the *DSM* (i.e., "psychoneurotic reactions" in *DSM-I*, "hysterical neurosis" in *DSM-II*).
   b. Recent work demonstrates a strong association among somatization, dissociation, and a history of sexual abuse.

2. Clinically, dissociative symptoms are often found in patients with somatization disorder. Some odd symptoms (e.g., picking at skin, pulling own hair) may be mechanisms a particular individual has learned to keep from dissociating.

E **Major depression**

1. A strong tendency exists for **major depression** to present with **somatic complaints** in some cultures, with patients at the same time denying symptoms of depression (e.g., headaches, malaise, abdominal pain in some Asian and Native American cultures). In most of these cases, patients respond well to treatment for major depression.

2. **Major unipolar depression** can manifest atypically, with symptoms resembling almost all of the somatoform disorders, particularly if psychotic and melancholic features are present.

3. In the United States, **hypochondriasis** and **body dysmorphic preoccupations** are not uncommon as features of a major depression.

4. For reasons that remain unclear, major depression is commonly missed and incorrectly treated in primary medical care settings.

5. **Depression concurrent with chronic pain** is quite common. In some studies, up to 87% of patients with chronic pain suffer from major depression.

6. Somaticized presentations seem to be more common in **unipolar depression** than in bipolar depression. Some investigators propose that no somatization disorder is present in the depressed phase of bipolar disorder.

F **Anxiety disorders**

1. **Panic disorder** frequently occurs acutely, with symptoms resembling a myocardial infarction or a pulmonary embolus. Somatic preoccupations with heart disease, seizure disorders, and brain tumors are quite common, chronically, as patients grope for an explanation of their alarming symptoms.
   a. Some studies report that patients with panic disorder have comorbid rates of mitral valve prolapse on echocardiogram of between 10% and 20%. Other studies find no increase in prevalence of mitral valve prolapse compared with the general population.
   b. Cardiovascular causes of death increase the risk of premature death in patients with panic disorder.

2. Patients with **OCD** frequently have health-related preoccupations and rituals that may involve contamination fears and excessive handwashing.

3. **Posttraumatic stress disorder** (PTSD) may involve physical health preoccupations, depending on the nature of the psychological trauma.

G **Psychotic disorders**

1. Occasionally, patients with **schizophrenia** and **schizophreniform disorder** may have primarily somatic hallucinations and delusions. These hallucinations tend to be bizarre enough to be dis-

tinguished easily from symptoms of somatoform disorders (e.g., one's organs are being squeezed by someone's telepathic powers).

2. **Mood congruent hallucinations** and **delusions** involving the body rotting or having cancer are common in patients with psychotic depressions.

3. Distinguishing **folk beliefs** from psychotic and somatoform disorders may be difficult. If other members of the culture or subgroup share the belief system, beliefs should not be called "psychotic."

   a. **Culture-bound somatic syndromes** include **koro,** a syndrome primarily affecting Asian men, in which patients believe that the penis is shrinking into the body, with death as the expected result; and **dhat** in India, in which anxiety and concerns with the discharge of semen are associated with beliefs about weakness and exhaustion.

   b. In the United States, **health-related subcultures** have beliefs about such health topics as the cause of disease, nutrition, vitamin use, and crystals. On occasion, these beliefs lead to behaviors that can cause major health problems and even psychotic symptoms (e.g., fat-soluble vitamin overdose, scopolamine poisoning from too much herbal tea).

   c. Patients with limited information about health, physiology, and anatomy sometimes present with physical complaints that are grossly incorrect. This aspect should be seen as an educational problem rather than as a psychotic symptom in the absence of other symptoms of psychotic disorders.

4. Patients with **psychotic physical delusions** and **hallucinations** generally respond to the treatment of the specific psychotic disorder producing the symptom.

H Other psychiatric disorders

1. **Personality disorders** may manifest as a variety of physical preoccupations, concerns, and symptoms of a psychological etiology.

   a. Patients with **antisocial personality disorder** are likely to produce symptoms of malingering when legal cases promise substantial potential reward, when they can escape the legal consequences of their acts, or when they can otherwise experience profits through "secondary gain."

   b. Patients with **borderline personality disorder** may create injuries or harm themselves in ways that may resemble factitious disorder or malingering. However, the motivation does not appear to be adopting a sick role but rather relieving psychological distress through the self-mutilating act.

   c. Patients with **histrionic and narcissistic personality disorders** magnify symptoms of physical illnesses as a means of making themselves the center of attention and ensuring what they believe to be adequate commitment from the health care provider.

2. Patients with **social phobias** and **avoidant personality disorder** may avoid health care settings because of fears about having to disrobe and talk to a physician. They may even postpone treatment of very serious illnesses (e.g., myocardial infarctions, cancer).

V SPECIFIC SOMATOFORM AND RELATED DISORDERS

A Somatization disorder

1. **Epidemiology.** Approximately 1% of women have somatization disorder, and the ratio of women to men is 10:1. It is thought to be less common in individuals with higher education. Prevalence and incidence differ among cultures and ethnic groups.

2. **Etiology**

   a. Recent studies suggest a significant **genetic component** to somatization disorder. It has been linked to a high incidence of:

   (1) Alcoholism and other substance-use disorders in first-degree male relatives

   (2) Antisocial personality disorder in first-degree male relatives

   (3) Somatization disorder in first-degree female relatives

   b. **Adoption studies** of female children of somatizing women showed a markedly increased rate of somatization disorder compared with control groups.

    c. Environmental influences are suggested by an increased rate of somatization disorder when children are raised in chaotic circumstances involving parental divorce, poverty, and alcoholism.

    d. Evidence of **dysfunction on neuropsychiatric tests** has led some investigators to hypothesize that patients have an impaired ability to screen out somatic sensations.

    e. Secondary gains of the sick role may provide a learned component of the disorder.

3. Associated features

    a. Excessive medical evaluations with frequent consultation with multiple physicians

    b. Unnecessary invasive diagnostic procedures and surgery

    c. Anxiety and depressive symptoms, which are common in this population

    d. A wide range of associated interpersonal difficulties, including marital and parenting problems

    e. Substance abuse, including prescribed medications

    f. Suicidal ideation, particularly in patients with substance abuse problems and depression

    g. Sexual function impairment (i.e., lack of interest in sex, specific sexual dysfunctions)

4. Differential diagnosis. Disorders to be ruled out include major depression, general medical conditions, schizophrenia, panic disorder, and hypochondriasis.

5. Treatment. Therapy is often frustrating for physicians, who should expect and accept their own feelings of frustration and anger when managing patients with this condition. Somatization disorder is best conceptualized as a lifelong disorder rather than a curable condition. Symptoms tend to fluctuate with stress in patients' lives. General principles of treatment include:

    a. Regular appointments so that patients are assured of an ongoing, supportive relationship with one physician. Appointments should focus on life stresses and the patient's functioning rather than on symptoms. Recent studies have shown that supportive treatment reduces use of health services (e.g., emergency department visits), hospital days, and physician charges. Periodic visits should include a limited but reasonable examination of new symptoms.

    b. Consolidation of care with one physician to minimize medications, reduce surgery, and limit diagnostic evaluations to a reasonable level.

    c. Avoidance of unnecessary surgery. Surgical procedures should be considered only for clear indications. Physicians should thoughtfully consider the expected gains compared with the potential complications. Frequently, the initial surgery is followed by multiple subsequent surgeries for "adhesions."

    d. Avoidance of habit-forming medications. Little or no medication should be given for questionable indications.

    e. Appropriate evaluation of new symptoms when they occur. Patients with somatization disorder are still at risk for organic illness.

    f. Adequate use of antidepressant medications. Outcome studies demonstrate a much improved result for patients with somatization disorder who have depressive symptoms, in contrast to patients with the disorder but without depressive features.

    g. Use of monoamine oxidase (MAO) inhibitors. These agents are reported to be very effective in some patients with somatization disorder.

B **Conversion disorder** (non–*DSM-IV* criteria)

1. Clinical presentation

    a. Associated features. Conversion disorder involves the unconscious "conversion of a psychological conflict" into a loss of physical functioning, which suggests a neurologic disease or other disease. The symptom is temporally related to a psychosocial stressor.

        (1) An **additional psychiatric diagnosis** (e.g., adjustment disorder, schizophrenia, personality disorder) can be made in 30% to 50% of patients.

        (2) Conversion disorders are also seen in patients with real organic physical illness.

        (3) *La belle indifference,* in which patients exhibit little concern over the symptoms, is sometimes present. However, it is not a reliable sign of conversion alone because patients with a physical illness may be stoic about their condition.

        (4) Modeling is common. Patients may unconsciously imitate the symptoms observed in important individuals in their lives.

    b. **Symptoms.** Although most conversion symptoms are transient, some can have a chronic course and result in a significant disability. Also, symptoms may be inconsistent with known pathophysiology such as a stocking-glove anesthesia. Patients classically present with an acute loss of function, which suggests neurologic disease. Symptoms may be bizarre or unusual, including:

        (1) Paresthesias and anesthesias

        (2) Gait disturbances (e.g., astasia, abasia)

        (3) Paralysis

        (4) Loss of consciousness and seizures

        (5) Aphonia

        (6) Vomiting

        (7) Fainting

        (8) Visual disturbances (e.g., blindness, tunnel vision)

2. Epidemiology. Incidence and prevalence are not known with certainty; however, conversion disorder seems to be less common now than in the past, and it may present with less classic symptomatology than was seen previously. Conversion disorder is seen more frequently in low socioeconomic classes, and some cultures have much greater rates of conversion disorder than others. Although the disorder occurs more commonly in women, it is seen in men as well. Onset is usually in adolescence through the twenties; however, it can occur at any age.

3. Etiology. Causes are thought to be psychological.

    a. **Two mechanisms** have been described that explain the gains experienced by patients with conversion disorder.

        (1) The **primary gain** is that the internal conflict is kept from consciousness.

        (2) The **secondary gain** is reinforcement from the environment (e.g., a patient who avoids unpleasant duties because of the symptoms). Some secondary gain is seen in almost all illnesses, however.

    b. **Other causes** that have been postulated include the following:

        (1) Less powerful individuals gain control over the environment by the elaboration of symptoms (i.e., the concern and attention of others are focused on the patient).

        (2) Symptoms are learned and are then reinforced by the reactions of those around patients.

        (3) Symptoms are seen more frequently in patients with brain injuries and other neurologic defects, which suggests a physiologic contribution.

4. Differential diagnosis. It is important to note that between 15% and 30% of patients diagnosed as having conversion disorder have an undiagnosed physical illness (e.g., MS, other neurologic conditions). Approximately 20% of cases initially diagnosed as conversion disorder have been later diagnosed as somatization disorder.

5. Prognosis. A good prognosis is associated with:

    a. Good premorbid functioning

    b. Acute onset

    c. An obvious stressful precipitant

6. Treatment

    a. **Attention to the possibility of organic disease is critical.** However, workups should be based only on objective findings. First, organic causes of the symptom must be considered and ruled out. If an organic condition such as intoxication with anticonvulsants is present, treatment of the organic condition may often lead to the resolution of the conversion symptom.

    b. Stressful events in patients' lives should be evaluated, and appropriate intervention such as psychotherapy or family therapy should be provided. Associated psychiatric illness (e.g., depression) should be treated, which may involve pharmacologic approaches.

    c. The patients' symptoms have a psychological basis, but confronting patients with this fact is not helpful. Some patients come to understand the symbolic aspect of the symptom and gain conscious mastery of the conflict. However, most patients are receptive to the explanation that the disorder is a reaction to stress and to the reassurance that the condition will resolve over time. These interventions may allow patients to let go of symptoms without losing face.

d. Suggestion during hypnosis or an amobarbital (Amytal) interview that the symptoms will improve can result in dramatic resolution. Symptom substitution, suggested in the psychodynamic literature, is relatively rare in actual practice.

C **Pain disorder**

1. **Clinical presentation.** Patients complain of pain for which there is no demonstrable physical cause or pain that is excessive given the known organic pathology. Generally, this disorder results in significant impairment and inability to function.

   a. Clinical differentiation of pain disorder from chronic pain itself may be difficult, and the distinction between pain disorder and chronic pain itself may not be terribly useful in daily practice. In both pain disorder and chronic pain, accepting the patient's pain is a good starting place for treatment. Individual differences in pain threshold, depressive and anxiety symptoms, and physical pathology that may have been missed dictate caution in making this diagnosis. As patients with pain disorder are followed over time, an organic cause of the pain becomes clear in a portion of the group.

   b. In some cases, **psychological factors** appear to play a role in the symptoms such as:

      (1) Secondary gain because of financial compensation

      (2) Avoidance of objectionable work

      (3) Control of significant others

   c. In other cases, there is little indication of psychological factors.

   d. Most cases of chronic pain involve both physical and psychological contributions, which can lead to:

      (1) Problems with the physician–patient relationship

      (2) Multiple physical examinations

      (3) Unnecessary surgery

      (4) Substance abuse

2. **Epidemiology. Incidence and prevalence** are unknown. However, pain disorder is a common condition in primary care settings. The disorder occurs more frequently in women than in men.

3. **Etiology**

   a. Psychological factors

      (1) Patients may have learned as children to express emotions physically instead of verbally.

      (2) Patients may be unconsciously reinforced by the sick role.

      (3) When compensation for injury is an issue, patients may be consciously or unconsciously reinforced for illness behavior.

      (4) Many patients report histories of deprivation, neglect, or abuse, which may make them more vulnerable as adults.

      (5) Many patients have a history of working at an early age, holding physically demanding jobs, and centering their lives around work.

   b. Physical theories

      (1) Endogenous opiate substances (endorphins) in the brain, which raise the pain threshold, may be altered genetically, developmentally, or secondarily to stress, making these individuals more prone to continued pain.

      (2) Monoamine neurotransmitters (particularly serotonin) appear to be involved in pain inhibitory fibers in the brain stem. This neurotransmitter system may be altered genetically, developmentally, or secondarily to stress, which results in continued pain perception. This hypothesis is supported by patients' responsiveness to tricyclic antidepressants.

      (3) A possible genetic component is suggested by the increased incidence of first-degree relatives with:

         (a) Chronic pain

         (b) Depression

         (c) Alcohol dependence

         (d) Substance abuse

4. **Differential diagnosis** (see IV E). This disorder requires a thorough diagnostic workup to rule out organic pathology. Other disorders to be ruled out include hypochondriasis, somatization,

depression with somatic symptoms, and schizophrenia. When secondary gain (e.g., financial compensation) is evident, conscious simulation of the pain symptom (i.e., malingering) must be considered. When the assumption of the role of a patient is repeatedly the goal of the consciously produced symptom, factitious disorder must be considered. Also, personality and cultural attributes must be taken into consideration; for example, a dramatic, histrionic presentation of organic pain should not be confused with somatoform pain disorder.

5. **Prognosis**
   a. **Duration of illness.** The longer the duration, the less likely the chance of functional recovery. Very few patients with chronic pain of greater than 5 years' duration improve.
   b. **Age.** The older the patient, the less likely the chance of recovery.
   c. **Secondary gain.** The more reinforcement (financial, social, or otherwise) for the symptom, the less likely the chance of recovery. Many clinicians who treat patients with chronic pain refuse to treat their patients with pending litigation because of the poor outcome under these circumstances.
   d. **Coexisting personality disorder** is also a negative prognostic factor.
   e. Prominent depressive features are considered a good prognostic feature if patients consent to treatment for the depression. (Surprisingly, few patients actually consent.)

6. **Treatment.** This condition is notoriously difficult to treat; although many patients can make significant improvements in functioning, few are cured.
   a. **Medications**
      (1) **Chronic narcotic use,** paradoxically, is not helpful in chronic pain because patients become habituated to the narcotics, which results in a loss of the analgesic effect and a vulnerability to withdrawal symptoms. Because of the peaks and valleys of short-acting narcotic blood levels, these agents can actually exacerbate chronic pain symptoms. Detoxification can improve pain symptoms. For a minority of patients with chronic pain who appear to require chronic narcotic treatment, a long-acting preparation such as methadone is preferable.
      (2) **Sedative–hypnotics** depress the nervous system and increase pain perceptions as well as inactivity. Therefore, they should be avoided.
      (3) **Antidepressants** may be useful. From 50% to 60% of patients report improvements in sleep, sense of well-being, and pain perception with tricyclic antidepressants (up to 87% in some studies). Some controversy exists in terms of what doses of antidepressants to use. Doses lower than antidepressant doses may be adequate for treatment of chronic pain (e.g., 75 to 125 mg/day amitriptyline or equivalent) versus an antidepressant dose (150 to 225 mg/day for adults). Antidepressant doses must be adjusted carefully because of the other medications these patients may be taking.
   b. **Therapies**
      (1) **Psychotherapy** may be useful. Supportive approaches are useful in helping patients deal with life stresses that may exacerbate pain symptoms. Cognitive and interpersonal therapy are indicated if patients have prominent depressive or anxiety symptoms.
      (2) **Behavioral therapy** focuses on reinforcing wellness instead of sick role behavior. Although this approach may not affect patients' perception of pain, it is effective in improving the level of patient functioning. By reducing the secondary gain from the symptoms, patients may devote less attention to the pain.
      (3) **Family therapy** is a useful adjunctive approach when family dynamics reinforce a patient's sick role and undermine attempts to improve functional capacity.
      (4) **Group therapy,** where available, is a useful adjunct in supporting patients' efforts to improve functional capacity.
   c. **Multidisciplinary approaches,** which are usually available in pain clinic settings, allow a comprehensive treatment plan, which some patients may need to maximize their functioning. It may involve the previously mentioned strategies, as well as:
      (1) Physical therapy
      (2) Occupational therapy
      (3) Biofeedback training
      (4) Relaxation techniques

        (5) Hypnosis

        (6) Acupuncture

        (7) Neurosurgical ablation of pain tracts

        (8) Transcutaneous electrical stimulation

7. Prevention

    a. Information about preventing pain disorder is inadequate. However, some pain experts suggest that, paradoxically, inadequate treatment of acute pain may lead to the development of chronic pain. These experts suggest adequate prescription of narcotics after surgery or physical trauma, but they avoid chronic narcotic prescriptions.

    b. Adequate screening and treatment of major depression and other psychiatric disorders are helpful in people whose pain complaints extend beyond the expected time or severity after surgery or trauma.

D **Hypochondriasis**

1. Clinical presentation. Patients are chronically preoccupied with fears that they have an illness despite thorough evaluation and reassurance from the physician that no organic problems can be found.

    a. Normal physical sensations such as sweating and bowel movements **are misinterpreted. Minor ailments** such as cough or backache **are exaggerated.** Minor physical symptoms are interpreted as being of sinister health significance, and vigilance may become a form of auto-suggestion. The fear and misperception become a cyclic, self-reinforcing pattern. For example, patients may believe that a cough or a mole is cancerous, and close observation of the cough or mole convinces patients that the fear is realistic.

    b. "Doctor shopping" is common and is a frustration for both patients and physicians. Simple reassurance that the feared symptom is not serious is interpreted by a particular patient as evidence that the treating physician is not taking the situation seriously. The patient then seeks another doctor.

    c. Anxious and depressed mood as well as obsessive-compulsive features are commonly observed and suggest a good prognosis with treatment of the primary condition.

    d. Impairment can be mild or so severe as to result in invalidism.

    e. In general, these patients do not accept the idea that they have a psychiatric disorder.

2. Epidemiology

    a. As many as 1% of the population may be hypochondriacal, and the condition is commonly seen in medical practice. Equal numbers of men and women are affected.

    b. Usual age of onset is between age 20 and 30 years, but patients most commonly present to the physician in their forties and fifties.

3. Etiology. Patients with primary hypochondriasis may have been raised in homes with excessive concern about illness or little parental warmth except when children were ill. Hypochondriasis that occurs in the course of another psychiatric illness is thought to be a part of the familiar symptoms that develop in the primary illness (e.g., the foreboding of anxiety, the hopelessness of depression, or the delusional beliefs of schizophrenia). **Cognitive and behavioral theories** suggest the cyclic pattern of fear, vigilance, and distorted reasoning, which are also common to the development of phobias.

4. Differential diagnosis. Other conditions that must be ruled out are:

    a. Depression

    b. Panic attacks

    c. OCD

    d. Schizophrenia

    e. Somatization disorder

    f. Actual physical pathology

    g. Personality disorders (if comorbid condition, a poor prognostic feature)

5. Treatment

    a. Physician reaction to hypochondriacal patients is often negative. Physicians who are unaware of such feelings may act on them in an antitherapeutic way such as overprescribing medication or performing unnecessary diagnostic procedures.

b. Physicians should acknowledge that patients are concerned and want assistance early in treatment. A sympathetic, educational approach to patients is ideal. As soon as rapport is established, screening for other conditions, particularly depression, anxiety, and OCD, should be undertaken. Regular follow-up appointments to evaluate new symptoms are often helpful and reassuring.

c. It may be necessary to prescribe medication; however, patients should be told that it will help but not "cure" the ailment. Narcotics and other habit-forming drugs should not be prescribed in the absence of physical pathology (although hypochondriacal patients can also get broken legs, for example, which should be treated normally).

d. **Pimozide** is reported to be dramatically effective in some patients with hypochondriasis of a delusional intensity, but this agent is not approved for this use in the United States. (It is approved in the United States only for the treatment of Tourette's disorder.)

E Body dysmorphic disorder

1. **Clinical presentation.** The hallmark of this disorder is preoccupation with some imagined defect in the body, usually of the face. Usually a history shows frequent visits to doctors, especially dermatologists or plastic surgeons. Depressive mood and obsessive compulsive traits are common.

2. **Epidemiology. Incidence and etiology** are unknown. Even epidemiologic studies admit probable underestimation of the prevalence of the disorder because most of these patients have shame about reporting their symptoms.

3. **Differential diagnosis**
   a. If the symptom is of delusional intensity, it should be classified as a **delusional disorder, somatic subtype,** which may be responsive to antipsychotic medication.
   b. Major depression and schizophrenia should be ruled out. This process may be difficult if distorted ideas about the body reach delusional proportions. Many patients with body dysmorphic disorder have symptoms such as ideas of reference related to their symptoms.
   c. Recent evidence suggests strong links between OCD and body dysmorphic disorder, and suggests that they sometimes co-occur.
   d. Anorexia nervosa and body dysmorphic disorder should be differentiated.
   e. Personality disorders in the context of this disorder represent a poor prognostic feature.

4. **Treatment**
   a. Invasive diagnostic procedures or unnecessary surgery should be avoided. When reconstructive surgery is undertaken, patients are unlikely to be satisfied with the results.
   b. There are some reports of medication treatment with antidepressants (SSRIs and MAO inhibitors) and neuroleptics (pimozide) being therapeutic.
   c. There are anecdotal reports of behavior therapy and dynamic psychotherapy being effective; an educational–supportive approach has been reported to have some success.

F Environmental illness A relatively new phenomenon, environmental illness is a polysymptomatic disorder that some experts believe is associated with immune system dysfunction and allergy-like sensitivity to many compounds in food and air. Early studies suggest an association with increased somatic, mood, and anxiety symptoms indicative of personality disorders. Clinicians working with affected patients report very high levels of depression and anxiety in this population. This phenomenon may represent the emergence of a new culture-bound disorder in the United States and Europe, as was found with people who compulsively exercise to the point of physical damage.

VI DISSOCIATIVE DISORDERS

A Clinical presentation This group of four disorders is known for their disruptions in consciousness, memory, identity, or perception of the environment.

1. **Dissociative amnesia** is an inability to recall important personal information usually of a traumatic nature that is not ordinary forgetfulness.

2. **Dissociative fugue** is characterized by sudden, unexpected travel away from home with an inability to recall one's past and failure to recall personal information. Sometimes with the assumption of a new identity.

3. **Dissociative identity disorder** is the presence of two or more distinct identities or personality states that recurrently take control of the individual's behavior.

4. **Depersonalization disorder** is a recurrent feeling of being detached from one's mental processes or body with intact reality testing.

B **Epidemiology and etiology**   Limited for this group of disorders. Dissociative amnesia, dissociative identity disorder, and depersonalization disorder tend to occur more often in women. Dissociative amnesia, dissociative fugue, and dissociative identity disorder tend to occur after some traumatic event.

C **Treatment**   Limited for this group of disorders. Hypnosis and drug-assisted interviews with short-acting barbiturates (e.g., sodium amobarbital) may help recover lost memories. Psychotherapy may help to address issues surrounding the underlying events.

VII   FACTITIOUS DISORDER

A **Clinical presentation**   Patients are in voluntary control of their symptoms in that, although their behavior is deliberate, what precipitates this behavior is not.

1. **Symptoms.** Patients may complain of pain in a range of circumstances such as when they feel no pain or after self-inflicted infection such as that arising from self-injection with feces or saliva, which can develop into life-threatening illness. The medical knowledge of patients is often highly sophisticated. By complaining of bizarre or unusual symptoms, these patients may encourage invasive diagnostic procedures such as laparotomy or angiography. Patients may lie about any aspect of their history with a dramatic flair (**pseudologia fantastica**). Narcotic abuse and addiction are associated findings in about half of these patients.

2. **History.** At hospital admission, the patient's behavior is disruptive and demanding. Symptoms change as workups prove negative. Eventually, patients are confronted with evidence of faking, and they usually react angrily and leave against medical advice. This pattern of behavior can become chronic and involve multiple admissions to different hospitals. It is then called **Münchausen syndrome.**

B **Epidemiology**   The disorder may seem to be more common than it actually is because a single patient may interact with many physicians in different hospitals. It usually begins in adulthood and is a lifelong condition.

C **Etiology**   Although an illness or operation in early childhood may be a contributing factor, the disorder is considered to be entirely psychological. There may have been an experience with a physician in early life through a family relationship or through illness. A significant portion of these patients are employed in the health care field as paraprofessionals. Masochism has been considered an important feature in patients who seek unnecessary surgery. The illness has also been conceptualized as a variant of the borderline syndrome in that the physician becomes the perpetual object of transference; patients continually reenact with the physician the disordered relationship with their parents. Object loss or fear of loss is frequently reported as a precipitant of an episode. Studies indicate relatively frequent electroencephalogram (EEG) abnormalities in this group, suggesting some central nervous system (CNS) dysfunction.

D **Differential diagnosis**

1. **Physical illness.** A patient with a true physical disorder may present the symptoms with an unusual or dramatic flair that makes the physician suspicious of faking and that is more likely to occur if the patient also has a personality disorder, including one of the following types:
   a. Histrionic
   b. Borderline
   c. Schizotypal

2. **Somatization disorder.** The symptoms are not under patients' voluntary control, and patients do not usually insist on hospitalization. Conversion disorder may also be present.

3. **Hypochondriasis.** The essential feature of this disorder is the patient's preoccupation with the illness in general rather than with symptoms. The symptoms are not under the patient's voluntary control. Hypochondriasis starts later in life than factitious disorder, and patients with hypochondriasis are less likely to insist on hospital admission or submit to dangerous diagnostic procedures.

4. **Malingering.** Although it is difficult to differentiate between malingering and factitious disorder, the goals in malingering are clear to both patients and physicians, and the symptoms can be stopped when they no longer serve an end. In patients with factitious disorder, the goal of the behavior seems to be the patient role itself, in contrast to other secondary gain features of malingering.

E Treatment Patients with factitious disorder with physical symptoms rarely receive psychiatric treatment. The reactions of the treatment team are usually strongly negative, and this countertransference must be examined. Until patients are willing to face the reality of a psychiatric illness and agree to psychiatric hospitalization or treatment, the prognosis is likely to be poor. The therapeutic approach is one of management rather than cure, and unnecessary diagnostic procedures should be avoided. Patients should be confronted in a calm, noncondemning, indirect manner. There should be minimal expectation that patients admit the deception. Treatment must involve coordination with other treatment providers. The focus of therapy is usually underlying dynamic issues. When medication is used, it should target specific comorbid conditions and symptoms such as depression.

F Factitious disorder by proxy (Münchausen's by proxy) Currently, this disorder is classified as factitious disorder not otherwise specified in the *DSM-IV*. In this condition, intentional production of symptoms occurs in individuals who are under the care of other persons. Perpetrators desire to attain the sick role by proxy. There are *DSM-IV* research criteria for the disorder.

VIII MALINGERING

A Clinical presentation Malingering **is not considered a mental disorder or an illness.** Malingering individuals fully and deliberately fake or exaggerate illness with the conscious intent to deceive others. Their reasons for faking illness (e.g., monetary and legal concerns) can be understood by examining the circumstances affecting these individuals rather than their psychological constitutions. Individuals are often evasive and uncooperative on examination, and a marked discrepancy appears between their claimed disability and the physical findings. Individuals who malinger may have an antisocial personality disorder (see Chapter 2: IV A).

B Epidemiology True malingering is rarely seen. Physicians are more likely to misdiagnose this condition in patients with one of the somatoform disorders because they have a negative reaction to patients and are unable to see that patients are not consciously faking another disorder such as hypochondriasis.

C Differential diagnosis In **factitious disorder** with physical symptoms, the patient's goals cannot be clearly understood as they can in the case of malingering, even though the patient is voluntarily causing the symptoms of illness.

D Treatment Because malingering is not an illness, it has **no medical or psychiatric treatment.**

IX PLACEBO RESPONSE

A Definition This condition has been defined as any effect attributable to a medication, procedure, or other form of therapy but not to the specific pharmacologic property of that therapy.

B Epidemiology All medical treatments can show the effects of nonspecific curative factors, or placebo effects. For instance, 30% to 40% of patients in pain respond as well to placebos as they do to morphine. No particular personality type responds to a placebo (e.g., a histrionic patient is no more likely to have a placebo response than is any other patient).

C **Significance** Physicians use the placebo response (mistakenly) to help differentiate "real" from "psychological" symptoms in their patients. The placebo response is a powerful aspect of most medical care. It operates commonly, even when the physician is unaware of it. However, **it does not differentiate physical from psychological symptoms.** Recent findings suggest that the placebo response to pain is a **physiologic phenomenon.** Placebo response can be blocked by a narcotic antagonist, naloxone, which suggests that the analgesic effect of a placebo may be based on the action of endorphins, the naturally occurring opioid substances in the brain, which increase the pain threshold.

BIBLIOGRAPHY

American Psychiatric Association: *Diagnostic and Statistical Manual of Mental Disorders,* 4th ed. Washington, DC, American Psychiatric Association Press, 1994.

DeLeon J, Bott A, Simpson GM: Dysmorphophobia: Body dysmorphic disorder or delusional disorder, somatic subtype? *Compr Psychiatry* 30:457–472, 1989.

Fallon BA, Schneir FR, Narshall R, et al: The pharmacotherapy of hypochondriasis. *Psychopharmacol Bull* 32:607–611, 1996.

Folks DG, Ford CW, Houck CA: Somatoform disorders, factitious disorders, and malingering. In *Clinical Psychiatry for Medical Students,* 3rd ed. Edited by Stoudemire A. Philadelphia, Lippincott-Raven, 1998, pp 343–381.

Jellinek MJ, Herzog DB: The somatoform disorders. In *Textbook of Child and Adolescent Psychiatry,* 2nd ed. Edited by Wiener JM. Washington, DC, American Psychiatric Press, 1997, pp 431–436.

Kent DA, Thomasson K, Coryell W: Course and outcome of conversion and somatization disorders. *Psychosomatics* 36:138–144, 1995.

Leamin MH, Plewes J: Factitious disorders and malingering. In *Essentials of Clinical Psychiatry,* 3rd ed. Edited by Hales RE, Yudofsky SC. Washington, DC, American Psychiatric Press, 1999, pp 439–451.

Martin RL, Yutzy SH: Somatoform disorders. In *Essentials of Clinical Psychiatry,* 3rd ed. Edited by Hales RE, Yudofsky SC. Washington, DC, American Psychiatric Press, 1999, pp 413–437.

Nernzer ED: Somatoform disorders. In *Child and Adolescent Psychiatry: A Comprehensive Textbook,* 2nd ed. Edited by Lewis M. Baltimore, Williams & Wilkins, 1996, pp 693–702.

Phillips KA: Body dysmorphic disorder: Diagnosis and treatment of imagined ugliness. *J Clin Psychiatry* 57(suppl):61–65, 1996.

Riding J, Munro A: Pimozide in the treatment of monosymptomatic hypochondriacal psychosis. *Acta Psychiatr Scand* 52:23–30, 1975.

Sadock BJ, Sadock VA: *Kaplan & Sadock's: Synopsis of Psychiatry,* 9th ed. Baltimore, Williams & Wilkins, 2003.

Weaver RC, Rodnick JE: Type A behavior: Clinical significance, evaluation, and management. *J Fam Pract* 23:255–61, 1986.

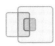 *Study Questions*

Directions: *Each of the numbered items or incomplete statements in this section is followed by answers or by completions of the statement. Select the ONE lettered answer or completion that is BEST in each case.*

1. A 53-year-old Asian man is brought to the clinic believing that his penis is shrinking into his body. He now has no energy. He thinks that he may eventually die from this problem. Which one of the following diagnoses is most appropriate?

- A Conversion disorder
- B Major depression
- C Psychotic disorder not otherwise specified
- D Somatization disorder
- E Diagnosis deferred on Axis 1

2. A 54-year-old mechanic has been unable to work for 2 years because of chronic back pain caused by lifting a heavy toolbox. Repeated neurologic and neuroradiologic examinations reveal muscle spasm and pain in the L4–L5 area, which occasionally is referred in the expected distribution. No herniations, tears, or fractures have been found. Which one of the following would be a single best intervention for this patient?

- A Antidepressants
- B Anti-inflammatory agents
- C Benzodiazepines
- D Family therapy
- E Narcotic analgesics

3. A 55-year-old woman is seen on a medical service for complaints of abdominal pain. The physician notes a history of lifelong poor health and multiple past somatic complaints. Which of the following is the best treatment strategy?

- A A trial of monoamine oxidase (MAO) inhibitors
- B Placement on long-term benzodiazepine medications
- C Immediate transfer to the psychiatry service
- D Appointments in the outpatient medicine clinic for periodic evaluations of the patient's symptoms by the same attending physician
- E A trial of neuroleptic medication to control the delusional aspects of the illness

4. A 63-year-old man presents with a preoccupation with his bowel movements. He is convinced that this irregularity, which did not begin until during the past year, represents an occult cancer. Repeated examinations and a lower gastrointestinal series reveal no abnormalities. No occult blood is present in the stool. Which of the following is the most likely diagnosis?

- A Conversion disorder
- B Hypochondriasis
- C Major depression
- D Panic disorder
- E Somatization disorder

5. A 38-year-old woman sees her internist to be checked for colon cancer. She reports recent constipation and a family history of colon cancer. She denies other symptoms, and her organic workup is negative. She becomes irritated when she is reassured about her physical health and believes the evaluation was not complete. Which of the following statements about the patient is most likely to be correct?

- A Her disorder affects women more often than men.
- B She perceives her bodily functions more acutely than others.
- C Medication will cure her disorder.
- D Narcotic analgesics are the treatment of choice.
- E It is unlikely that she will seek another medical opinion.

6. A 35-year-old woman presents with a 10-year history of numerous physical complaints with negative organic workups. Given her most likely diagnosis:

- Ⓐ There is a high incidence of a family history of alcoholism in male relatives in this disorder.
- Ⓑ There is a high incidence of somatization disorder in female relatives in this disorder.
- Ⓒ There is an increased rate of this disorder in persons raised in chaotic settings.
- Ⓓ All of the above
- Ⓔ None of the above

7. What should treatment of body dysmorphic disorder include?

- Ⓐ Surgery
- Ⓑ SSRIs
- Ⓒ Long-term psychotherapy
- Ⓓ All of the above
- Ⓔ None of the above

8. Patients with somatization disorder

- Ⓐ are often underevaluated medically.
- Ⓑ commonly experience anxiety and depressive symptoms.
- Ⓒ have no need for evaluation of medical symptoms.
- Ⓓ often require use of benzodiazepines.
- Ⓔ are rarely frustrating to treat.

9. Many patients with conversion disorder

- Ⓐ have comorbid body dysmorphic disorder.
- Ⓑ with an obvious stressful precipitant have a poor prognosis.
- Ⓒ respond to benzodiazepines.
- Ⓓ are later diagnosed with a physical illness that explains their symptoms.
- Ⓔ intentionally produce their symptoms.

10. Conversion disorder symptoms

- Ⓐ are culturally sanctioned.
- Ⓑ affect voluntary motor or sensory function.
- Ⓒ are not associated with stressors.
- Ⓓ are intentionally produced.
- Ⓔ are rarely comorbid with another psychiatric diagnosis.

11. The following diagnoses occur more frequently in women than in men.

- Ⓐ Conversion disorder
- Ⓑ Pain disorder
- Ⓒ Somatization disorder
- Ⓓ All of the above
- Ⓔ None of the above

12. In factitious disorder,

- Ⓐ Symptoms are not under the patient's voluntary control.
- Ⓑ The primary goal of the symptoms is secondary gain.
- Ⓒ The physician may become the perpetual object of transference.
- Ⓓ Substance addiction is rare.
- Ⓔ None of the above

13. What does malingering involve?

- Ⓐ Consciously faking an illness
- Ⓑ The intent to deceive others
- Ⓒ No medical or psychiatric treatment
- Ⓓ All of the above
- Ⓔ None of the above

14. The placebo response

[A] helps to differentiate "real" from "psychological" symptoms in patients.

[B] to pain is a physiologic phenomenon.

[C] is more likely to occur in a histrionic patient.

[D] is a minimal part of most medical treatment.

Directions: *Each set of matching questions in this section consists of a list of seven lettered options followed by several items. For each numbered item, select the ONE lettered option that is most closely associated with it. Each lettered option may be selected once, more than once, or not at all.*

QUESTIONS 15–20

Match the following symptoms to the disorder most likely to be associated with it.

[A] Conversion disorder

[B] Dissociative fugue

[C] Dissociative identity disorder

[D] General medical condition

[E] Major depression

[F] Panic disorder

[G] Somatization disorder

15. Unilateral temporal headache, parietal headache, or both

16. Sudden loss of sensation and flaccid paralysis of the entire left arm in a 20-year-old woman

17. General malaise in a 50-year-old man with a negative workup

18. Complaints of episodic chest tightness and breathing difficulty in a 28-year-old woman with a negative workup

19. Chronic, multiple system physical complaints in a 40-year-old woman with a negative organic evaluation

20. 32-year-old woman who disappeared 5 years ago after the accidental death of her child shows up in a town 100 miles away with a new identity and no memory of her previous life

QUESTIONS 21–23

Match the following symptoms to the medical condition most likely to be associated with it.

[A] Depressive symptoms

[B] Schizophreniform disorder symptoms

[C] Panic disorder symptoms

21. Paroxysmal atrial tachycardia

22. Toxic delirium

23. Hypothyroidism

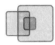

Answers and Explanations

1. The answer is E [*IV G 3 a*]. Without culture-specific information, the clinician has no idea whether this man's beliefs are associated with those of his culture. In this case, the culture-bound somatic syndrome, koro, accounts for his feelings. It is commonly assumed that his complaint is a symptom of psychosis and that treatment with a neuroleptic agent will be beneficial. Not only would this not help him, but it also exposes him to unnecessary additional risk. Although the patient may be depressed, his depression may have been triggered by his belief that he will die. The symptoms do not follow the pattern of a conversion or somatization disorder. In this case, the clinician's best choice is to defer the diagnosis and to seek consultation from another member of the culture, ideally a health care provider or traditional healer.

2. The answer is A [*V C 6*]. One would never treat a patient on the basis of such limited information or limit treatment to a single intervention. However, given the chronicity of the pain, the disproportionate level of disability, and the stability of the condition, antidepressants would probably be the best choice. The only bad choice of the group would be a narcotic analgesic. Although effective in the treatment of patients with acute pain, the role of narcotics in chronic pain is quite limited. The chances are that this patient would become habituated without long-term benefit from narcotics. The doses of antidepressant are controversial; some clinicians believe that a nonantidepressant dose is adequate, but others advocate an antidepressant dose.

3. The answer is D [*V A 5 a*]. The best treatment strategy involves continuity of care as the most important aspect of patient care. At each scheduled visit, the physician conservatively evaluates new symptoms, attempts to keep the patient away from exploratory or nonindicated surgery, and avoids giving the patient narcotics and other habituating medications. Any medication should be prescribed only in the context of an ongoing relationship with a single doctor to avoid "doctor shopping" and multiple prescriptions of habituating medications. Monoamine oxidase (MAO) inhibitors should be considered only with adequate informed consent after the physician knows the patient well. Benzodiazepines should be used with caution because of the propensity for patients with somatization disorder to become habituated and to use them in greater than prescribed amounts. Transfer to the psychiatry service will likely be opposed by the patient, who will view it as a rejection and evidence of lack of competence of the medical service. The patient is likely to try to get another doctor to diagnose and treat her condition adequately. Neuroleptic medications should be avoided because they are unlikely to produce substantial benefit, yet they run the risk of producing tardive dyskinesia.

4. The answer is C [*IV B 4; V A, B, D*]. Major depression is the likely diagnosis on the basis of prevalence in the population, patient age, and patient symptoms. The most significant issue is the age of onset. For all of these disorders except major depression, onset beyond age 35 years is very unusual. It is likely that the patient is facing retirement, which may be a major stressor and a threat to his identity. Hypochondriasis is a possibility. However, if it is hypochondriasis, this condition is likely to be secondary to major depression, which receives diagnostic priority. Given the monosymptomatic nature of his presentation, somatization disorder is not possible. Conversion disorder is highly unlikely. Conversion symptoms are usually neurologic in focus and usually represent a sensory or motor loss. No evidence of a panic disorder is present, and the patient's age does not support this diagnosis.

5. The answer is B [*V D 1*]. The patient most likely has hypochondriasis; she is preoccupied with a fear of cancer despite a thorough negative evaluation and reassurance by her physician. With hypochondriasis, normal physical sensations are often misinterpreted. Affected individuals seem to perceive their body functions more acutely than others and attribute their symptoms to serious disease. Men and women are equally affected. Medication does not "cure" hypochondriasis. Habit-forming medications such as narcotic analgesics should not be prescribed in the absence of physical pathology. Patients with hypochondriasis commonly "doctor shop."

6. The answer is D [*II A, V A 1, 2*]. Given the onset before age 30 years, involvement of multiple organ systems, a long history of symptoms, and negative organic workups, the likely diagnosis is somatization disorder. Recent studies suggest both genetic (as in A and B above) and environmental (as in C above) components in somatization disorder.

7. The answer is B [*V E 1, 4*]. There are some reports of antidepressants (SSRIs) being effective in treating patients with body dysmorphic disorder. Surgery should be avoided. Patients are not usually satisfied with reconstructive surgery. There is no evidence for the use of long-term psychotherapy. Anecdotal reports show behavior therapy, dynamic therapy, and educational-supportive therapy to be effective.

8. The answer is B [*V A 2, 3, 4, 5*]. Patients with somatization disorder commonly experience symptoms of anxiety and depression. They often receive excessive medical evaluations with frequent consultations with multiple physicians. There should be appropriate medical evaluation done of any new symptoms. The physician should avoid prescribing habit-forming medications. Patients with somatization disorder are often frustrating for physicians to manage.

9. The answer is D [*V B*]. Between 15% and 30% of patients diagnosed with conversion disorder have an underlying physical illness that is later diagnosed. Between 30% and 50% of patients with conversion disorder have a comorbid psychiatric diagnosis, but there is no specific association with body dysmorphic disorder. A good prognosis is associated with an obvious stressor, acute onset, and good premorbid functioning. There is no evidence to support the use of benzodiazepines in patients with conversion disorder. One criterion of conversion disorder is that the symptoms are not intentionally produced.

10. The answer is B [*II C; V B 1*]. One criterion of the diagnosis of conversion disorder is the presence of a voluntary motor or sensory function symptoms or deficit. Culturally sanctioned symptoms are not diagnosed as conversion disorder. A psychosocial stressor usually precipitates conversion symptoms. By definition, conversion symptoms are not intentionally produced. Conversion disorder is comorbid with another psychiatric diagnosis 30% to 50% of the time.

11. The answer is D [*V A 1, B 2, C 2*]. Pain disorder, conversion disorder, and somatization disorder all occur more frequently in women than in men. Hypochondriasis occurs equally in men and women.

12. The answer is C [*II H, VII A, C*]. The physician may become the perpetual transference object in factitious disorders. Symptoms are voluntarily produced by the patient for the primary goal of being in the patient role. Addiction occurs in about half of these patients.

13. The answer is D [*II J, VIII A, D*]. By definition, malingering involves intentionally faking an illness or symptoms with the intent to deceive others for secondary gain. Because it is not an illness, malingering does not require any medical or psychiatric treatment.

14. The answer is B [*IX*]. Evidence suggests that the placebo response to pain is physiologically based. Physicians *mistakenly* think that the placebo response can differentiate real from psychological pain. No particular personality type is more likely to respond to a placebo. The placebo response is a powerful aspect of most medical care.

15–20. The answers are 15-D [*I E; III C 3 a; IV A 4*], 16-A [*II A 4; IV D; V B*], 17-E [*IV E*], 18-F [*IV F 1*], 19-G [*V A*], and 20-B [*VI A 2*]. Unilateral presentations of headache usually represent organic pathology, specifically migraine headaches. It is also possible that on the basis of the limited data, several other forms of organic illness might be the cause. It is unlikely to be a conversion symptom or a symptom of somatization disorder because of the unilateral presentation, and it is not likely to be the headache associated with depression, which is commonly bifrontal, nor the occipital headache of muscular headache associated with anxiety. The sudden onset of a sensory and motor loss in the left arm could be caused by a neurologic illness (e.g., multiple sclerosis, stroke, cervical injury) but would be unlikely given the overlapping distribution of the sensory and motor losses, which do not follow more specific nerve distributions. If it is a conversion symptom, it could also be associated with somatization disorder. However, the unexplained joint problems are much more characteristic of somatization disorder, leaving conversion disorder as the best diagnosis in this case.

A unilateral headache is unusual in either depression or somatoform disorders. General malaise could easily be caused by any number of medical illnesses, ranging from hypothyroidism to hypokalemia. However, general malaise is also a common complaint in patients with major depression, making this the best answer.

Complaints of difficulty breathing and tightness in the chest can certainly be caused by general medical conditions such as myocardial infarction. The episodic nature of the complaint makes an arrhythmia possible, as well as several more exotic conditions. However, the age of the patient and the type of presentation make this case relatively typical of early panic disorder.

Chronic multiple organ system physical complaints in a woman with a negative organic evaluation is most likely to be somatization disorder. This condition, which is more common in women, is a chronic multiple system disorder.

Conversion disorder includes voluntary motor or sensory function rather than multiple organ systems. Major depression does not usually involve multiple organ systems. Panic disorder involves discrete panic attacks. A general medical condition is unlikely to involve multiple organ systems or have a negative organic evaluation.

Dissociative fugue includes the elements of sudden travel away from home sometimes after a traumatic event and with loss of memory. Individuals have been known to assume new identities. Dissociative identity disorder involves the incorporation of more than one distinct personality states into one individual usually secondary to a traumatic event or events.

21–23. **The answers are 21-C, 22-B, and 23-A [*I E*].** Medical conditions can cause psychiatric symptoms resembling almost any psychiatric disorder. Common examples are paroxysmal atrial tachycardia resembling panic disorder; toxic delirium mimicking schizophreniform disorder; and hypothyroidism mimicking depression.

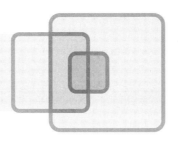

chapter **9**

Sexual and Gender Issues

MARGARET A. SHUGART

I **NORMAL SEXUAL RESPONSE**

A **General issues**

1. **Sexuality is a part of the human condition** and involves all aspects of the biologic, psychological, and social framework. It concerns not only the mental and physical aspects of an individual's life but also the cultural, social, and religious aspects as well. Much has been learned since 1990 about the complexity of human sexuality, and many earlier ideas have been supplanted by these new understandings.

2. **Assessment of sexual functioning by the physician** should be a routine part of the complete medical evaluation, but it is often not done because of anxiety or discomfort on the part of the physician. Psychiatrists may also be less eager than in the past to inquire about sexual functioning. Media attention to sexual abuse by trusted caregivers may cause some physicians to fear that questions about sex will be misperceived by the patient. However, to understand sexual disorders, the physician must be comfortable with sexual issues and must understand normal sexual function, including the stages of sexual response.

B **Stages of sexual response** Physiologic studies have greatly increased the understanding of both healthy and impaired sexual functioning. The sexual response cycle is divided into four phases in the *Diagnostic and Statistical Manual of Mental Disorders,* 4th edition (*DSM-IV*), as well as by Masters and Johnson (1970): desire or appetitive, excitement, orgasm, and resolution. Other aspects of the sexual response cycle from physiologic studies are listed in the following sections.

1. **Desire or appetitive phase (phase 1)**
   a. The desire to have sexual activity and fantasies about sexual activity rather than physiology are the primary components of this phase.

2. **Arousal**
   a. **Physical stimulation** of the genitals, bowel, or bladder may produce an involuntary sexual response via spinal reflex through sacral parasympathetics.
   b. **Psychic stimulation** is mediated through a complex neural pathway involving at least the limbic system, the hypothalamus, and the lateral spinal cord.
   c. **Physiologic response**
      (1) **Erection and lubrication** are influenced by several **neurotransmitter systems.**
         (a) **Cholinergic nerves** were previously believed to be responsible for erection in men and pelvic vasocongestion in women. The failure of atropine (an anticholinergic) to block these responses suggests that cholinergic nerves are only partially responsible for this response.
         (b) The ability of β_2-adrenergic stimulants and α-adrenergic blocking agents to enhance erection suggests that **adrenergic neurons** are involved in sexual arousal and focuses attention on vascular mechanisms of arousal in both sexes.
         (c) **Vasoactive intestinal polypeptide (VIP)** is found in high concentrations in male and female erectile tissues and may enhance cholinergic neurotransmission, accounting for the inability of atropine to block vasocongestion and erection.
         (d) **Dopaminergic systems** in the central nervous system (CNS) facilitate arousal.

(2) **Vascular mechanisms** for vasocongestion and erection have been the focus of recent attention.

  (a) **Classic studies** suggest that polsters, which are pads located between erectile bodies and arterioles, may permit increased blood flow into erectile tissues.

  (b) **Recent studies** focus on the role of pelvic musculature in controlling both arterial inflow and venous outflow as primary mechanisms for erectile tissue function.

3. **Excitement (phase 2)**

  a. **Men.** Approximately 10 to 30 seconds after stimulation, erection of the penis begins as blood flow into the erectile tissue increases.

    (1) **Physiologic changes.** The urethral meatus dilates, the testes elevate slightly, skin temperature increases, the heart rate increases to 100 to 180 beats per minute, and diastolic pressure increases by 10 to 40 mm Hg.

    (2) **Measurement of arousal.** Penile tumescence (as measured by plethysmometry) is considered the most reliable measure of arousal state.

  b. **Women**

    (1) **Physiologic changes.** The breasts increase in size, and the nipples become erect. The labia majora and minora engorge with blood and spread. The clitoris lengthens. The skin flushes, and skin temperature increases. Heart rate and blood pressure increase.

    (2) **Measurement of arousal.** Physiologic changes may not correlate with a subjective sense of arousal. Arousal in women may be most reliably measured by vaginal blood photometric devices.

4. **Plateau**

  a. **Men.** The testicles elevate and become engorged with blood. Secretions from the Cowper gland appear on the glans of the penis. These secretions contain viable sperm. The scrotum thickens and loses all the skin folds. There is general muscle tension and hyperventilation.

  b. **Women.** The clitoris becomes very sensitive and retracts. The labia deepen in color. The orgasmic platform develops, in which the outer third of the vagina narrows because of swelling and muscle tension and the inner two thirds lengthen and widen. The vagina becomes lubricated, general muscle tension increases, and there is hyperventilation.

5. **Orgasm (phase 3)**

  a. **Men.** The sensation of ejaculating inevitably occurs before orgasm. The muscles of the perineum contract rhythmically, and the prostate gland, seminal vesicles, and urethra also contract, causing the emission of semen.

  b. **Women.** There may be a variety of experiences in women. The orgasmic platform contracts rhythmically, and the rectal and urethral sphincters close. The controversy of whether there are one or two types of female orgasms (i.e., clitoral and vaginal) remains unresolved.

6. **Resolution (phase 4)**

  a. **Men.** Detumescence of the penis occurs. There is general muscle relaxation. The testes become uncongested and descend. There is a refractory period during which the man cannot have an erection. The length of the refractory period increases from approximately 1 or 2 minutes in adolescents to several hours in older men.

  b. **Women.** There is a general relaxation. Vasocongestion is lost, and the labia return to their original size, shape, and color. The inner vagina remains distended for several minutes. Women do not have a refractory period and are able to achieve another orgasm immediately.

II   NORMAL SEXUAL FUNCTION AND GENDER IDENTITY DEVELOPMENT

A **Definitions**

1. **Gender identity** is the psychological sense of being masculine or feminine rather than the biologic state of being masculine or feminine.

2. **Gender role** is the social behavior that allows others to categorize the person as male or female.

3. **Sexual orientation** describes the object of a person's sexual impulses.

4. **Sexual identity** refers to biologic sexual characteristics, such as genitalia, hormonal composition, and secondary sexual characteristics.

B Sexual development

1. **Sexual differentiation.** The early embryo is undifferentiated sexually. The Y chromosome is necessary for the development of complete male genitalia. H-Y antigen is responsible for the development of testes. Testicles secrete fetal androgen. The development of male genitalia in utero depends on fetal androgen. However, male-appearing genitalia may be formed in the presence of high levels of fetal androgens in chromosomally XX fetuses. If the fetus is XX and is not exposed to excessive androgens, female external genitalia develop. Genetic problems and changes in hormones during embryonic development may lead to intersex conditions, hermaphroditism, pseudohermaphroditism, and other conditions that are beyond the scope of this chapter.

   a. **Androgens** are produced by the fetal testicles and adrenal glands. Androgens influence the organization of the developing brain, which later influences "male" behavior.

   b. Among other effects, **testosterone** may be associated with changes in brain structure, including the relative size increase of the nondominant hemisphere and of the interstitial nuclei of the anterior hypothalamus, and in reduction in intrahemispheric connections.

   c. **Estrogen.** It previously was believed that only androgens were important in sexual differentiation of the brain (i.e., a developing brain without androgen exposure would develop into a "female" brain). It is now known that estrogen also has a masculinizing effect on the brain and appears to be necessary for the normal development of both male and female brains.

2. **Gender designation.** An infant is assigned a gender on the basis of genitalia and is reared with all of the parents' and society's attitudes regarding that gender. Gender identity appears to be set by age 3 years.

C Sexual development and gender identity theories   In humans, behavior that is masculine or feminine appears to be determined more by learning and culture than by biology. Theories about the development of sex roles have undergone major revisions in recent years.

1. **Sexual development theories**

   a. **Prenatal factors.** In addition to chromosomal makeup, the amount of androgen present or absent in the fetus determines whether male or female genitalia will develop. Testes begin to develop at the fetal age of 6 weeks if fetal testicular androgens are present. External genitalia are morphologically complete by 14 weeks of fetal life.

   b. **Infancy (0 to 18 months).** Masturbation is common and normal between the ages of 15 and 19 months. Parental attitudes about the infant's gender influence the parents' interaction with the infant. For example, encouragement of aggressive behavior, rough play, and role-related social play may all be affected by attitudes regarding sexual roles.

   c. **Toddler (18 months to 3 years).** According to some theories, core gender identity is set by the end of the toddler years. Major developmental tasks of this phase include emergence of control over bodily functions. Children become aware of the anatomic differences between the genders.

   d. **Preschool (3 to 6 years).** Masturbation appears to be recognized as pleasurable by the child. The child appears to be aware of anatomic differences as they relate to gender roles. Some theorists believe that gender role is largely determined during this period.

   e. **School age (6 years to adolescence).** Little is known about sexuality during this period. It formerly was called "latency" age because of what appeared to be a lack of sexual development and new sexual behavior in the age group. However, identity issues related to gender, peer group, and self-esteem are clearly issues in this age group.

   f. **Adolescence.** A great deal of sexual behavior occurs during adolescence, including experimentation with heterosexual, homosexual, and masturbatory experiences. Peer group identity, which is of major importance in adolescents, may contribute to the types of sexual experiences to which the adolescent is exposed. On average, whereas boys report having had their first sexual experience at age 15.7 years, girls report having their first sexual experience at age 16.2 years. Recent studies suggest that adolescents in the United States are engaging in sexual behaviors at earlier ages, with almost two-thirds of boys and half of girls reporting their age of first sexual intercourse before 17 years.

   g. **Adulthood.** Changes in gender role, relationships, and expressed sexual orientation may occur throughout much of the life cycle. For example, a middle-aged man or woman may "come out" as gay in relation to a midlife existential crisis, or a previously isolated person may find a relationship that kindles or rekindles sexual behavior.

  h. Late adulthood. Sexual behavior continues throughout the life cycle. Although the deleterious effects of medical illnesses on sexual function may increase with age, it is not normal for sexual functioning to stop in the elderly.

2. **Psychodynamic theories** follow the thinking of Sigmund Freud and subsequent psychoanalysts.
  a. Much has been written about how disturbances of certain phases of development affect the formation of sexual identity and paraphilias. There is a lack of prospective research supporting many of these ideas, and they have largely been abandoned by psychoanalysts.
  b. **Newer schools of thought** also explain both normal and pathologic sexuality as effects of developmental problems, but they emphasize different psychodynamic models (e.g., separation–individuation, formation of a stable self). For example, a patient suffering from borderline personality disorder may demonstrate "polymorphous perversity" in having indiscriminate sex of many types because of an unstable self, seeking intense relationships at any cost.

3. **Learning theory models** are associated less with the developmental phase than with patterns of imitation, fantasy, and reinforcement. For example, according to these models, when a child is able, he may **imitate the gender role behavior** of individuals of either the same gender or opposite gender encountered in his environment.
  a. Patterns of positive, negative, or absent **reinforcement of these behaviors** may lead to gender role–specific patterns of behavior.
  b. Likewise, in adolescence or later, a person may be exposed to a sexual stimulus (either internally or externally generated) and may masturbate using the fantasy as a stimulus for arousal. If the pattern is not interrupted, a cycle of self-reinforcing, erotic orientation can be created.
  c. For example, an adolescent who has an experience experimenting with sex with younger children may masturbate to this fantasy and, over time, consolidate a pedophilic sexual orientation. This model has been particularly useful in understanding the more unusual paraphilias as well as socially sanctioned, "normal" sexual orientation.

4. **Biologic theories.** Much of the research over the past decade has focused on the biology of sexuality and sexual behavior. Current controversies focus on whether neuroanatomic and endocrinologic differences exist between persons of homosexual and heterosexual orientation. The extent to which endocrine and neuroanatomic differences between men and women contribute to a wide range of social and sexual behaviors has also been controversial.
  a. **Attempts to show biologic differences between persons of heterosexual and homosexual orientation have been inconclusive.**
    (1) **Family pedigree and twin studies** suggest that male homosexuality may have some genetic component, although data in this area are not extensive.
    (2) **LeVay's finding** of smaller anterior hypothalamic nuclei in homosexual men and women than in heterosexual men is subject to methodologic concerns raised by LeVay himself.
    (3) **Early reports of higher testosterone levels in heterosexual** than in homosexual men have not been proved. The finding may have resulted from higher marijuana use by the homosexual men in the sample.
    (4) **Early reports of higher luteinizing hormone (LH) response** to estrogen administration in homosexual men than in heterosexual men (similar to the LH response in women) were not replicated in later studies.
    (5) Theories that persons of homosexual orientation are more associated with maternal stress (and possibly maternal high levels of stress hormones) have not survived well-designed studies of recent years.
    (6) **Animal models** of homosexuality, particularly in studies of rats, have fallen into disrepute for a number of methodologic reasons.
  b. **A variety of hormones regulate the aspects of sexuality in both men and women.**
    (1) **Men.** In a number of experiments in men, the administration and withdrawal of testosterone are clearly associated with frequency of sexual thoughts and desires but not with erectile function. In aging men, the levels of testosterone and human chorionic gonadotropin (hCG) decrease, and the levels of estrogen, LH, and follicle-stimulating hor-

mone (FSH) increase. Reportedly, prolactin decreases and luteinizing hormone–releasing hormone (LHRH) increases sexual desire and functioning.

    (2) Women

        (a) Androgens are associated with increased coital frequency, higher sexual gratification ratings, and more intense and prolonged responses to erotic stimuli. However, androgens are also associated with fewer sexual partners, lower partner-related activity, and higher masturbation frequency.

        (b) There is some evidence that **progesterone** decreases and estrogen increases sexual interest. Progesterone also appears to have behavioral effects; low levels of this hormone are associated with postpartum sadness and "blues" in some women.

        (c) Estrogen is responsible for "masculinizing" sexual behavior in animal models. In humans, estrogen stimulus produces an LH response in women but not in men. Estrogen may be responsible for a number of human behaviors—there have been reports of exogenous estrogen precipitating panic attacks in some women and creating a sense of well-being in others.

        (d) Prolactin levels are, at least indirectly, associated with reduced interest in sex.

    5. Social factors. Social groups may be formed based on the sexual orientation of their members, for example, homosexuals or sadomasochists. There is remarkably little psychiatric literature about these groups and their role in the lives of the individuals in the groups. This may be a result of persecution by religious or political groups of people with certain sexual orientations and a resulting reluctance on the part of these people to speak.

III   SEXUAL AND GENDER IDENTITY DISORDERS

The sexual and gender identity disorders as defined in the *DSM-IV* are now a larger group than described under earlier diagnostic systems. The *DSM-IV* does not describe all the sexual disorders and gender identity disorders encountered in clinical practice, however. The *DSM-IV* has a more descriptive approach, and it contains less discussion of presumed etiology than was common in earlier diagnostic approaches. The *DSM-IV* diagnostic groups include the following disorders:

A Sexual dysfunctions

    1. Hypoactive sexual desire disorder is an absence or deficiency of sexual fantasies and a lack of desire for sexual activity that is persistent or recurrent. The judgment of deficiency or absence is made by the clinician, who accounts for factors that affect sexual function, including the person's age and the context of his or her life (i.e., issues of interpersonal conflict, grief, isolation).

      a. The disturbance causes marked distress or interpersonal difficulty.

      b. The sexual dysfunction is not better accounted for by another Axis I disorder (e.g., major depressive episode, panic disorder, somatization disorder) and is not caused exclusively by direct physiologic effects of a substance (drug of abuse, medication), or a general medical condition.

    2. Sexual aversion disorder is a persistent or recurrent extreme aversion to and avoidance of all (or almost all) genital sexual contact with a partner.

      a. The disturbance causes marked distress or interpersonal difficulty.

      b. The sexual dysfunction is not better accounted for by another Axis I disorder.

    3. Female sexual arousal disorder is a persistent or recurrent inability to attain or to maintain an adequate lubrication-swelling response until completion of the sexual activity.

      a. The disturbance causes marked distress or interpersonal difficulty.

      b. The sexual dysfunction is not better accounted for by another Axis I disorder, a substance of abuse, a medication, or a general medical condition.

    4. Male erectile disorder is a persistent or recurrent inability to attain or to maintain an adequate erection until completion of the sexual activity.

      a. The disturbance causes marked distress or interpersonal difficulty.

      b. The erectile dysfunction is not better accounted for by another Axis I disorder, a substance (drug of abuse, medication), or a general medical condition.

5. **Female orgasmic disorder** is a persistent or recurrent delay in or an absence of orgasm after a normal sexual excitement phase. Women exhibit wide variability in the type and intensity of stimulation that triggers orgasm. The diagnosis of female orgasmic disorder should be based on the clinician's judgment that the woman's orgasmic capacity is less than would be reasonable for her age, her degree of sexual experience, and the adequacy of sexual stimulation she receives.
   a. The disturbance causes marked distress or interpersonal difficulty.
   b. The sexual dysfunction is not better accounted for by another Axis I disorder, a substance (drug of abuse, medication), or a general medical condition.

6. **Male orgasmic disorder** is a persistent or recurrent delay in or absence of orgasm after a normal sexual excitement phase. The clinician accounts for the man's age when judging that the sexual activity is adequate in focus, intensity, and duration.
   a. The disturbance causes marked distress or interpersonal difficulty.
   b. The sexual dysfunction is not better accounted for by another Axis I disorder, a substance (drug of abuse, medication), or a general medical condition.

7. **Premature ejaculation** is ejaculation that occurs with minimal sexual stimulation before, on, or shortly after penetration and before the man wishes it. This disturbance persists or recurs. The clinician must account for factors that affect the duration of the excitement phase, including age, novelty of the sexual partner or situation, and recent frequency of sexual activity.
   a. The disturbance causes marked distress or interpersonal difficulty.
   b. The sexual dysfunction is not better accounted for by the direct effects of a substance (drug of abuse, medication).

8. **Dyspareunia (not caused by a general medical condition)** is a recurrent or persistent genital pain associated with sexual intercourse. This condition can occur in both men and women.
   a. The disturbance causes marked distress or interpersonal difficulty.
   b. The disturbance is not caused exclusively by vaginismus or lack of lubrication and is not better accounted for by another Axis I disorder (except another sexual dysfunction). It also is not caused exclusively by the direct physiologic effects of a substance (drug of abuse, medication) or a general medical condition. Medications associated with dyspareunia include amoxapine and thioridazine.

9. **Vaginismus (not caused by a general medical condition)** is a recurrent or persistent involuntary spasm of the musculature of the outer third of the vagina that interferes with sexual intercourse.
   a. The disturbance causes marked distress or interpersonal difficulty and is not better accounted for by another Axis I disorder (except another sexual dysfunction) or a general medical condition.

10. **Subtypes of sexual dysfunction** include:
    a. **Lifelong type.** Present since the onset of sexual functioning
    b. **Acquired type.** Has its onset after a period of normal functioning
    c. **Generalized type.** Not limited to certain types of stimulation, situations, or partners
    d. **Situational type.** Limited to certain types of stimulation, situations, or partners
    e. **Sexual dysfunction caused by psychological factors.** The subtype diagnosed when psychological factors are judged to have the major role in the onset, severity, exacerbation, or maintenance of the condition and when a general medical condition or substances (drug of abuse, medication) are not the cause.
    f. **Sexual dysfunction caused by combined factors.** Diagnosed when psychological factors as well as a general medical condition or substance contribute to the sexual dysfunction but none of the factors are sufficient separately to account for it

11. **Sexual dysfunction caused by a general medical condition.** This category represents clinically significant sexual dysfunction that results in marked distress or interpersonal difficulty and predominates in the clinical picture. Evidence from the history, physical examination, or laboratory findings suggests that the sexual dysfunction is fully explained by the direct physiologic effects of a general medical condition. The disturbance is not better accounted for by another mental disorder (e.g., major depressive disorder). The type of dysfunction as well as the particular medical condition responsible for the dysfunction should be specified.

12. **Substance-induced sexual dysfunction** is clinically significant sexual dysfunction with marked distress or interpersonal difficulty predominating in the clinical picture. The disturbance is not better accounted for by a sexual dysfunction that is not substance induced.
    a. Evidence from the history, physical examination, or laboratory findings suggests that the sexual dysfunction is fully explained by substance use by either of the following:
       (1) The symptoms of criterion A, which develop during or within 1 month of substance intoxication
       (2) Medication use that is etiologically related to the disturbance
    b. The type of dysfunction should be specified (e.g., substance-induced sexual dysfunction with impaired desire).

13. **Sexual dysfunction not otherwise specified** includes sexual dysfunctions that do not meet the criteria for any specific sexual dysfunction (e.g., absence of subjective erotic feelings despite physiologically normal arousal and orgasm).

B **Paraphilias** Paraphilias involve recurrent, intense, sexually arousing fantasies, sexual urges, or behaviors generally involving nonhuman objects, the suffering or humiliation of oneself or one's partner, or children or other nonconsenting persons, and occur over a period of at least 6 months. Paraphilias almost always occur in men.

1. **Exhibitionism.** Over a period of at least 6 months, recurrent, intense, sexually arousing fantasies, sexual urges, or behaviors involving the exposure of one's genitals to an unsuspecting stranger occur. The fantasies, sexual urges, or behaviors cause clinically significant distress or impairment in social, occupational, or other important areas of functioning.

2. **Fetishism.** Over a period of at least 6 months, recurrent, intense, sexually arousing fantasies, sexual urges, or behaviors involving the use of nonliving objects (e.g., female undergarments) occur.
   a. The fantasies, sexual urges, or behaviors cause clinically significant distress or impairment in social, occupational, or other important areas of functioning.
   b. The fetish objects are not limited to articles of female clothing used in cross-dressing or to devices designed for the purpose of tactile genital stimulation.

3. **Frotteurism.** Over a period of at least 6 months, recurrent, intense, sexually arousing fantasies, sexual urges, or behaviors involving touching and rubbing against a nonconsenting person occur. The fantasies, sexual urges, or behaviors cause clinically significant distress or impairment in social, occupational, or other important areas of functioning.

4. **Pedophilia.** Over a period of at least 6 months, recurrent, intense, sexually arousing fantasies, sexual urges, or behaviors involving sexual activity with a prepubescent child or children (generally age 13 years or younger) occur. The fantasies, sexual urges, or behaviors cause clinically significant distress or impairment in social, occupational, or other important areas of functioning.
   a. The pedophile is at least 16 years of age and at least 5 years older than the child or children in criterion A.
   b. **Subtypes** include:
      (1) Sexually attracted to boys only
      (2) Sexually attracted to girls only
      (3) Sexually attracted to both genders
      (4) Limited to incest
      (5) Exclusive type (attracted only to children)
      (6) Nonexclusive type

5. **Sexual masochism.** Over a period of at least 6 months, recurrent, intense, sexually arousing fantasies, sexual urges, or behaviors occur that involve the act (real, not simulated) of being humiliated, beaten, bound, or otherwise made to suffer. The fantasies, sexual urges, or behaviors cause clinically significant distress or impairment in social, occupational, or other important areas of functioning.

6. **Sexual sadism.** Over a period of at least 6 months, recurrent, intense, sexually arousing fantasies, sexual urges, or behaviors occur that involve acts (real, not simulated) in which the psychological or physical suffering (including humiliation) of the victim is sexually exciting to the person with this disorder. The fantasies, sexual urges, or behaviors cause clinically significant distress or impairment in social, occupational, or other important areas of functioning.

7. **Transvestic fetishism.** Over a period of at least 6 months, a heterosexual male has recurrent, intense, sexually arousing fantasies, sexual urges, or behaviors involving cross-dressing, which cause clinically significant distress or impairment in social, occupational, or other important areas of functioning. This disorder is coded as **transvestic fetishism with gender dysphoria** if the man has persistent discomfort with gender role or identity.

8. **Voyeurism** occurs over a period of at least 6 months and is a recurrent, intense, sexually arousing fantasies, sexual urges, or behaviors involving the act of observing an unsuspecting person who is naked, in the process of disrobing, or engaging in sexual activity. The fantasies, sexual urges, or behaviors cause clinically significant distress or impairment in social, occupational, or other important areas of functioning.

9. **Paraphilia not otherwise specified** is reserved for paraphilias that do not meet the criteria for any of the specific categories (e.g., telephone scatologia [obscene phone calls], necrophilia [corpses], zoophilia [animals]).

C **Gender identity disorders**

1. **Gender identity disorder** is a strong and persistent cross-gender identification, not merely a desire for any perceived cultural advantages of being the other sex, and persistent discomfort with one's sex or sense of inappropriateness in the gender role of one's sex.
   a. **Symptoms** manifest as:
      (1) Insisting that one is of the other sex
      (2) Cross-dressing
      (3) Preferring opposite-sex roles in play
      (4) Having an intense desire to play games stereotypical of the opposite sex
      (5) During childhood, strongly preferring playmates of the other sex
      (6) During adolescence and adulthood, having a conviction that one has feelings typical of the other sex
      (7) Stating a desire to be of the other sex
      (8) Frequently passing for the other sex
   b. The patient has a persistent discomfort with his or her sex or sense of inappropriateness in the gender role of that sex. During childhood, a boy may assert that his testicles or penis will disappear or that he would be better without them; a girl may reject urinating in the sitting position. During adolescence and adulthood, the disturbance is manifested by symptoms such as a preoccupation with getting rid of primary and secondary sex characteristics or believing that he or she was born the wrong sex.
   c. The disturbance is not concurrent with a physical intersex condition (i.e., an inconsistency between genitalia and chromosomal makeup or external genitalia is inconsistent with internal structures).
   d. The disturbance causes clinically significant distress or impairment in social, occupational, or other important areas of functioning.
   e. **Subtypes** are classified according to whether the disorder occurs in children, adolescents, or adults, and whether the person is sexually attracted to males, females, both sexes, or neither sex.
   f. Cross-dressing is commonly known as **transvestism** (not a *DSM-IV* term).
   g. A person with **transsexualism** (a term commonly still in use but not in *DSM-IV*) has a persistent preoccupation with becoming a member of the opposite sex.

2. **Gender identity disorder not otherwise specified** includes conditions of gender identity disorder that are not classifiable as a specific gender identity disorder (e.g., intersex conditions with gender dysphoria; transient, stress-related cross-dressing behavior; persistent preoccupation with castration or penectomy without a desire to acquire the sex characteristics of the other sex).

D **Sexual disorder not otherwise specified** is a diagnosis of exclusion made when a sexual disturbance does not meet any criteria for a specific sexual disorder and is neither a sexual dysfunction nor a paraphilia. This diagnosis may apply to feelings of inadequacy concerning sexual performance or other traits related to gender role or to persistent and marked distress about sexual orientation.

E Diagnosis of sexual and gender identity disorders

1. **The sexual complaint** may be elicited in response to a question about the patient's chief complaint or by asking sexual history screening questions. If the patient has a complaint, it is necessary to **obtain baseline information,** including:
   a. Subjective distress
   b. Frequency of occurrence
   c. Effect of the condition on other areas of the patient's functioning

2. **Sexual history.** A thorough discussion of sexual functioning is particularly necessary for patients whose medical problems (e.g., diabetes, heart disease) predispose them to sexual problems. A sexual history should be taken at the time of the complete patient history and physical examination or the initial psychiatric interview.
   a. **If sexuality is related to the presenting illness,** the physician should ask, "How has your sexual functioning been affected by the illness?" or "Many patients experience changes in sexual functioning as a result of this problem. How has it affected you?" The physician should convey openness and a willingness to discuss the subject of sex.
   b. **If sexuality is not addressed during the history of the presenting illness,** it can be reviewed during the **review of systems.**
      (1) **Pathology** involving the genital organs, including sexually transmitted disease, pain, and discharge should be evaluated as well as the interest in and capacity for sexual functioning.
      (2) If a sexual dysfunction is present, a detailed sexual history is needed for further evaluation, addressing the following points:
         (a) First childhood awareness of sexuality, including attitudes and punishment
         (b) Problems with gender identity
         (c) First sexual experience, including masturbation
         (d) Age of and reaction to puberty, including menarche in women
         (e) History of sexual abuse
         (f) Patient knowledge about sex and how knowledge was acquired
         (g) First experience with a sexual partner, including intercourse
         (h) Homosexual, sadomasochistic, and other experiences and interests
         (i) Current sexual functioning, including frequency and satisfaction
         (j) Questions about extramarital partners if the patient is married
   c. **Problems that may be uncovered** in the sexual history include:
      (1) Concern about normal sexuality or sexual development secondary to the patient's lack of knowledge or misinformation
      (2) Sexual aspects of a pervasive problem in the relationship with the sexual partner
      (3) Sexual problems that result from the presenting medical or surgical problem
      (4) Primary sexual dysfunction that needs further evaluation and treatment

F Etiology and differential diagnosis

1. **Medications** prescribed for medical and psychiatric conditions may have obvious or subtle effects on sexual functioning.
   a. **Antihypertensive agents,** through antiadrenergic effects, can impair erectile function in men and lubrication in women.
   b. **Tricyclic antidepressants, monoamine oxidase inhibitors,** and **antipsychotics,** through anticholinergic effects, can impair erectile function in men and lubrication in women.
   c. **Antipsychotics,** through dopamine-blocking effects, can impair arousal and orgasm.
   d. **Serotonin reuptake inhibitors,** through serotonergic effects, can inhibit sexual desire, arousal, and orgasm.
   e. **Steroids, estrogens,** and **spironolactone,** through antiandrogenic effects, can decrease sexual desire.
   f. **Fluphenazine, thioridazine,** and **amoxapine** have been reported to be associated with painful orgasm (dyspareunia).
   g. **Trazodone, chlorpromazine,** and **clozapine** have been associated with priapism.

2. **Substances of abuse** are common causes of sexual dysfunction.
   a. **Alcohol.** Acutely, alcohol may have a culture-related, disinhibiting effect on sexual behavior. However, alcohol often causes acute sexual dysfunctions, impairing performance in both men and women, and can have negative long-term effects (e.g., testicular atrophy).
   b. **Cocaine** may increase sexual behavior and interests acutely because of dopaminergic effects. With long-term use, however, cocaine decreases interest and performance because of depletion of CNS dopamine stores.
   c. **Amphetamines** have an effect similar to that of cocaine.
   d. **Sedative hypnotics** produce a range of sexual dysfunctions during states of intoxication and withdrawal. Despite the propensity to inhibit sexual response, benzodiazepines are prescribed at times for anxiety related to sexual performance. Such prescribing should be reconsidered.
   e. **Narcotics** produce sexual dysfunction with long-term use, possibly as a result of dopamine depletion.

3. **General medical conditions** may account for more than 50% of complaints of certain sexual dysfunctions, such as impotence in men.

4. **Psychiatric disorders** that may cause sexual dysfunction or performance problems include the following:
   a. **Major depression**
   b. **Panic disorder with agoraphobia**
   c. **Somatization disorder**
   d. **Bipolar disorder**
   e. **Personality disorders**

G Treatment

1. **Sexual dysfunctions**
   a. **Evaluation** is the first, most critical, step in devising a treatment plan. A **complete physical examination** and, if appropriate, **urologic or gynecologic examinations** are indicated. **Substance abuse and psychiatric screening examinations** are the next steps in the evaluation.
   b. **Education** may be among the most effective available treatments for general sexual dysfunctions. The clinician should gently assess the patient's knowledge of sexual function and beliefs about sex. Interventions should be tailored to the information deficits identified.
      (1) Patients may need to learn the stages of sexual arousal to solve misinterpretation problems.
      (2) A couple may need to be taught details of sexual activity to eliminate the cause of their sexual "dysfunction."
      (3) Teaching each partner about the sexual responses of both sexes often is a major step in helping couples deal with sexual dysfunction.
      (4) Desensitizing the discussion of sexual issues for individuals and couples by teaching language for discussing sex is a useful communication tool for sexual partners or for the therapist and patient.
      (5) **Specific physiologic and anatomic education** may be helpful for some patients. For example, some patients may not know that most women cannot have an orgasm without some clitoral stimulation. These patients can be taught that in some women, sexual positions that pull down on the labia minora can provide strong, indirect stimulation of the clitoris. Often, this type of simple suggestion solves much of a patient's or couple's sexual dysfunction.
   c. **Communication training** of the couple to enable them to talk about sex and about their own wishes and needs can lead to greater intimacy. Getting both partners to agree to tell the other what they enjoy and what they find unpleasant is a critical step in working with the couple (if they can agree to express needs and wishes in a nonthreatening manner and learn to accept feedback nondefensively). Steps to better communication include the following:
      (1) **Exploration of cultural and religious beliefs**
      (2) **Examination of the "goals" of sex,** which can lead to a productive renegotiation of these goals
      (3) **Teaching the couple to talk during sex,** which is often a major step in resolving minor difficulties
   d. **Behavioral therapy** is another effective group of techniques for "simple" sexual dysfunctions. Behavioral interventions usually involve education and a behavioral technique designed to address a specific problem.

(1) **Relaxation training** may be helpful for both men and women whose dysfunction is related to anxiety.

(2) **Sensate focus (male).** Couples are instructed to explore noncoital caressing, focusing on the discovery and enjoyment of sensual feelings. These exercises should have a pleasuring quality rather than a demanding quality. This allows rediscovery of sensual feelings, which may have been suppressed by the sexual problem.

    (a) **Managing anxiety.** Fear of failure and pressure to perform are common in men with erectile dysfunction. Prohibition of intercourse during sensate focus sessions removes this anxiety and allows the patient a feeling of success in enjoying arousal.

    (b) **Regaining confidence.** As sensate focus exercises continue, the stop–start technique may be used. After the erection has occurred, the couple ceases the sexual stimulation and allows the erection to subside. They then continue the pleasurable activity, which allows recurrence of the erection. With this technique, the man gains a sense of control of his own arousal level.

    (c) **Gradual resumption of coitus.** As the couple feels more confident, gradual approximation of coitus can occur. The man first achieves vaginal containment of the penis but then withdraws so that anxiety is managed and the sense of success can continue. As the couple feels confident, active thrusting can be added with stopping and starting as needed to control anxiety.

(3) **Sensate focus (female).** Exercises initially are used for the woman to explore her own sensuality. The activities are designed to progress at the patient's own rate and to be nondemanding.

    (a) The woman starts by touching her skin, breasts, and genitals and noticing the pleasurable sensations. She then progresses to caressing her genitals while noting pleasurable sensations. She is then encouraged to explore clitoral and vaginal sensations and masturbation. A vibrator may be used to provide a high level of stimulation and assist in the experience of orgasm.

    (b) **Anxiety management.** Prohibiting orgasm during sensate focus exercises reduces performance anxiety. Relaxation techniques, hypnosis, and, occasionally, antianxiety agents may be used.

    (c) **Strengthening the pubococcygeal muscles** is associated with a high rate of orgasmic competence. This is accomplished by having the woman consciously tighten the pelvic floor muscles several times a day.

    (d) **Experiencing orgasm with a partner.** After the woman has gained confidence in her ability to experience orgasm by herself, she then learns to experience it with a partner. The woman is encouraged to educate her partner about activities that she finds stimulating. She is thus given permission to obtain pleasure for herself in the relationship.

e. **Combined educational and behavioral techniques.** Most physicians use the **P-LI-SS-IT model** developed by Jack Annon for the treatment of sexual dysfunction. For several sexual dysfunctions, these techniques may be effective in approximately 90% of cases.

(1) **Permission (P).** The physician's relaxed manner and interest facilitates the discussion of sexual concerns, normalizing these concerns and providing permission to discuss them. Approval and permission for enjoyment of sexual activity should be conveyed. The authority of the physician's role contributes to the effectiveness of this approach.

(2) **Limited information (LI).** In the many cases of sexual dysfunction that result from lack of information or misinformation about sex, the physician can reassure as well as educate the patient about "normality" by providing limited information about anatomy and physiology.

(3) **Specific suggestions (SS).** This type of intervention requires physician skill, and the level of intervention depends on the complexity of the problem. Masters and Johnson, among others, have developed therapy programs for couples that use short-term behavior approaches. After an extensive history is taken and physical and laboratory examinations are conducted, the couple is taught sensate focusing.

(4) **Intensive therapy (IT).** Patients who do not respond to the basic therapy described in *permission, limited information,* and *suggestion* may require psychotherapy and should be referred accordingly. In these cases, there usually are more complex problems in the relationship or associated psychopathology.

    (a) **Relationship problems** may be addressed for the individual patient through **interpersonal therapy** or **psychodynamic therapy.** Trouble with sexual relationships usually extends to other nonsexual relationships in the patient's life (e.g., a fear of abandonment may infiltrate relationships with coworkers, friends, and extended family).

        (i) The therapist may focus on overcoming the fear of abandonment by exploring past relationships, exploring feelings about current relationships, and testing the reality of assumptions about these relationships.

        (ii) Psychodynamic approaches may focus on the patient's fears and feelings about the therapist to illustrate the patient's relationship problems with people in general.

    (b) **Cognitive therapy** may be particularly useful for anxious and depressed patients, whose routine styles of thinking create a pattern of incorrect interpretations of events and expectations (see Chapter 4: III B).

f. Couples therapy (conjoint therapy). As with individual psychotherapy, couples therapy has a long history of use in the treatment of sexual dysfunctions, starting with Masters and Johnson. Some of the issues that may be dealt with in couples therapy include the following:

    (1) Communication problems

    (2) Conflict management, in which rules for productive arguing are set

    (3) Power and control issues, which are solved by power-sharing arrangements or, if needed, individual psychotherapy

g. Group therapy is reported to be effective for people with sexual dysfunctions. People with similar problems gain a great deal from sharing with each other.

h. Medications. In some cases of sexual dysfunction, the clinician may take advantage of a secondary effect of a medication, and in other cases, the medication may be prescribed for its direct effects on sexual performance.

    (1) Estrogen replacement is indicated for inadequate lubrication, atrophy of the vaginal epithelium and related pain on intercourse, and other symptoms associated with menopause. Oral and topical estrogens are effective and are commonly prescribed for these conditions.

    (2) Testosterone is widely prescribed in the United States for both men and women. This anabolic steroid increases sexual interest and functioning in testosterone-deficient men and in women.

        (a) Men. Testosterone has no beneficial effects in men with normal testosterone levels; in fact, it may reduce secretion of endogenous testosterone. Its use may stimulate existing testicular and prostatic cancers in men.

        (b) Women. For some women, testosterone may have virilizing effects, which may preclude its use.

        (c) Although there is a clear use for testosterone in clinical practice, it should be used with more care than is often currently practiced.

    (3) Sildenafil (Viagra), **Tadalafil** (Cialis), and **Vardenafil** (Levitra) are prescribed for erectile dysfunction in men. These medications affect all four phases of the sexual response. Their mechanism of action is as a selective inhibitor of cyclic guanosine monophosphate (cGMP)-specific phosphodiesterase type 5(PDE5), enhancing the effect of nitrous oxide in the corpus cavernosum.

    (4) Yohimbine is a central α_2-antagonist that stimulates postsynaptic norepinephrine effects. It has been shown to be effective in the treatment of some cases of male impotence; however, it can cause cardiac problems and anxiety.

    (5) LHRH, also known as **gonadotropin-releasing hormone (GnRH),** is a hypothalamic hormone with controversial uses. Its effects are very complex, including improving sexual characteristics in hormonally deficient men and inhibiting its own effects if used chronically in high doses. When used in pulsatile doses, it stimulates ovulation in women and testosterone production in men. By increasing testosterone production in men, it may increase sexual interest in testosterone-deficient men.

    (6) Dopaminergic medications have a variety of effects on sexual performance. In some cases, L-**dopa** is reported to enhance sexual performance in older men, as is **bromocriptine.** The *dopaminergic antidepressant* **bupropion** has been shown to improve both sexual drive and performance in men and women, but it increases the speed at which ejaculation is reached in men. Dopamine-blocking medications (e.g., neuroleptic medications) increase the time to achieve ejaculation and may interfere with sexual interest. Dopamine inhibits prolactin secretion and may cause amenorrhea in women.

(7) **Serotonergic medications** may increase prolactin secretion, decrease sexual interest, and increase time to ejaculation. Whereas patients taking serotonergic medications often find these effects disturbing, patients with premature ejaculation and depression may consider these effects beneficial.

(8) **Phenylethylamine,** a substance found in chocolate, has sexually stimulating effects in rats. Its precise effects in humans are unknown.

(9) **Bupropion**-treated patients with depression may experience prosexual effects, including increased libido, increased level of arousal, and increased intensity and duration of orgasm.

2. **Gender identity disorders**

   a. **Psychotherapy.** Pervasive identity problems can sometimes cause confusion and doubt about sexual and gender roles.

   (1) For example, patients with **borderline personality disorder** may have histories of a variety of paraphilias and sexual dysfunctions.

   (2) In other cases, the patient may experience specific **conflicts about sexuality** (e.g., patients whose parents had rigid morals and condemned sex, patients with homosexual wishes who try to perform heterosexually).

   (3) In patients with **secondary gender identity disorder,** the fluctuations in the patient's dissatisfaction with his or her assigned sex allows the clinician to get a sense of the permanent versus temporary issues of the patient's gender identity.

   (a) For example, the patient may be most rejecting of his or her gender in relation to conflicts with a significant person or as a result of a depressive illness.

   (b) In such cases, helping the patient to cope better with relationships or treating the depression may give the psychiatrist a better sense of the stable versus unstable parts of the patient's gender identity issues.

   b. **Behavioral therapies for children with primary gender identity disorder** involve a number of methods of reinforcing desired gender-specific behaviors without reinforcing nondesired behaviors.

   (1) Techniques range from therapeutic communities to specific rewards for desired behaviors.

   (2) Many of these techniques are highly effective for modifying patterns of gender-specific play and behavior. Critics argue that they may not alter "core identity" as a person of the other sex. There is little evidence that psychotherapy, pharmacotherapy, or other psychiatric interventions can reverse established patterns of gender dysphoria in people with primary gender identity disorder.

   (3) Long-term outcome data for these approaches are sparse.

   c. **Psychodynamic and psychoanalytic approaches for children with gender identity disorder** focus on establishing appropriate parenting roles for parents whose relationships with each other and with the child are disordered.

   (1) For example, the therapist may help strengthen the role of the father (who reportedly is usually the weak parent) in relation to the mother.

   (2) Another therapeutic task may be to help the child form a sense of self that is separate from the mother, father, and others in the environment.

   d. **Gender reassignment surgery** may be indicated for patients with a stable, long-term dissatisfaction with their assigned gender.

   (1) Male-to-female reconstruction surgery is performed approximately four times more often than female-to-male reconstruction.

   (2) As expected, many patients with primary gender identity disorder adapt well after surgery. Perhaps unexpectedly, a number of those with secondary gender identity disorders also do well after surgery. In general, patients who are otherwise well adapted psychologically before surgery tend to be well adapted after surgery.

   (3) Patients with gender identity disorder and other concurrent psychiatric disorders (e.g., borderline personality disorder) may have an increased risk of suicide after surgery when they discover that the surgery does not solve all of their problems.

(a) **Ethical problem.** The psychiatrist can encourage the patient to prepare for surgery if he or she suspects that the patient is at risk for suicide because of gender crisis. Or the psychiatrist can encourage the patient to postpone surgery until the patient has reduced comorbid factors, so that the risk of suicide will be decreased after surgery. The latter option often is viewed by the patient as paternalism, however.

(b) The psychiatrist may be confronted with the problem of having to continue estrogen therapy for a patient who has no intention or means of having gender reassignment surgery. In some cases, the patient prefers the halfway changes of estrogen therapy to either a purely male or female state.

    (i) Some clinicians believe that supporting patients in a halfway state is humane and appropriate.

    (ii) Other clinicians are concerned about the medical risks of this practice and may believe that this halfway state is not adaptive.

3. **Paraphilias.** Generally, treatment outcomes for patients with paraphilias are not impressive, mainly because this patient population often does not want treatment.

    a. **Psychodynamic and psychoanalytic approaches** do not seem to provide significant results in patients with paraphilias.

    b. **Behavioral therapies** consisting of aversive conditioning, penile plethysmometry to measure arousal, and other techniques have been the mainstay of treatment for convicted sexual offenders for more than a decade. Unfortunately, the positive results first reported from these techniques tend to be only temporary.

    c. **Pharmacologic treatments** have included female sex hormones (progestin derivatives), antiandrogens, and, more recently, serotonin reuptake inhibitors. However, these treatments appear to reduce sexual drive rather than alter the patient's focus of sexual interest. As a result, these treatments may be most effective in hypersexual patients.

    d. **Multimodal treatment** currently is the treatment of choice for patients with paraphilias.

        (1) There appears to be an almost pervasive lack of appropriate social skills among many patients with paraphilias. Group therapy is often included in the therapeutic program to teach social skills and empathy for other people. Patients in these programs may also be given medications and may be involved in individual therapy, behavioral therapy, or other structured programs. Coexisting psychiatric diagnoses also are treated.

        (2) Treatment outcomes are not impressive, particularly when public systems are overwhelmed by the number of patients, limited funds, and high political expectations for positive outcomes in patients who do not want treatment.

IV PREMENSTRUAL DYSPHORIC DISORDER (*DSM-IV*), PREMENSTRUAL SYNDROME (PMS), OR LATE LUTEAL PHASE DYSPHORIC DISORDER (*DSM-III*-R)

A Definition This disorder has been relegated to criteria sets and axes provided for further study in the *DSM-IV*, implying that it is no longer an official diagnosis. Researchers question whether it is a distinct entity, a cultural belief pattern, or an artifact of other disorders, particularly affective disorders. PMS is defined as **physical or psychological symptoms that begin the week before menstruation and resolve shortly after the onset of menstrual flow.** The symptoms must be of such severity that they impair functioning.

B Diagnosis To make this diagnosis, symptoms must be charted prospectively because retrospective reports have been shown to be invalid. Up to 80% of women who complain of PMS do not meet the criteria when prospective charting is used.

1. Most women who complain of PMS without meeting the charting criteria exhibit an affective disorder, anxiety disorder, or substance abuse disorder. Of the women whose cyclical symptoms are verified by prospective charting, a subgroup meets the criteria for other *DSM-IV* diagnoses and should receive treatment for those disorders.

2. The diagnosis of PMS should be reserved for women with cyclic symptoms who do not meet other psychiatric diagnostic criteria.

C **Symptoms**   Women who expect to have PMS symptoms are more likely to report symptoms, whether or not the symptoms are actually premenstrual. Although a multitude of symptoms have been described for PMS, typical complaints include:

1. **Psychological complaints**
   a. Tension
   b. Irritability
   c. Depression
   d. Anxiety
   e. Affective lability
   f. Food cravings
   g. Concentration difficulty
   h. Lethargy

2. **Physical complaints**
   a. Breast tenderness
   b. Weight gain
   c. Bloating
   d. Fatigue

D **Etiology**   The cause of PMS is not well established.

1. Theories about an imbalance of estrogen and progesterone levels have not been validated.
2. There is an increasing interest in the effect of **female gonadal hormones** on CNS monoamine activity, particularly serotonin.
3. **Thyroid abnormalities** that meet the rigorous definition of PMS have been noted in some groups.
4. **Endorphin activity** may be altered by the menstrual cycle.
5. **Aldosterone** levels may be elevated, leading to water retention.
6. **Prostaglandin** levels may be elevated, leading to water retention, pain symptoms, and dysphoria.

E **Treatment**   Because the etiology of PMS is unclear, various empirical approaches are used.

1. **Education.** The patient can be taught to recognize her cyclic fluctuations and anticipate problems. The process of charting the symptoms is helpful in promoting self-awareness.
2. **Nonspecific approaches**
   a. **Diet** should consist of regular, small meals low in sodium, sugar, and caffeine.
   b. Substance use, especially of alcohol, should be avoided.
   c. **Regular physical exercise** reduces tension and stress.
3. **Medications** have been shown to be helpful for some patients.
   a. **Bromocriptine** is useful in alleviating breast tenderness.
   b. **Diuretics** are useful for weight gain and edema.
   c. **Prostaglandin inhibitors** are useful for dysmenorrhea pain. Some patients report that prostaglandin inhibitors help with mood, although this has not been tested.
   d. **Ovulation suppressants** (e.g., oral contraceptives) are useful for some patients.
   e. **Antianxiety medication** is useful for alleviating symptoms of tension and irritability.
   f. Progesterone suppositories were a popular treatment for PMS, but numerous well-designed studies have proved them to be no more effective than placebo.
   g. **Pyridoxine (vitamin B$_6$)** and **magnesium supplementation** were popular, but their efficacy is unclear.
   h. **Selective serotonin reuptake inhibitors** may have specifically beneficial effects on PMS. Fluoxetine (Sarafem) has been approved for the treatment of premenstrual dysphoric disorder.

BIBLIOGRAPHY

Althof SE, Levine SB, Corty EW, et al: A double-blind crossover trial of clomipramine for rapid ejaculation in 15 couples. *J Clin Psychiatry* 56(9):402–407, 1995.

American Psychiatric Association: *Diagnostic and Statistical Manual of Mental Disorders*, 4th ed. Washington, DC, American Psychiatric Association, 1994.

Anand KJS, Nemeroff CB: Developmental psychoneuroendocrinology. In *Child and Adolescent Psychiatry: A Comprehensive Textbook,* 2nd ed. Edited by Lewis M. Baltimore, Williams & Wilkins, 1996, pp 64–86.

Becker JV, Johnson BR, Kavoussi RJ: Sexual and gender identity disorders. In *Essentials of Clinical Psychiatry,* 3rd ed. Edited by Hales RE, Yudofsky SC. Washington, DC, American Psychiatric Press, 1999, pp 471–484.

Edinger M, Junker M, Knoll C, et al: Social networks of gay men in the era of AIDS. *Int Conf AIDS* 9(2):900, 1993.

Ellison JM: Exercise-induced orgasms associated with fluoxetine treatment of depression. *J Clin Psychiatry* 57(12):596–597, 1996.

Fagan PJ, Schmidt CW: Psychosexual disorders. In *Clinical Psychiatry for Medical Students,* 3rd ed. Edited by Stoudemire A. Philadelphia, Lippincott-Raven, 1998, pp 481–506.

Feiger A, Kiev A, Shrivastava RK, et al: Nafazodone versus sertraline in outpatients with major depression: Focus on efficacy, tolerability, and effects on sexual function and satisfaction. *J Clin Psychiatry* 57(suppl 2):53–62, 1996.

Gagnon M, Layton S, Messiet C: Sexual dysfunction and selective serotonin reuptake inhibitors. *Biol Psychiatry* 44(5):374, 1998.

Goldblum DS, Kennedy SH: Adverse interaction of fluoxetine and cyproheptadine in two patients with bulimia nervosa. *J Clin Psychiatry* 52(6):261–262, 1991.

Grimes JB: Spontaneous orgasm with the combined use of bupropion and sertraline. *Biol Psychiatry* 40:1184–1186, 1996.

Jacobsen FM: Fluoxetine-induced sexual dysfunction and an open trial of yohimbine. *J Clin Psychiatry* 53(4): 119–122, 1992.

LeVay S: A difference in hypothalamic structure between heterosexual and homosexual men. *Science* 253(5023): 1034–1037, 1991.

Marans S, Cohen DJ: Child psychoanalytic theories of development. In *Child and Adolescent Psychiatry: A Comprehensive Textbook,* 2nd ed. Edited by Lewis M. Baltimore, Williams & Wilkins, 1996, pp 156–170.

Masters WH, Johnson VE: *Human Sexual Inadequacy.* Boston, Little Brown, 1970.

Miller NS, Gold MS: The human sexual response and alcohol and drugs. *J Subst Abuse Treat* 5(3):171–177, 1988.

Modell JG, Katholi CR, Modell JD, DePalma RL: Comparative sexual side effects of bupropion, fluoxetine, paroxetine and sertraline. *Clin Pharmacol Ther* 61(4):476–487, 1997.

Offer D, Schonert-Reichl KA, Boxer AM: Normal adolescent development: Empirical research findings. In *Child and Adolescent Psychiatry: A Comprehensive Textbook,* 2nd ed. Edited by Lewis M. Baltimore, Williams & Wilkins, 1996, pp 278–290.

Perelman MA: Commentary: Pharmacological agents for erectile dysfunction and the human sexual response cycle. *J Sex Marital Ther* 24(4):309–312, 1998.

Sadock BJ, Sadock VA: *Kaplan & Sadock's: Synopsis of Psychiatry,* 9th ed. Baltimore, Williams & Wilkins, 2003.

Saks BR: Identifying and discussing sexual dysfunction. *J Clin Psychiatry Monograph* 17(1):4–8, 1999.

Sarwer DB, Durlak JA: A field trial of the effectiveness of behavioral treatment for sexual dysfunctions. *J Sex Marital Ther* 23(2):87–97, 1997.

Segraves RT: Antidepressant-induced sexual dysfunction. *J Clin Psychiatry* 59(suppl 4):48–54, 1998.

Sussman N: The role of antidepressants in sexual dysfunction. *J Clin Psychiatry Monograph* 17(1):9–14, 1999.

Walker PW, Cole JO, Gardner EA, et al: Improvement in fluoxetine-associated sexual dysfunction in patients switched to bupropion. *J Clin Psychiatry* 54(12):459–465, 1993.

Werry JS: Brain and behavior. In *Child and Adolescent Psychiatry: A Comprehensive Textbook,* 2nd ed. Edited by Lewis M. Baltimore, Williams & Wilkins, 1996, pp 86–95.

Wilson RE: The nurse's role in sexual counseling. *Ostomy Wound Manage* 41(1):72–78, 1995.

Zucker KJ, Green R: Gender identity and psychosexual disorders. In *Textbook of Child and Adolescent Psychiatry,* 2nd ed. Edited by Wiener JM. Washington, DC, American Psychiatric Press, 1997, pp 657–676.

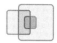

Study Questions

Directions: *Each of the numbered items or incomplete statements in this section is followed by answers or by completions of the statement. Select the ONE lettered answer or completion that is BEST in each case.*

1. A 38-year-old man presents to his family physician complaining that he has had no interest in sex for the past 4 months. There have been no significant changes in his life circumstances in the past year (e.g., divorce, death in the family, loss of job). With no additional information, what is the most likely cause of this patient's loss of interest in sex?

- A Generalized anxiety disorder
- B Major depressive episode
- C Paranoid schizophrenia
- D Personality disorder
- E Sexual aversion disorder

2. A 47-year-old woman presents to her primary care physician complaining of pain during intercourse. The pain has become increasingly problematic over the last 6 months. What should be the first item in the differential diagnosis?

- A Atrophic vaginitis
- B Dyspareunia
- C Major depression
- D Somatization disorder
- E Vaginismus

3. A 25-year-old man is brought to the emergency room by the police. He has been rubbing his penis against unsuspecting young women in the subway. He was apprehended by the police and became suicidal, saying that his arrest would ruin his job and his relationship with his family. What is the most likely diagnosis?

- A Frotteurism
- B Major depression
- C Paraphilia not otherwise specified
- D Pedophilia
- E Voyeurism

4. A 30-year-old man presents with a 15-year history of dressing in women's clothing in order to become sexually aroused. He reports being comfortable with his male gender identity. What is the most likely diagnosis?

- A Gender dysphoria
- B Gender identity disorder
- C Paraphilia
- D Transsexualism
- E Transvestic fetishism

5. Which one of the following reactions is associated with the plateau phase of sexual response?

- A Erection of the penis begins.
- B The refractory period occurs.
- C The breasts enlarge in size.
- D The clitoris retracts.
- E The testicles descend.

Directions: *The set of matching questions in this section consists of a list of four to 26 lettered options (some of which may be in figures) followed by several numbered items. For each numbered item, select the ONE lettered option that is most closely associated with it. To avoid spending too much time on matching sets with large numbers of options, it is generally advisable to begin each set by reading the list of options. Then for each item in the set, try to generate the correct answer and locate it in the option list, rather than evaluating each option individually. Each lettered option may be selected once, more than once, or not at all.*

QUESTIONS 6–10

Match each of the behavioral effects with the corresponding substance.

- [A] Dopamine
- [B] Estrogen
- [C] Progesterone
- [D] Prolactin
- [E] Testosterone

6. Inhibits prolactin secretion

7. In high levels, inhibits sexual interest and performance

8. Is responsible for inducing asymmetric fetal brain development

9. Is necessary for the normal development of both male and female brains

10. In low levels, is associated with the postpartum "blues"

QUESTIONS 11–15

Match each of the possible effects with the corresponding medication or other substance most likely responsible for the effect.

- [A] Alcohol
- [B] Amoxapine
- [C] Antihypertensive
- [D] Serotonin reuptake inhibitor
- [E] Trazodone

11. Increased time to ejaculation

12. Dyspareunia

13. Priapism

14. Testicular atrophy with long term use

15. Decreased erectile function in males

Answers and Explanations

1. The answer is B [*III A 1–2*]. A major depressive episode is the most likely cause of the patient's loss of interest in sex. On a statistical basis, with a recent onset of the problem and no major life events, depression is the most likely cause of this symptom. The diagnosis of sexual aversion disorder requires ruling out Axis I disorders; therefore, sexual aversion disorder is a less appropriate choice for the starting point in the differential diagnosis.

2. The answer is A [*III A 8–9*]. On a statistical basis and on the basis of the patient's age, the physician may suspect that menopause may have decreased this woman's circulating estrogen levels, resulting in atrophic vaginitis. However, the physician must perform a pelvic examination before making a diagnosis because of the possibility that a neoplasm or other disease may be causing the pain. Diagnoses such as dyspareunia and vaginismus require that general medical conditions be excluded before making these diagnoses. Although dyspareunia is a symptom of somatization disorder, a late onset of the symptom is unusual in a patient suffering from somatization disorder. There is no information given about multiple physical complaints as in somatization disorder.

3. The answer is A [*III B 3*]. This case is a typical example of frotteurism, although the patient is at the upper limit of the usual age range. Voyeurism involves watching rather than touching. Major depression is unlikely because there is no evidence that the patient was depressed before the police arrested him. His suicidal impulses are most likely in response to his current situation, although they still must be taken very seriously.

4. The answer is E [*III B 7 and III C 1*]. Transvestic fetishism usually begins in childhood or early adolescence and involves sexual urges to dress in clothing of the opposite gender as a means of sexual arousal. Gender identity disorder and gender dysphoria are not correct because the man is comfortable with his male gender identity. Transvestic fetishism is a paraphilia, but transvestic fetishism is more specific diagnosis and, therefore, this is the "best" answer. The answer "transsexualism" is not correct because the man does not desire to be a female.

5. The answer is D [*I B*]. The clitoris retracts during the plateau phase in women. In men, the erection of the penis **begins** in the excitement phase. The breasts enlarge in women in the excitement phase. The testicles descend and the refractory period in men occurs during the resolution phase.

6–10. The answers are 6-A, 7-D, 8-E, 9-B, and 10-C [*II B 1, II C 4, and III F 2*]. Dopamine inhibits prolactin secretion. Hyperprolactinemia is characterized by a markedly diminished interest in sex and a reduction in sexual performance in both men and women. Hyperprolactinemia can be the result of medications, neoplasms, and other conditions. Testosterone is believed to be the agent responsible during and after fetal development for the increase in the size of the nondominant hemisphere and for the reductions in interhemispheric connections commonly found in male brains. Estrogen appears to be necessary for the normal development of the brain in both boys and girls. Low levels of progesterone are associated with postpartum "blues" in some women.

11–15. The answers are 11-D, 12-B, 13-E, 14-A, and 15-C [*III F 1*]. Serotonin reuptake inhibitors can increase time to ejaculation through their serotonergic effects. Dyspareunia has been reported with amoxapine, and priapism has been reported with trazodone. Long-term alcohol use can lead to testicular atrophy in men. Use of antihypertensive medications can lead to decreased erectile function through the antiadrenergic effects.

chapter 10

Eating Disorders

NIOAKA N. CAMPBELL

Eating disorders are defined as severe disturbances in eating behavior in the revised fourth edition of the *Diagnostic and Statistical Manual of Mental Disorders,* 4th edition, text revision (*DSM-IV-TR*), and include anorexia nervosa, bulimia nervosa, and eating disorder not otherwise specified.

I ANOREXIA NERVOSA

Anorexia nervosa is an eating disorder characterized by a refusal to maintain a minimally normal body weight, fears and preoccupations with gaining weight, and a disturbance of body image.

A Diagnostic criteria (Table 10–1)

B Epidemiology

1. **Onset.** The average age of onset of the illness is the midteens, with the most common age between 14 and 18 years. The onset may be preceded by a period of mild obesity or mild dieting.

2. **Incidence and prevalence.** Anorexia is estimated to occur in 0.5% to 1% of adolescent girls. It occurs 10 to 20 times more often in girls than boys. It seems to be more frequent in developed countries. Whites have the highest rate of occurrence. The disorder is more often found in higher socioeconomic classes and among young women in professions such as modeling and dance that require thinness.

C Clinical features and associated findings

1. **Behavioral features** are varied but commonly include:
   a. Overactivity
   b. Obsessions and rituals connected with food and food preparation
   c. Purging (self-induced vomiting), diuretic or laxative abuse
   d. Secretiveness
   e. Extreme behavioral rigidity and inflexibility
   f. Preoccupations and distortions regarding body image and weight

2. **Associated findings** that accompany the illness are listed in Table 10–2. In general, these findings reflect metabolic slowing, fluid and electrolyte disturbances, alterations in multiple endocrinologic axes, and organic brain symptoms.

4. **Comorbidity** with other psychiatric disorders is associated with anorexia nervosa in some cases.
   a. **Depression** is associated with approximately 65% of patients with anorexia nervosa.
   b. **Social phobias** are associated with up to 34% of cases.
   c. **Obsessive-compulsive disorder (OCD)** is associated with approximately 26% of the cases of anorexia nervosa. Perfectionistic traits in other areas of life may overlap with compulsivity in eating behavior as well.

5. **Clinical subtypes.** There are two identifiable subtypes recognized by the *DSM-IV-TR*, both with specific historic and clinical features.
   a. The **binge eating–purging type** exists in up to 50% of individuals with anorexia nervosa. These individuals may have a history of a heavier body weight as well as family members who

TABLE 10–1 *DSM-IV-TR* **Diagnostic Criteria for Anorexia Nervosa**

Refusal to maintain weight at or above minimal weight for age and height (85% of ideal body weight or developmentally expected body weight)

Fear of gaining weight or becoming obese, even when significantly underweight

Disturbed body image, such that appropriate body weight is perceived as excessive or low body weight is perceived as appropriate

Amenorrhea in postmenarcheal (absence of at least three consecutive menstrual cycles)

Two distinct types:

Restricting: Weight maintained largely by caloric restriction

Bingeing/purging: Both binge eating and purging (vomiting; use of laxatives, diuretics, enemas) occur during the current episode

are obese. Patients may be more extroverted or present with the disorder later in life. They are more likely to be associated with substance use, impulse control, and personality disorders. **Suicide** is higher in these patients than in the restricting subtype. Some patients may purge without binge eating.

    b. The **restricting** subtype is characterized by strict self-starvation and calorie restriction. Obsessive-compulsive traits may often be associated with food and preparation. Individuals with both subtypes may exercise excessively.

  6. Medical complications (Table 10–3)

D **Etiology and pathogenesis**   Although no single cause is known, biological and psychosocial factors are implicated in the etiology of anorexia nervosa.

  1. Biological factors include comorbidities with certain mental disorders, neuroendocrine abnormalities, and genetic factors that occur with increased frequency in patients with anorexia.

    a. Mental illnesses such as unipolar and bipolar mood disorders occur at an increased rate in anorectic patients. These illnesses tend to occur later in life and are not causative with anorexia nervosa. As already noted, (I C 5 a), there is a higher rate of suicide in specific subtypes of anorexia.

    b. Neuroendocrine dysfunction

      (1) Alterations in catecholamine activity within the central nervous system (CNS) may account for some of the clinical features of the illness. Because most of these changes normalize after weight gain, causality is difficult to determine.

      (2) Hypothalamic–pituitary axis dysfunction may account for some of the endocrine abnormalities that occur in individuals with anorexia. Serotonin, dopamine, and norepinephrine are neurotransmitters involved in the hypothalamus associated with eating behaviors.

      (3) Other factors that may be involved include corticotrophin-releasing factor (CRF), neuropeptide Y, thyroid-stimulating hormone, and gonadotropin-releasing hormone.

    c. Genetic studies involving twin pairs suggest heritability in the transmission of anorexia nervosa. A review of clinic-based samples revealed concordance rates as high as 55% in monozygotic twins versus 5% in dizygotic twins. Population-based samples also indicate heritability.

TABLE 10–2 **Associated Findings in Anorexia Nervosa**

Peripheral edema

Lanugo hair development

Skin changes (dryness, scaling, yellow tinge caused by carotinemia)

Lowered metabolic rate (bradycardia, hypotension, hypothermia)

Normal thyroid-stimulating hormone levels; low T3 syndrome

Normal or overstimulated adrenal axis; possible loss of diurnal variation in cortisol

Normal serum protein and albumin concentrations

Impaired regulation in growth hormone levels; increased basal levels

TABLE 10-3 Medical Complications of Anorexia Nervosa

Organic brain symptoms (cognitive slowing, apathy, dysphoria)
Gastric dilatation and rupture if bingeing and purging
Constipation, bloating, abdominal pain
Hematologic changes (anemia, leukopenia)
Endocrinologic changes, cold intolerance
Menstrual irregularities, amenorrhea
Electrocardiogram changes
Osteoporosis
Cachexia (loss of fat and muscle mass, inability to maintain core temperature)

2. **Psychological factors** include proposed theories in the etiology of anorexia nervosa.
   a. **Fear of sexuality** is a classic theory that holds that anorectic patients fear impregnation and fantasize that impregnation may occur orally. Therefore, they defend themselves by not eating. A corollary with this theory is that affected adolescents starve themselves to remain prepubertal for fear of sexuality, menarche, and pregnancy.
   b. **Parent–child conflict** involves the **transactional theory** that purports how a series of conflicts may cause slight changes in the family system. In turn, these changes may lead to a new and more deviated series of interactions. The child's request to not eat or refusal to eat is overridden by the parent's need to feed the child. Eventually, the child becomes dependent on the environment for cues concerning this and other areas of self-regulation.
   c. **Dysfunctional family** dynamics may involve the **family system model** that considers parent–child interactions and asserts that family systems seek to maintain equilibrium. Changes in any part of the system cause disequilibrium and require compensatory changes elsewhere. An adolescent's attempt to begin the process of separation and emancipation in an overinvolved family or to exert developmentally appropriate autonomy and self-control in a rigid, autocratic family is seen as disrupting the family system. Therefore, the regression of the child from normal adolescent strivings to a preadolescent developmental posture (through the symptoms of anorexia nervosa) represents an accommodation within the family system, resulting in a more tenable, albeit pathologic, equilibrium.
      (1) **The mother–daughter relationship** may play a role in the etiology. Mothers of anorectic girls often are controlling, allowing their daughters little autonomy. Mothers of anorectic girls may also be fragile in terms of feminine identity and self-esteem, perceiving their pubescent daughters as competitive and threatening. Regression of the child to prepubertal body morphology may serve to relieve this disequilibrating force in the family system.
      (2) **Fathers** of anorectics often are obsessive-compulsive. They may participate in quasi–weight control activities, such as distance running, and may transmit their attitudes about weight to their daughters. ("Obligate running" among boys and men has been considered by some to be a male equivalent to anorexia nervosa.) Fathers of anorectic girls may also be fearful of their own sexual impulses toward their daughters, which are heightened by the girls' pubertal development.
   d. **Temperament** is a factor that may be associated in the etiology of anorexia. Many anorectics are high achievers with above average intelligence. They may tend toward rigid self-control and affective constriction. Interpersonal conflict is more likely expressed through passive-aggressive modalities than through direct confrontation.

E **Differential diagnosis**
   1. **Medical conditions.** The differential diagnosis for unexplained weight loss in adolescence is included. An adequate medical assessment for illnesses that may account for weight loss must include consideration of the following:
      a. **Addison's disease** may present as weight loss, anorexia (loss of appetite), vomiting, and electrolyte and endocrine abnormalities (low sodium concentration, high potassium concentration, and suppressed serum cortisol levels). Listlessness and depression are common findings, in contrast to the hyperactivity of anorexia nervosa.

b. **Hypothyroidism** may present as intolerance to cold, constipation, bradycardia, low blood pressure, and skin changes similar to those seen in anorexia nervosa (i.e., dry, scaling skin). Obsessional food handling, weight loss (and accompanying fear of weight gain), and hyperactivity are not usual, however.

c. **Hyperthyroidism** presents as elevated vital signs, hyperactivity, and sometimes weight loss. However, patients with hyperthyroidism are usually not obsessive about food.

d. **Any chronic illness** (e.g., Crohn's disease, ulcerative colitis, rheumatoid arthritis, tuberculosis) can cause progressive weight loss but should be readily identifiable as a physical disorder.

e. **Neoplasms, especially CNS tumors** (e.g., tumors of the hypothalamus or third ventricle), can cause endocrine malfunction with accompanying weight loss of either a primary or secondary nature. Other symptoms of the tumor, such as visual disturbances or panhypopituitarism, should be evident.

f. **Superior mesenteric artery syndrome** can cause vomiting and anorexia. The mechanism apparently involves compression of the duodenum by the superior mesenteric artery, particularly when the patient is supine and especially in individuals who are thin. When found concomitantly with anorexia nervosa, it is often difficult to ascertain whether superior mesenteric artery syndrome is primary (causative) or secondary to the weight loss of anorexia nervosa.

2. **Psychiatric conditions**

   a. **Schizophrenia.** Although schizophrenics may be delusional about food, the delusions are more bizarre than those seen in anorectics (e.g., "There's poison in this" versus "This will make me fat"). Other features of schizophrenia should be present.

   b. **Bulimia nervosa** involves binge eating, usually followed by some form of purging, in a patient who otherwise maintains a normative weight. Patients with bulimia rarely lose 15% of their body weight.

   c. **Depression** often is accompanied by anorexia. In this case, the anorexia is a so-called "vegetative" sign of depression, and a depressed mood is usually pronounced.

   d. **Hysterical noneating** can be distinguished by the absence of a morbid concern with weight and calories.

F **Treatment**

1. **Medical assessment** of the anorectic patient must consider the potentially lethal complications of starvation such as metabolic disturbances, fluid and electrolyte disturbances, and cardiac arrhythmias. Management should always begin with the assessment and treatment of these potentially life-threatening medical complications. Intervention for a medical emergency is sometimes necessary; therefore, immediate assessment requires a determination of how much weight has been lost and over what period of time, as well as an assessment of cardiac, metabolic, and hydration status. Only when medical stability has been attained does treatment for the underlying psychologic disorder begin.

2. **Screening tools** have been developed, including the Eating Attitudes Test (EAT) and the SCOFF (acronym based on questions). These tools have shown some success in epidemiologic studies regarding identification and assessment.

3. **Psychotherapeutic modalities**

   a. **Individual psychotherapy** is a useful adjunct to other treatment modalities but is rarely effective alone. **Psychoanalysis** can be particularly ineffective in patients with anorexia nervosa if it is the only treatment intervention. Such therapies can foster a regression in patients, which, in treatment, is useful only when the patient has the ability and strength to pull out of the regression at the end of the session. Neither treatment provides enough structure for the patient; anorectics may need to be watched and instructed for most of the day.

      (1) Initially, therapeutic work should be aimed at forming an alliance with the patient to work on particular problems. The focus need not include weight or eating habits as long as physiologic stability is maintained.

      (2) Gaps in the patient's ego should be clarified. For example, when the patient is obviously angry about something but is unaware of this, the isolation of affect may be addressed.

      (3) Transference reactions should be interpreted if and when they interfere with the patient's ability to work out and talk about problems.

(4) An empathic stance should be maintained with the patient at the same time that issues of physiologic stability and compliance with medical treatment are treated as nonnegotiable. A close partnership must be maintained among the patient, the psychiatrist, and the primary care physician in the collaborative management of these patients.

b. **Cognitive-behavioral therapy (CBT)** as an adjunct can be used in the treatment of anorexia nervosa, although no large sample size studies have yet shown effectiveness in this illness. Monitoring feelings of food, intake, feelings, emotions, relationships and behaviors is essential. Cognitive restructuring identifies automatic thoughts and core beliefs, and behavioral problem solving for coping strategies replaces former maladaptive patterns.

c. **Group therapy.** Peer interaction and feedback should be sought and emphasized because adolescents often pay more attention to their peers than to adults. Adolescents respond to peers with more trust and less suspicion, such that the perception of empathy is enhanced. In addition, the realization that others share the same symptoms helps adolescents feel less isolated. Although many types of groups have been used, self-help groups have been increasing in number and prominence.

d. **Family therapy.** Some form of **family intervention is nearly always indicated,** especially for adolescents. Styles of family interaction should be clarified, and projections and vicarious pleasures that family members derive from the patient's symptoms should be interpreted and restructured. Individual therapy for either or both of the parents may be indicated; when marital issues contribute to the symptomatology of the child, marital therapy for the parents may also be indicated. Parent education concerning the normal developmental tasks and transitions of adolescence may be necessary. In general, the family should be allied with the staff, working toward patient improvement.

e. **Hospitalization.** In some cases, the patient cannot be treated effectively within the dysfunctional home environment and adequate, less restrictive alternatives are not available. **Out-of-home placement** is indicated if the patient loses weight despite outpatient intervention, if the patient is suicidal, or if vomiting and purging is causing serious medical complications.

(1) **Therapeutic approach** reflects the understanding that anorectics have a propensity to deny and conceal the severity of their condition.

(a) Careful attention must be paid to the **accuracy of weight measurements.** Serial weights should be obtained at the same time of day, on the same scale, in the same garb (preferably a hospital gown only), and after voiding. Attempts to pad weight artificially by drinking large quantities or concealing objects on the body are typical.

(b) **Splitting** (pitting one staff member against another) and manipulations concerning eating are common and should be discussed at staff meetings and with the patient. Flexibility among members of the treatment team with regard to the treatment plan is important.

(2) **Behavioral techniques** may be necessary with refractory adolescents.

(a) The patient should be **weighed every other day.** Urine should be **monitored regularly for ketones,** sometimes as often as daily before every meal.

(b) **Alimentation** should be provided by a nasogastric tube if the patient steadfastly refuses to eat and should be readministered if the food is vomited. **Hyperalimentation** may be provided through a central intravenous line if these measures fail.

(c) Patient privileges (e.g., freedom to leave the ward versus confinement in a locked unit) should be tied to the behavioral approach and commensurate with the patient's ability to regulate activity and eating. Such a program may take the following form:

(i) The patient's weight, not the eating behavior, amount of exercise, or vomiting, should be the target symptom. Reinforcers should be tied to weight fluctuation.

(ii) As soon as the patient is stable medically and has some weight reserve, urine can be monitored for ketones before every meal as part of a behavioral treatment approach. Monitoring ketones provides information about starvation state, provides the patient with immediate feedback, and offers the opportunity to alter the starvation state immediately. If the patient's urine contains ketones, activities and privileges should be completely restricted until urine reverts to normal.

    f. Medications. There is no pharmacologic treatment established for anorexia nervosa. Medications may be useful therapeutic adjuncts, but only when targeted at specific, underlying symptoms.

        (1) Cyproheptadine may be of some value because it has appetite-stimulating properties.

        (2) Antidepressants may benefit when depressive symptoms are prominent. Some studies have reported that fluoxetine may result in weight gain and be of some benefit in reducing relapse after weight is restored. Further studies are needed in this area.

        (3) Prominent anxiety symptoms should be treated with **anxiolytics.**

        (4) When eating and food preparation are excessively ritualized or other symptoms of OCD are present, medications to target these symptoms may prove beneficial.

        (5) Because of potentially severe side effects, **antipsychotic medication** should be used only when the patient suffers from a psychotic illness.

        (6) In cases of anorexia associated with major depression, some studies have shown improvement with electroconvulsive therapy (ECT).

G Prognosis On average, 25% of patients will have a relatively complete recovery; 50% may demonstrate partial improvement (some may undergo a period of obesity); and another 25% continue to demonstrate bizarre eating habits, weight loss, and a severe disease course. About half of patients will have some symptoms of bulimia during their illness.

    1. Positive prognostic indicators include early onset of disease, decreased denial of a problem, gaining self-esteem, and admitting to feeling hungry.

    2. Negative prognostic indicators include a long disease course; a schizoid personality; family conflict; and recurrent bulimia, vomiting, and laxative abuse.

    3. Mortality rates are reported to be 5% to 18%. Death is caused by electrolyte abnormalities, suicide, cardiac arrhythmias, or sudden rehydration and weight gain complications.

II BULIMIA NERVOSA

Bulimia nervosa is an eating disorder characterized by ravenous overeating while feeling out of control, followed by guilt, depression, and anger at oneself. Recurrent compensatory behaviors such as purging accompany the overeating. Additionally, a body weight within the normal range is maintained.

A Diagnostic criteria are listed in Table 10–4. Bulimia nervosa patients fall into two distinct categories:

    1. Patients with the **purging type** engage in regular vomiting and use of diuretics or cathartics.

    2. Patients with the **nonpurging type** compensate for high-calorie binges with subsequent caloric restriction or exercise; they do not regularly purge.

B Epidemiology

    1. Onset. Bulimia nervosa is often later in adolescence than in anorexia nervosa. It may occur even in early adulthood.

    2. Incidence and Prevalence. Bulimia nervosa is very common, existing in gradations from mild (perhaps a variant of normal) to severe. Prevalence is 1% to 3% in industrialized countries. It is

---

TABLE 10–4 *DSM-IV-TR* **Criteria for Bulimia Nervosa**

Two distinct types ("purging" and "nonpurging")
Recurrent episodes of bingeing, characterized by:
- Consumption of a quantity of food that exceeds what a normal person would eat during a given time period, under similar circumstances
- A feeling of not having control over eating during the episode

Recurrent inappropriate weight-controlling behavior (e.g., self-induced vomiting, use of cathartics, excessive exercise)
Bingeing and inappropriate weight-controlling behavior, both at least twice weekly for 3 months
Self-evaluation unduly influenced by body shape and weight
Disturbance does not occur exclusively during episodes of anorexia nervosa

TABLE 10–5   Associated Findings in Bulimia Nervosa

Ingestion of high-calorie food
Bingeing episodes occur in secret
Wide fluctuations in weight
Persistent overconcern with weight and body shape
Attempts to lose weight (through dieting, exercise, or use of cathartics, diuretics, enemas)
Bingeing episodes terminated by sleep, abdominal pain, social interruption, or self-induced vomiting
Lengthy phases of normal eating

more common than anorexia nervosa and may be present in up to 5% to 10% of college-age females. The disorder is many times more common in females than in males.

C **Clinical features and associated findings**

1. **Behavioral features.** Individuals with bulimia nervosa have an increased frequency of mood and anxiety symptoms, substance use disorders, and personality disorders. Other symptoms of impulsivity, such as stealing, are common. Stealing may be necessary to support an expensive eating habit.

3. **Associated findings** are listed in Table 10–5.

4. **Medical complications** are listed in Table 10–6.

D **Etiology** Very little is known about the cause of the disorder, although biological, psychological, and social factors may be considered.

1. **Psychological theories**
   a. Bulimia could be caused by a need to take in something orally, perhaps as a substitution for some degree of maternal deprivation. Conflict concerning separation from a maternal figure may be played out in ambivalence toward food. Generally, this ambivalence is ego dystonic for the patient.
   b. Patients with bulimia nervosa may have histories of difficulty separating from caretakers and may use their own bodies as transitional objects.
   c. Bulimia may be a disorder of self-regulation. There are high rates of coexistent substance use disorders, impulsivity, and stealing.

2. **Biologic factors** may include neurotransmitters such as serotonin and norepinephrine, which are linked to satiety in the hypothalamus. Elevated endorphins have been identified in some patients after purging that may relate to reported feelings of satisfaction after the behavior. Genetic studies have demonstrated increased frequency of this illness in first-degree relatives.

E **Differential diagnosis**

1. **Prader-Willi syndrome** is characterized by continuous overeating, obesity, mental retardation, hypogonadism, hypotonia, and diabetes mellitus.

2. **Klüver-Bucy syndrome.** Objects are examined by mouth, and hypersexuality and hyperphagia are characteristic. Visual agnosia, compulsive licking and biting, and hypersensitivity to stimuli are common as well. The condition may result from temporal lobe dysfunction.

TABLE 10–6   Medical Complications of Bulimia Nervosa

Metabolic abnormalities (e.g., hypokalemia, hypochloremic alkalosis)
Parotid gland swelling
Dental erosion and caries
Menstrual irregularities
Gastric dilatation and rupture
Chronic sore throats and esophagitis
Anemia
Neuropsychiatric symptoms (seizures, neuropathies)

3. **Kleine-Levin syndrome** manifests as hyperphagia and hypersomnia, both of which occur in spurts of 2 to 3 weeks at a frequency of two or three cycles per year. Loss of sexual inhibitions may occur as part of the syndrome. This disorder is more common in men and may represent a limbic or hypothalamic dysfunction.

4. **Hypothalamic lesions** or other **CNS tumors** should be considered.

5. **Anorexia nervosa.** Binge eating and purging cannot occur solely during the episodes of anorexia nervosa. This would fall under a subtype of anorexia.

6. **Binge eating in obesity** represents a pattern of overeating that is not terminated by purging and is not accompanied by a preoccupation with body shape.

7. **Epileptic seizures**

F Treatment   Patients with bulimia nervosa are more amenable to outpatient treatment than are those with anorexia nervosa because those with bulimia tend to be less secretive regarding their behaviors.

1. **Individual psychotherapies** of psychodynamic, behavioral, and cognitive orientations have been used in the treatment of this population with some success. However, a specific form of **CBT** is identified as the benchmark and most effective primary treatment for this illness. The efficacy data are based on 18 to 20 strictly manual based sessions over a 6-month period. The goals of these sessions focus on:
   a. Identifying and interrupting the binge–purge cycle of behavior
   b. Addressing the patient's distorted and dysfunctional thoughts regarding food, weight, behaviors and self image while instituting a change in these beliefs.

2. **Antidepressant medications,** including selective serotonin reuptake inhibitors (SSRI) and tricyclic antidepressants (TCAs), have been shown to be effective, with up to 22% abstinence of behavioral symptoms in some studies. Combination treatment with CBT and antidepressants may be the most effective modality. Lithium, carbamazepine, and phenytoin are indicated only if comorbid mood disorders are identified.

3. **Hospitalization** is indicated for the management of serious medical complications, for relentless bingeing and purging (several times daily), and for severely depressed or suicidal bulimic patients.

G Prognosis   Bulimia nervosa tends to result in better outcomes than in anorexia nervosa, with more than half of patients who are in treatment reporting improvement in binge eating and purging. Bulimia is a chronic illness, with a varied course and differing prognostic outcomes. In a 10-year study of the disorder, approximately half of the patients had a full recovery.

III   EATING DISORDER NOT OTHERWISE SPECIFIED

Eating disorder not otherwise specified is the *DSM-IV-TR* category for disorders of eating that do not meet criteria for any specific eating disorder. This category includes patients with some but not all criteria for anorexia nervosa or bulimia nervosa. Binge-eating disorder without inappropriate compensator behaviors is also included in this category.

BIBLIOGRAPHY

American Academy of Pediatrics, Committee on Adolescence, Policy Statement. Identifying and treating eating disorders. *Pediatrics;* 111(1):204–211, 2003.

American Psychiatric Association: *Diagnostic and Statistical Manual of Mental Disorders,* 4th ed, text revision. Washington, DC: American Psychiatric Association, 2000.

American Psychiatric Association, Work Group on Eating Disorders: Practice guideline for the treatment of patients with eating disorders (revision). *Am J Psychiatry* 157(1 supp l):1–39, 2000.

Halmi KA: Eating disorders. In *Kaplan and Sadock's Comprehensive Textbook of Psychiatry,* 7th ed, vol 2. Edited by Sadock BJ, Sadock VA. Baltimore, Lippincott Williams & Wilkins, 2000, pp 1663–1676.

Keel PK, Herzog DB. Long-term outcome, course of illness, and mortality in anorexia nervosa, bulimia nervosa, and binge eating disorder. In *Clinical Handbook of Eating Disorders, An Integrated Approach.* Edited by Brewerton TD. New York, Marcel Dekker, 2004, pp 97–116.

Steiner H, Lock J: Anorexia nervosa and bulimia nervosa in children and adolescents: A review of the past 10 years. *J Am Acad Child Adolesc Psychiatry* 37:352–359, 1998.

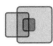

Study Questions

Directions: *Each of the numbered items or incomplete statements in this section is followed by answers or by completions of the statement. Select the ONE lettered answer or completion that is BEST in each case.*

1. A 15-year-old girl presents to the emergency room with severe weight loss. On physical examination, she is cachectic, with a weight of 68 lb. Her heart rate is 36 bpm, and her blood pressure is 72/50 mm Hg. Her height is 5 feet 3 inches. What should be the first intervention?

- A Evaluate the family to determine the family's dynamics.
- B Immediately administer a high-protein and high-carbohydrate diet via a nasogastric tube.
- C Draw blood for a serum electrolyte determination and then start intravenous feeding.
- D Arrange to have the patient admitted to the psychiatric service.
- E Arrange for electroconvulsive therapy.

2. The Prader-Willi syndrome is characterized by which constellation of symptoms?

- A Overeating, mental retardation, and stealing food
- B Hypersexuality, overeating, and mouthing objects
- C Binge eating interspersed among lengthy phases of normal eating
- D Overeating and hypersomnia
- E Overeating, weight loss, and heat intolerance

3. Which treatments have shown improvement in the symptoms of anorexia in preliminary studies?

- A Antidepressants
- B Antipsychotics
- C Cyproheptadine
- D Electroconvulsive therapy
- E All of the above

4. A 17-year-old young woman is referred by her dentist for evaluation after she was found to have severe caries and bilateral parotitis. She is 5 feet 5 inches tall and weighs 116 pounds. She is a talented gymnast and a straight-A student. Her serum potassium is 3.1 mEq/L. What is the most likely diagnosis?

- A Addison's disease
- B Anorexia nervosa
- C Bulimia nervosa
- D Rumination disorder
- E Superior mesenteric artery syndrome

5. Which symptom of bulimia nervosa must be invariably present to establish diagnosis?

- A Episodic purging behaviors
- B Periods of binge eating
- C Periods of excessive exercising
- D Periods of fasting
- E Wide fluctuations in weight

6. What percentage of weight loss below ideal body weight is necessary to diagnose anorexia nervosa?

- A 10%
- B 15%
- C 20%
- D 25%
- E 30%

7. What mortality rate for anorexia nervosa has been reported in most studies?
   - [A] 1% to 8%
   - [B] 5% to 18%
   - [C] 20% to 25%
   - [D] 25% to 35%
   - [E] >35%

8. Which of the following is not associated with bulimia nervosa?
   - [A] Mood symptoms, anxiety symptoms, substance use, or personality disorders
   - [B] Cognitive behavioral therapy is the current treatment of choice, alone or in combination with medication management
   - [C] Parotid gland enlargement
   - [D] Highest mortality rate of eating disorders
   - [E] Metabolic alkalosis

9. All of the following are characteristics of anorexia nervosa EXCEPT:
   - [A] Onset is most common in the midteens
   - [B] Up to 20 times more frequent in females than males
   - [C] Prevalence is equivalent regardless of race or ethnicity
   - [D] More prevalent in developed countries
   - [E] Often associated with professions that require thinness

Answers and Explanations

1. The answer is C [*I F 1, G 3*]. Anorexia nervosa may be a life-threatening illness. Significant mortality accompanies this condition, most commonly caused by the metabolic or cardiac complications secondary to starvation. The first intervention with anorectic patients should always be an assessment of the medical state by drawing blood for serum electrolyte determination, followed by supportive or emergency medical intervention, such as starting intravenous feeding. Too-rapid hydration or weight gain should be avoided because it may lead to further complications and even death. A high-protein and high-carbohydrate diet administered by nasogastric tube would not correct fluid and electrolyte problems quickly. Evaluation and treatment of the individual and family dynamics are always secondary to emergency medical management.

2. The answer is A [*II E 1–3*]. The Prader-Willis syndrome is characterized by ravenous overeating and is accompanied by obesity, mental retardation, and hypotonia. It is probably caused by a hypothalamic lesion. Examining objects by mouth, hypersexuality, and hyperphagia are attributed to the Klüver-Bucy syndrome, and overeating and hypersomnia are associated with the Kleine-Levin syndrome. Binge eating interspersed with lengthy phases of normal eating may be seen in individuals with bulimia nervosa and may be associated with wide fluctuations in weight. The constellation of increased appetite, weight loss, and heat intolerance suggests hyperthyroidism.

3. The answer is E [*I F 3 f*].

4. The answer is C [*Table 10–6, I E*]. Frequent exposure of the teeth, parotid salivary gland, and esophagus to gastric acid (as occurs in the purging type of bulimia nervosa) can result in irritation, inflammation, and damage to each of these tissues. Individuals with Addison's disease may present with weight loss, but it occurs in conjunction with hyperkalemia rather than hypokalemia. Superior mesenteric artery syndrome can cause vomiting and anorexia, but this usually occurs after substantial weight loss. Anorexia nervosa cannot be diagnosed until weight is at or below 85% of ideal body weight. Rumination disorder, in which food is repeatedly regurgitated and rechewed, is an uncommon disorder of infancy and early childhood that rarely progresses into adulthood except in individuals with mental retardation or pervasive developmental disorders.

5. The answer is B [*Table 10–4*]. The diagnosis of bulimia nervosa requires both recurrent episodes of binge eating and recurrent, inappropriate, compensatory behaviors aimed at preventing weight gain. Prevention of weight gain may be achieved by fasting, excessive exercise, or purging behaviors such as self-induced vomiting or laxative or diuretic abuse. Individuals with bulimia nervosa vary according to which weight management method they use. Wide fluctuations in weight are common but not invariable.

6. The answer is B [*Table 10–1*]. Refusal or inability to maintain weight at or above 85% of ideal body weight is necessary for the diagnosis of anorexia nervosa.

7. The answer is B [*I G 3*]. Most studies report mortality rates ranging from 5% to 18%.

8. The answer is D [*Table 10–5, 6, II F G*]. Bulimia nervosa tends to result in better outcomes than in anorexia nervosa, with more than half of patients who are in treatment reporting improvement in binge eating and purging. Associated findings do include parotid gland enlargement, metabolic alkalosis, and increased comorbidity with other Axis I and Axis II disorders.

9. The answer is C [*I B*]. Anorexia occurs 10 to 20 times more often in females than males. It seems to be more frequent in developed countries and in higher socioeconomic classes. Whites have the highest rate of occurrence. The disorder is often found among young women in professions such as modeling and dance that require thinness.

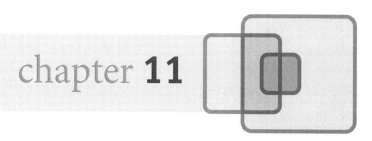

chapter 11

Impulse Control Disorders

NIOAKA N. CAMPBELL

Impulse control disorders are varying illnesses characterized by patients' failing to resist an impulse to perform an act that is harmful to themselves or others. The *Diagnostic and Statistical Manual of Mental Disorders,* 4th edition, text revision (*DSM-IV-TR*), lists several disorders in this category, which are not included in any other diagnostic heading, as **impulse control disorders not elsewhere classified.**

I   INTERMITTENT EXPLOSIVE DISORDER

A Diagnostic criteria

1. **Repeated, discrete episodes of loss of behavioral control characterized by aggression toward persons or property** are the hallmark of this disorder. Commonly, the aggression assumes the form of a physical assault or as destruction of property.

2. **Precipitating events** may be variable or absent and **are disproportionately insignificant** compared with the extent of the aggressive behavior.

3. Whether the disorder exists independently from the conditions that must be ruled out in a differential diagnosis is controversial. Consequently, the condition may best be considered a **characteristic symptom constellation deriving from multiple etiologies.**

B Epidemiology   Intermittent explosive disorders are more common in men than in women. Whereas men with these disorders are reportedly more likely seen in correctional facilities, women are more likely seen in mental health facilities.

C The **differential diagnosis** includes a variety of psychological and organic etiologies. Regardless of the etiology, victimization by or exposure to violence and aggressive behavior may contribute to the expression of this disorder.

1. **Psychodynamic etiologies** may include the outbursts as a mechanism of defense against possible **narcissistic** injury. Situations that directly or indirectly represent earlier deprivation or trauma may evoke the destructive hostility.

2. **Organic etiologies** may include seizures (especially with temporal lobe foci), psychoactive substance intoxication, structural lesions (trauma, infarct, tumor, hemorrhage, abscess), normal-pressure hydrocephalus, central nervous system infection, metabolic disorders (hypoglycemia), and hormone disturbances (elevated androgen levels). Genetic studies have shown that first-degree relatives have higher rates of depression, impulse control, and substance use disorders.

3. The disorder may be differentiated from or comorbid with personality disorders (especially antisocial and borderline), psychotic disorders (schizophrenia), mood disorders (manic episodes), and disruptive behavior disorders (conduct and attention deficit hyperactivity disorder).

D Treatment is best aimed at the underlying condition or conditions.

1. **Combination treatment** of medication management and psychotherapy has the best yet limited success. Incarceration, institutionalization, seclusion, and restraint are measures that may control yet not alter behaviors.

2. **Behavior modification** techniques have met with only modest success, as have conventional psychotherapies.

3. Various **psychosurgical procedures** have been applied, although these are currently used rarely and are reserved for the most dangerous, refractory cases.

4. A variety of **medications** have also been used with some symptomatic benefit. Mood stabilizers (e.g., lithium), anticonvulsants (e.g., phenytoin, carbamazepine, valproic acid), β-blockers (e.g., propranolol), sedative-hypnotics, and selective serotonin reuptake inhibitors (SSRIs; e.g., fluoxetine, sertraline, paroxetine) have shown favorable responses in appropriately selected cases.

II KLEPTOMANIA

A **Diagnostic criteria**

1. **Multiple episodes of impulsive stealing in the presence of pertinent negatives.** Specifically, the stealing is not:
    (1) For monetary value or to satisfy a personal need
    (2) An expression of anger, retribution, or retaliation
    (3) Symptomatic of an underlying psychotic disorder (e.g., in response to a hallucination or delusion)

2. Individuals experience a **mounting sense of tension or anxiety before the stealing episode.** Pleasure, then, is derived from easing this internal tension or anxiety after gratifying the irresistible impulse to steal, not from the object(s) stolen. This contrasts sharply with shoplifting, robbery, burglary, and other stealing behaviors in which the secondary gain derives from the object or objects stolen. In fact, it is common for the objects stolen in kleptomania to be hidden, stored, discarded, returned, or given away.

B **Epidemiology and etiology** Kleptomania is believed to be extremely rare and more common in females than in males. Many reported cases must be carefully evaluated in light of the secondary gain afforded by conscious attempts to avoid criminal prosecution (malingering). Because the disorder is rare, little is known of its epidemiology or its etiology.

1. **Organic etiologies** related to behavioral disinhibition remain poorly understood. Differences in serotonin metabolism have been proposed. Genetic studies have shown an increased association with first-degree relatives and obsessive-compulsive disorder (OCD).

2. **Psychological etiologies** have been suggested, largely by psychoanalytic theorists who tend to view the behavior as an attempt to restore wishes, drives, and pleasures that were lost or at least frustrated during infancy and childhood. The symptoms tend to appear or worsen in times of increased stress.

C **Treatment** The literature is largely devoid of systematically controlled treatment studies and instead includes mostly single-case, anecdotal reports of either psychoanalytic or behavioral therapeutic modalities. SSRIs such as fluoxetine have shown effectiveness in some of these cases.

III PYROMANIA

A **Diagnostic criteria**

1. **Multiple episodes of willful and intentional fire setting in the presence of pertinent negatives.** Specifically, the fire setting is not:
    a. For financial gain (e.g., insurance reimbursement)
    b. An act of sociopolitical insurrection
    c. One of a series of related criminal activities
    d. An act of vandalism or an expression of retaliation or revenge
    e. A symptom of an underlying psychotic disorder

2. Individuals experience a **mounting sense of tension or anxiety before the fire-setting episode,** which may sometimes be in the form of a building sexual tension and excitement (**pyrolagnia**). Relief of tension and anxiety or sexual pleasure is derived when the fire-setting impulse is gratified as well as during the aftermath of the fire setting.

3. Afflicted individuals maintain an **obsessional preoccupation with fire** in much the same way individuals with eating disorders maintain obsessional preoccupations with food.

B **Epidemiology** Pyromania is a rare disorder that accounts for only a fraction of all cases of fire setting. The disorder appears to be more common in males than in females, and childhood onset is common. Individuals with pyromania appear to lack empathy of the physical destructiveness of their actions and consequences.

C **Etiology** Specific etiology tends to be obscured by the rarity of the disorder.

1. An underlying **organic factor** is suggested by long-standing observations of high rates of fire setting in organically impaired populations. Serotonergic and adrenergic involvement has also been postulated as biologic factors.

2. **Psychological theorists** have focused on the intrapsychic representation and meaning of fire. Such theories have emphasized issues related to sexuality, power, rage, and aggression as psychodynamic determinants, which may underlie this disorder.

D **Treatment** The nature of the disorder is such that "treatment" most often occurs in penal institutions. No systematically controlled studies have been applied in this population. Fire setting in children is a serious treatment consideration requiring supervision and family therapy. There is no clearly defined role for pharmacotherapy in this disorder unless an underlying organic state is identified.

IV PATHOLOGICAL GAMBLING

A **Diagnostic criteria**

1. **Chronic, progressive,** and **maladaptive gambling behavior,** as evidenced by:
   a. An obsessional, cognitive preoccupation with gambling
   b. Impaired personal, social, educational, and occupational functioning as a consequence of the gambling
   c. An overly determined, out-of-control quality that drives, perpetuates, and escalates the gambling despite the derivative functional impairment and adverse consequences
   d. There may be repeated efforts to control, cut back, or stop gambling.

2. In this context, pathological gambling may be viewed as a variant of an **addictive** disorder.

B **Epidemiology** Pathological gambling is a relatively common disorder. Approximately 3% of the adult population can be classified with this disorder, and it is considerably more common in men than in women. The prevalence is more common in areas where gambling is legal.

1. **Predisposing factors** may include extremes in parental discipline styles (either overly indulgent or overly rigid) and childhood exposure to parental gambling, parental substance abuse, or parental sociopathy.

2. **Associated conditions.** Associations between pathological gambling and mood disorders, anxiety disorders, substance use disorders, and personality disorders have been described.

C **Etiology** Only theories exist.

1. **Psychoanalytic theories** attempt to connect the behavior with various disturbances in psychosexual development (from the oral stage through latency) as well as with aggressive and libidinal drives.

2. **Behavioral theories** attempt to explain the behavior largely according to learning theory (i.e., that most pathological gamblers are exposed to the behavior and ultimately "learn" through patterns of reinforcement).

3. **Biological etiologies.** It has also been suggested that the behavior may be propagated through the activation of endogenous opioid systems or may be associated with serotonergic and noradrenergic receptor systems.

D **Treatment approaches** derive from the theoretic framework applied to explain the etiology. Both individual and group modalities have been applied.

1. The earliest **individual modalities** tended to be conventional psychodynamic approaches. Recently, **cognitive behavioral techniques,** including both aversive and desensitizing models, have been studied.

2. **Group modalities** have also played a more prominent role, particularly self-help groups such as Gamblers Anonymous, which have been structured consistently with a 12-step addictions model.

3. **Pharmacotherapy** efficacy has not yet been demonstrated in a significant role unless an underlying organic state has been identified. Early case reports have shown some improvement with fluoxetine.

V TRICHOTILLOMANIA

A **Diagnostic criteria**

1. **Recurrent episodes of pulling out one's own hair in quantities sufficient to result in identifiable hair loss** are the hallmark of this disorder.
   a. Trichotillomania must be distinguished from stroking, twirling, and fidgeting with hair, which may fall within a spectrum of normal behavior.
   b. Scalp hair most commonly is involved; facial hair, eyebrows, eyelashes, truncal hair, limb hair, axillary hair, and pubic hair may also be involved.

2. **Hair-pulling episodes are preceded by a sense of increasing internal tension and anxiety.** When the impulse to pull has been gratified, the individual experiences a pleasurable sensation or at least relief from the internal perception of tension and anxiety. Of note is that hair pulling in this context does not typically induce pain.

3. **Obsessional thoughts and other compulsive behaviors may be described.** In particular, specific rituals related to the disposition of the hair, including ingestion (**trichophagy**), may exist.

B **Epidemiology**   The prevalence of the condition is unknown. The disorder usually begins in childhood and is believed to affect females more frequently than males.

C **Etiology**   All etiologic theories are considered tentative and speculative at present.

1. One view holds that the behavior represents a form of **self-stimulation** in response to emotional deprivation. Significant disturbances in parent–child interactions are commonly described.

2. Other theorists emphasize the dimension of **self-mutilation** as a form of self-punishment in response to rejection, trauma, and loss.

3. Some features are consistent with a learned behavior, similar to the **habit disorders of childhood.** An association with OCD has been suggested.

4. Finally, it is possible that an underlying **organic substrate or substrates** may exist.

D **Treatment**

1. **Psychodynamic and behavioral individual approaches have been described.** Psychodynamic approaches were more common historically, but recently behavioral interventions have been discussed more frequently. Desensitization, aversion, and habit reversal have all been described. Therapeutic efficacy of all individual modalities has been limited.

2. **A variety of psychopharmacologic agents have been used.** Neuroleptics, anxiolytics, mood stabilizers, and anti-obsessional medications (clomipramine, fluoxetine) have met with only limited success. Some literature suggests that medications used to treat tic disorders may be of some benefit as well.

VI IMPULSE CONTROL DISORDER NOT OTHERWISE SPECIFIED

This is a diagnostic residual category within the *DSM-IV-TR,* including disorders of impulse control that do not meet specific criteria for an impulse control disorder. Disorders in this category include compulsive buying, Internet compulsion, cellular or mobile phone compulsion, repetitive self-mutilation, and compulsive sexual behavior.

BIBLIOGRAPHY

American Psychiatric Association: *Diagnostic and Statistical Manual of Mental Disorders,* 4th ed, text revision. Washington, DC, American Psychiatric Association, 2000.

Burt VK, Katzman JW: Impulse-control disorders not elsewhere classified. In *Kaplan and Sadock's Comprehensive Textbook of Psychiatry,* 7th ed, vol 2. Edited by Sadock BJ, Sadock VA. Baltimore, Lippincott Williams & Wilkins, 2000, pp 1701–1713.

Petry NM, Stinson FS, Grant BF: Comorbidity of DSM-IV pathological gambling and other psychiatric disorders: Results from the National Epidemiologic Survey on Alcohol and Related Conditions. *J Clin Psychiatry* 66: 564–574, 2005.

Potenza MN, Kosten TR, Rounsaville BJ: Pathological gambling. *JAMA* 286:141–144, 2001.

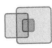

Study Questions

Directions: *Each of the numbered items or incomplete statements in this section is followed by answers or by completions of the statement. Select the ONE lettered answer or completion that is BEST in each case.*

1. The motive for fire setting in pyromania is most strongly associated with which of the following?

- [A] Psychotic delusions
- [B] Secondary gain
- [C] Tension reduction
- [D] Terrorism
- [E] Vandalism

2. Which statement is most accurate with regard to the role of environmental precipitants in the aggressive outbursts in intermittent explosive disorder?

- [A] They are variably present and proportionate to the aggression expressed.
- [B] They are variably present and disproportionate to the aggression expressed.
- [C] They are invariably present and proportionate to the aggression expressed.
- [D] They are invariably present and disproportionate to the aggression expressed.
- [E] They are unrelated to the aggression expressed.

3. A 28-year-old woman steals a valuable pocket watch from a jewelry store. She is most likely to suffer from kleptomania if she

- [A] anonymously mails the watch back to the jewelry store.
- [B] gives the watch to her boyfriend for a birthday gift.
- [C] sells the watch to help pay her house payment that is in arrears.
- [D] sells the watch and deposits the money into savings.
- [E] displays the watch in a showcase along with other artifacts in her home.

4. Which parental disorder would be most likely to contribute to the development of pathologic gambling in the parent's adolescent child?

- [A] Anxiety disorder
- [B] Attention deficit hyperactivity disorder
- [C] Bipolar disorder
- [D] Depressive disorder
- [E] Substance abuse

5. Which two impulse control disorders are more common in women than in men?

- [A] Trichotillomania and pyromania
- [B] Pyromania and intermittent explosive disorder
- [C] Intermittent explosive disorder and pathological gambling
- [D] Pathological gambling and kleptomania
- [E] Kleptomania and trichotillomania

Directions: *Each set of matching questions in this section consists of a list of four to 26 lettered options (some of which may be in figures) followed by several numbered items. For each numbered item, select the ONE lettered option that is most closely associated with it. To avoid spending too much time on matching sets with large numbers of options, it is generally advisable to begin each set by reading the list of options. Then, for each item in the set, try to generate the correct answer and locate it in the option list, rather than evaluating each option individually. Each lettered option may be selected once, more than once, or not at all.*

QUESTIONS 6–9

For each disorder listed below, select the association most consistent with it.

- [A] Addiction
- [B] Factitious symptoms

    C Irresistible urge
    D Obsessive-compulsive symptoms
    E Sexual excitation

6. Trichotillomania

7. Pathological gambling

8. Pyromania

9. Kleptomania

Answers and Explanations

1. The answer is C [*III A 1, 2*]. The motive for fire setting in individuals with pyromania is specifically not for secondary gain (e.g., to access insurance benefits), as an act of terrorism or political insurrection, or as an act of vandalism amid a constellation of delinquent behaviors. Neither is it in response to psychotic delusions or command auditory hallucinations. Rather, the motive for fire setting in individuals with pyromania is tension gratification and reduction, often of a sexual nature. Tension is relieved or sexual pleasure gratified only by indulging the impulse to set fires and its aftermath.

2. The answer is B [*I A*]. Multiple etiologies, including psychologic and organic states, likely underpin this disorder. Environmental precipitants are only variably present, but when present, they are disproportionately minor compared with the extent of the aggressive behavioral outburst. Nonetheless, precipitants may not be identifiable with each explosive outburst. Regardless of the underlying etiology, exposure to violence and aggression likely contributes to the behavior. Elevated androgen levels have been implicated in some cases.

3. The answer is A [*II A1, 2*]. Kleptomania is believed to be an extremely rare disorder. It is qualitatively different from most forms of stealing in that secondary gain is not derived from the object stolen, but rather from gratifying the impulse to steal. Consequently, the objects stolen often are returned to their owner. Many "cases" may be false-positives secondary to malingering in an attempt to avoid criminal prosecution. There is no clearly defined treatment for the disorder; all treatments are relatively speculative at this point.

4. The answer is E [*IV B 1, 2*]. Childhood exposure to parental gambling, substance abuse, and sociopathic or antisocial behavior have all been suggested as predisposing factors. Mood and anxiety disorders may occur along with pathological gambling as comorbid conditions; they have not been linked vertically, however. The impulsivity of attention deficit hyperactivity disorder (ADHD) may contribute to susceptibility to this disorder; however, parental ADHD has not been shown to predispose children to the development of pathological gambling.

5. The answer is E [*II B, V B*]. Most impulse control disorders occur more commonly in men than in women; however, kleptomania and trichotillomania appear to occur more commonly in women than in men.

6–9. The answers are: 6-D [*V C 3*], **7-A** [*IV A 2*], **8-E** [*III A 2*], and **9-C** [*II A 2*].

In addition to compulsive hair pulling, other obsessions or compulsions may be noted in trichotillomania. In addition, trichotillomania may be a symptom of an obsessive-compulsive disorder.

Pathological gambling has much in common with the addictive disorders. Both involve continuation of the maladaptive behavior despite chronic, progressive, adverse consequences. Likewise, peer support groups that use a 12-step approach have been of benefit in both disorders.

Pyromania often is precipitated by sexual tension that builds before setting a fire and that is gratified sexually both by setting the fire and during the aftermath of the fire.

Kleptomania must be distinguished from other forms of stealing by the distinction that the stolen object does not bring secondary gain or gratification as it does in other forms of stealing. When stealing brings secondary gain by way of the value of the object stolen, the attempt to invoke an "irresistible urge" as in true kleptomania more likely represents malingering as a means of avoiding criminal prosecution.

chapter 12

Child Psychiatry

JOSHUA T. THORNHILL IV

I INTRODUCTION

Child and adolescent psychiatry is the study and treatment of the mental, developmental, and behavioral problems of children. It overlaps with several pediatric subspecialties. An understanding of standard childhood development is essential to the understanding of childhood psychopathology because seemingly major difficulties may be normal at certain ages (e.g., negativism is usual at 2 years of age and again at adolescence but is problematic during the latency period and in adulthood).

A Overview of childhood psychopathology

1. **Most disorders are more common in boys** than in girls. This may reflect an inherent increased vulnerability of boys to stress and trauma.

2. **Psychopathology is usually the result of chronic, maladaptive interactions** between the child and the environment, often combined with some genetic, physiologic, or temperamental propensity toward developing a mental illness. Isolated traumatic events (e.g., a single episode of brief sexual fondling by a nonfamily member) can cause transient anxiety, anger, and depression; however, they generally do not cause psychopathology unless they generate long-lasting changes in the child's interactions with his or her environment.

3. **Misbehavior may be the result of conscious or unconscious prompting by the parents.** Children usually behave in a way that is consistent with their parents' desires.

B Developmental concepts

1. **Epigenesis.** There is a natural and unalterable sequence in which development must occur (e.g., in Freudian psychology, the anal period must follow the oral stage and cannot be reversed; in Eriksonian psychology, the autonomy stage must follow the stage of basic trust). Later stages are necessarily viewed as "advances" from earlier stages. In all individuals, there is a natural impetus toward development that progresses normally unless adversely influenced by extraneous variables. These variables may include in utero or perinatal insults, physiologic or genetic vulnerabilities, and a host of environmental stressors.

2. **Developmental continuities.** Some childhood personality traits and experiences may be "continuous" with and have ramifications for adulthood; others do not.
   a. For example, children who are abandoned at 3 years of age by their parents may feel depressed every time someone leaves them later in life. Children who experience persistent deprivation and neglect throughout childhood may manifest excessive dependency and neediness in their adult relationships. Thus, some childhood experiences may be "continuous" with adult behaviors or personality traits.
   b. Other characteristics, such as cognition and intellect, would be grossly oversimplified if they were thought of as continuous variables derived completely from experiences in early infancy because obvious genetic, physiologic, and individual differences (e.g., temperament) would be overlooked.
   c. In general, development is best viewed from a **multifactorial model** in which genetically determined capacities, individual differences in temperament, physiologic variables, and

environmental interactions all contribute. The relative weight of contribution from each of the variables differs for various personality traits and lines of development.

3. **Critical phases.** Particular phases of development must occur at certain ages.

   a. For example, a 4-year-old child who suffered a severe psychological trauma that arrested his development might not experience a normal oedipal period even though the trauma is overcome, and his development recommences at 7 years of age. This distorted oedipal phase might result in irrational fears of physical or psychological harm in competitive situations, a fear that could persist into adulthood. (This example is hypothetical; very little evidence for its inevitability is available.)

   b. The concept of critical phases has been largely supplanted by that of **"sensitive" phases** in which development is most efficient (although development with regard to a specific developmental task is not limited to that phase of development).

4. **Temperament.** Certain children are able to negotiate seemingly overwhelming psychological trauma with minimal overt effect on their subsequent personality development. Others, however, manifest marked symptomatology in the face of considerably less trauma and stress. This dimension of relative vulnerability and invulnerability is referred to as **temperament,** although it is poorly understood at present. What is known to be important is the match or fit between a child's needs and the ability of his environment and caregivers to meet those needs.

   a. For example, temperamentally difficult children may do well developmentally if they have highly competent parents, but they do poorly if they have limited or marginal parents.

   b. By contrast, children whose temperaments are characterized by flexibility and adaptability may demonstrate marked resiliency even in the face of recurrent and catastrophic life events.

C Approach to the child and adolescent patient

1. **The physician must be an advocate for the child** rather than for the parents. To do otherwise is to subject the child to the parents' wishes, even when they are unrealistic, inappropriate, or detrimental to the child. Nevertheless, child psychiatrists must deal respectfully and attempt to develop a working relationship with the parents. Often, the effectiveness of work with the child is measured by the effectiveness of the work with the parents. Ineffective work with the parents may substantially limit the therapeutic progress of the child.

   a. In general, parents should be seen frequently, especially at the beginning of treatment.

   b. Preadolescents should usually be seen alone, but in most cases, after the parents have been seen.

   c. An attempt should be made to communicate with the child patient by talking. If this is difficult, a small assortment of toys, including a dollhouse, paper and crayons, games, puppets, modeling clay, and building materials, can help a child communicate through play.

   d. Adolescents should usually be seen alone. Often, their emerging and developmentally appropriate autonomy should be supported by seeing them before their parents are seen. Use of unnatural slang to bridge the "generation gap" should be avoided. An attitude of sincerity and concern for the adolescent usually establishes rapport with the patient.

2. **The following should be observed during the patient interview:**

   a. The child's reaction to separation from the parents

   b. The child's behavior toward the interviewer (e.g., anxious, very open, shy)

   c. The child's perception of people in general (e.g., trustworthy or dangerous, reliable or neglectful, kind or hostile)

   d. The choice of verbal versus play communication

   e. The clarity of the child's thought processes

   f. The child's level of development (i.e., social, language, motor, psychosexual, cognitive, moral) and its appropriateness to the child's age

   g. The ability of the child to identify different affective states and to discharge these states in an age-appropriate manner

   h. The ability of the child to tolerate frustration and to control impulses. (In most cases, this may be observed through naturalistic circumstances such as setting a limit on an inappropriate behavior, declining an inappropriate request, announcing the end of a session, or requiring the child's assistance in cleaning up toys.)

    i. The child's perception of her- or himself (e.g., competent or ineffectual, master or victim) and the relative strength of his self-esteem

    j. The child's reaction to rejoining the parents after the interview

3. Gathering information from the child can be facilitated by requesting that the child:

    a. Make three wishes and elaborate on each wish.

    b. Make drawings and elaborate on each drawing. (Drawings of people and families are especially helpful.)

    c. Describe his or her family.

    d. Describe important nonfamily members.

    e. Describe favorite television shows, movies, and musicians, noting with whom the child identifies.

    f. Describe the problem that initiated therapy and how the family told the child of the appointment.

    g. Describe hopes and wishes for the future.

II   BONDING AND ATTACHMENT

A   Definitions

1. Bonding describes the **parent's affective relationship with the child.** Bonding develops over time. There appears to be no critical phase of bonding in humans such as that described in animal studies. Bonding likely commences long before the birth of the child and is apparent in the parents' attitudes, fantasies, and wishes for the child.

2. Attachment describes the **child's affective relationship with the parents.** Attachment, like bonding, develops over time. There is no critical phase for the development of attachment relationships, which may be formed at any time throughout the life cycle.

B   Assessment of bonding

1. The parents should be asked **when and how a name was chosen** for the child. This may suggest when they began planning for the new arrival. The name may also have special meaning. It may indicate how the family perceives the child or suggest attributions made to the child. For example, a son who is named after his father may be dealt with harshly by his mother when an acrimonious relationship exists between the parents.

2. It is important to determine what sort of **dreams and fantasies the parents had** about the child **during pregnancy.** Frequent, realistic, and hopeful reflection about the baby enhances the outcome related to bonding and attachment.

3. Likewise, it is important to determine **how the parents' relationship toward each other changed during the pregnancy.** The husband often assumes a maternal role toward his wife when she is pregnant. If, however, he begins abusing her, has affairs, or grows distant or uninvolved, a more difficult relationship between the parents and the new baby is likely. In addition, at this time, the parents' own unmet or inadequately met dependency needs and needs for nurture from childhood may complicate their relationships with each other and with their new child.

4. Parents should be questioned regarding their **early reactions to the child in the delivery room and in the nursery.** Ambivalence of the parents concerning their child may be communicated behaviorally. It is important, however, to distinguish ambivalence from uncertainty, anxiety, and lack of confidence, all of which are normal reactions to childbirth and are particularly common to first-time parents.

5. The parents should be asked **of whom the child reminds them.** This question assesses for transferences and preconceived attitudes about the infant. Inappropriate attributions to the child must be identified, clarified, disconnected from the child, and reconnected with the original object of attribution.

6. The mental health of the parents should be investigated. Depression, psychosis, personality disorders, and drug abuse are examples of problems that can distort the way the parent perceives, responds to, and interacts with the child.

7. Special problems are posed if the newborn spends extra time in the nursery because of illness (e.g., a child born 3 months premature who spends his first 2 months of life in a neonatal intensive care unit). A family with a child in the critical care nursery should be evaluated before discharge to ensure that the child will receive adequate care.

C **Disorders of bonding and attachment**

1. **Hospitalism** is an extreme example of failure of any affective relationship to develop.
   a. **Symptoms.** Affected infants suffer from:
      (1) Susceptibility to infection
      (2) Apathy
      (3) Retarded development
      (4) Failure to thrive
   b. **Treatment. Parents should be counseled to spend time with the newborn.** When the parents have not visited a sick infant or have been reluctant to see a newborn, a structured plan to facilitate parent–child interactions should be implemented.
      (1) There should be a **mandatory visitation** of the baby by the parents **of at least 12 consecutive hours.**
      (2) **Nursing support** should be available when the parents have questions.
      (3) **Psychiatric intervention** may be required when the parents' grief over a child's prematurity or illness is thought to contribute to the lack of parental involvement.
      (4) **Follow-up** in a special clinic for premature infants is indicated.
      (5) **Referral to a child protective agency** is necessary if the parents cannot demonstrate a bond to their child or when they do not understand their child's needs.
      (6) **Foster home placement** may be necessary to protect the child while attempts are made to correct parental deficits.

2. **Anaclitic depression** results when an attachment relationship is disrupted during a sensitive phase of development (e.g., 18 to 36 months; see V A 1).

3. **Child abuse** may occur if parents have not adequately bonded with the child. This may reflect a deficiency in the development of parental empathy. Not surprisingly, **premature infants** are at increased risk both for complications of bonding and attachment and, concomitantly, for child abuse and neglect [see II C 1 b (5)–(6)]. Psychopathology in either parent should be evaluated and treated.

4. **Vulnerable child syndrome** was originally described by Green and Solnit in 1964. These children, who have been ill and have recovered, have parents who may continue to treat them as though they are still vulnerable.
   a. **Symptoms** in this disorder derive from stifling and oppressive affective relationships of the parents with the child. Such children may later show a variety of psychological traits resulting from parental overprotectiveness, including:
      (1) Hypochondriasis
      (2) Hyperactivity
      (3) Separation anxiety
      (4) Learning difficulties
   b. **Management** of vulnerable child syndrome involves informing the parents that the child has recovered and is doing well. Surprisingly, parents may not realize this, and their attitude toward the child may change with this reassurance.
      (1) **If reassurance fails,** psychotherapy for the parents is indicated.
      (2) **If the child has internalized this sense of fragility and vulnerability** and it has become part the child's identity, psychotherapy for the child is indicated. Affective distance between the parents and the child must be increased, and the age-appropriate autonomy of the child must be reinforced.

5. **Separation anxiety** in toddlerhood and childhood may derive from ambivalent or insecure attachments formed during infancy.

III **FEEDING AND EATING DISORDERS OF INFANCY AND EARLY CHILDHOOD**

A **Pica** involves the persistent (for a period of at least 1 month) eating of nonfood products (e.g., dirt, clay, paper, plaster). This behavior is developmentally inappropriate and must be differentiated from the practice of mouthing inanimate objects, which is normal between 6 and 12 months of age.

1. **Epidemiology.** Pica may be more common in lower socioeconomic groups.
2. **Etiology**
    a. Children with **mental retardation** mouth objects more than normal children.
    b. **Nutritional deficiencies** may play a role in some cases. Deficiencies of both vitamins and minerals have been suggested. In particular, iron deficiency can cause a craving for ice and nonfood items.
    c. **Parent–child problems** (especially when repeated, traumatic separations are involved) are etiologic in some cases. In these cases, the ingestion most likely represents a response to deprivation and unfulfilled oral needs.
    d. A variety of **rare neurologic conditions** can cause children to mouth nonfood items (e.g., Klüver-Bucy syndrome).
    e. **Cultural factors** may play a role in some cases, in which the ingested substance is believed to have magical or medicinal properties.
3. **Complications** include **bezoars** and **lead poisoning,** which can present as a variety of neurologic and psychiatric manifestations. Lead poisoning is extremely dangerous and is more common in older homes with lead-based paint. Lead poisoning should be suspected in any child who has an encephalopathy or who exhibits unusual behavior (e.g., irritability, anorexia, decreased activity).
4. **Treatment** involves increasing the amount of stimulation the child receives. (Most cities offer infant-stimulation programs.) Psychotherapy for the child and parents may be necessary. Of course, dangerous objects should be removed from the child's environment, and any nutritional deficiencies should be corrected.

B **Rumination disorder** is a potentially fatal disorder that is most common in infancy and early childhood and is characterized by purposeful expulsion of previously ingested food followed by rechewing of the food. This usually occurs when the child is alone or is attended only peripherally. On extremely rare occasions, the disorder may be seen among adults, usually with coexistent bulimia nervosa or mental retardation.

1. **Epidemiology.** Rumination disorder is rare and may be decreasing in incidence.
2. **Etiology.** Although theories abound, the disorder often occurs in families in which the parents are psychosexually immature and either distant or overstimulating. Food and chewing may take on a transitional quality for the child and soothe the infant when alone, much like a special doll or blanket.
3. **Treatment**
    a. **Dyad (parent–child) interactions should be observed.** Cues that the parent gives the child to encourage regurgitation should be interpreted and eradicated.
    b. **In-depth psychotherapy of one or both parents** is often needed.
    c. The **infant's nutritional status** should be followed closely.

C **Feeding disorder of infancy or early childhood (failure to thrive)** is diagnosed when a child fails to gain or maintain weight at age-appropriate norms. Usually, the third percentile for age group is considered the threshold. Failure to grow in height sometimes accompanies this, but failure of head circumference growth occurs only in severe cases. In addition to the physical growth retardation, a characteristic emotional and behavioral constellation also may be observed. This constellation is described in the *Diagnostic and Statistical Manual of Mental Disorders,* 4th edition (*DSM-IV*), category of **reactive attachment disorder of infancy or early childhood** and is characterized by disturbed and developmentally inappropriate social relatedness. This may take the form of social unresponsiveness, withdrawal, and inhibition or excessive interpersonal familiarity and lack of appropriate social boundaries.

1. **Etiology**
    a. **Nonorganic failure to thrive.** Failure to thrive as a **psychiatric condition** has numerous causes and manifestations. The following list divides these causes by developmental phase but is not meant to be complete:
        (1) **Early infancy.** Before 8 or 9 months of life, a child is inactive and relies on parental feeding. Failure to thrive in this age range may indicate poor parenting or troubled parent–child interactions. Of note, "poor parenting" does not fairly encompass all parent–child interactional

problems that contribute to this disorder. Eating problems in infancy may also be caused by a lack of synchrony between the parent and the biologic rhythms (e.g., hunger) of the child. The parent may misinterpret certain cues from the infant and miss other cues altogether.

(2) **Late infancy.** After 8 months, failure to thrive may be secondary to anaclitic depression, poor parenting, or childhood psychosis.

(3) **Toddler stage.** The negativism associated with the "terrible twos" can also apply to eating. Children may refuse to eat in the service of autonomy. Sometimes this negativism may develop earlier, for example, in response to the parents' frantically forcing food on a 1-year-old child.

b. **Organic failure to thrive.** Several medical conditions can cause failure to thrive and should be evaluated. These include juvenile-onset diabetes mellitus, other endocrine disorders, and malabsorption syndromes.

2. **Treatment.** Any organic cause must be ruled out, and underlying medical disorders must be treated. Parent–child interactions should be evaluated carefully.

a. In some cases, **teaching the parents to recognize and respond to the cues of their child** is adequate intervention.

b. In other cases, **it may be necessary to hospitalize the child** to determine whether he or she can gain weight in a new environment.

c. When parental neglect is present, **child protective agencies** must be involved, to ensure that the child receives adequate care and that the services necessary to correct parental deficits are available. At times, custody of the child must be taken from the parents, and the child must be placed outside the home.

IV CHILDHOOD PSYCHOSES

A Autistic disorder

1. **Clinical data.** Autistic disorder is an illness in which the child is relatively unresponsive to other human beings, demonstrates bizarre responses to the environment, and has unusual language development. Autistic disorder most commonly begins before age 3 years. Autism is a symptom of several disorders (e.g., schizophrenia). As a symptom, autism refers to a preoccupation with the internal world of the individual to the exclusion of external reactivity.

a. Autistic children often treat other individuals indifferently, almost as though they are inanimate objects.

b. Language abnormalities include echolalia, pronoun reversals (e.g., use of the pronoun "you" when "I" is correct), mutism, qualitative abnormalities (e.g., a sing-song or monotonous quality), and general language delays.

c. Autistic children have a great need for consistency in their environment and may decompensate if, for example, furniture is rearranged. The cause of this need for sameness is unknown.

d. Social development is invariably abnormal.

2. **Diagnostic criteria** (Table 12–1)

3. **Epidemiology.** Although the disorder has an even socioeconomic distribution, it is more common in boys.

4. **Etiology.** A cold, distant mother figure was formerly thought to be responsible for the development of coldness and aloofness in the child (i.e., growing in an emotional vacuum leads to unrelatedness in the child). However, this theory has been replaced by the understanding that **organic rather than reactive pathology** underlies the disorder, although precise neuropathologic processes have not been determined. Genetic, congenital, immunologic, neuroanatomic, neurophysiologic, and biochemical aberrations have all been suggested.

5. **Associated findings**

a. **Abnormal auditory evoked potentials** (i.e., tracings of the transmission of sound stimuli from the brain stem to the cerebral cortex) are seen.

b. Imaging studies (e.g., computed tomography scans and magnetic resonance imaging) suggest possible **structural abnormalities.**

TABLE 12-1 Diagnostic Criteria for Autistic Disorder

Social interactional deficits, such as impairment in:
- Nonverbal communicative behaviors
- Peer relationships
- Taking the initiative in social interactions
- Interpersonal reciprocity within relationships

Communicative deficits, such as:
- Impairment in language development
- Impairment in conversational skills
- Use of repetitive or idiosyncratic language
- Impairment in the development of imaginative or imitative play

Behavioral deficits, such as:
- Consuming preoccupation with one or a few idiosyncratic areas of interest; otherwise, restricted breadth of interest in the surrounding environment
- Excessive need for routine; ritualized behaviors; inordinate resistance to change
- Stereotyped motor movements (e.g., hand flapping, rocking)
- Preoccupation with parts of objects

---

    c. Positron-emission tomography (PET) studies suggest possible **glucose utilization abnormalities.**

    d. **Decreased nystagmus** in response to vestibular stimulation occurs.

    e. **Developmental distortions** (i.e., qualitative abnormalities in development) above and beyond mere delays may occur.

6. **Differential diagnosis**
    a. Hearing deficits
    b. Visual deficits
    c. Mental retardation accompanied by global developmental delays (not focal social and language distortions and delays as in autism)
    d. Organic mental disorders (e.g., hepatic encephalopathy and congenital cytomegalovirus), which can mimic autism
    e. Tourette syndrome
    f. Fragile X syndrome
    g. Obsessive-compulsive disorder (OCD)
    h. Childhood schizophrenia
    i. Elective mutism
    j. Other pervasive developmental disorders (e.g., Rett's disorder, childhood disintegrative disorder, Asperger's disorder)

7. **Treatment**
    a. A **highly structured classroom setting** is important to help autistic children focus their attention on learning and communication tasks. Pragmatics, daily living skills, and a functional curriculum may take precedence over conventional academics. Precautions should be taken to ensure that the environment remains stable (e.g., predictable schedules, routines, personnel, and materials).

    b. **Psychotherapy for both the child and parents** may be of value in cases in which parental factors are considered to be complicating. Psychotherapy may also be indicated when the family is having trouble coping with the stress of having an autistic child.

    c. **Medication is rarely of value unless a specific indication is present.**
        (1) Some hyperactive autistic children may benefit from stimulant medication (e.g., fenfluramine or methylphenidate).
        (2) Obsessional features may respond to clomipramine or fluoxetine.
        (3) Mood instability may be improved with **mood stabilizers** such as lithium, valproic acid, and carbamazepine.
        (4) Self-stimulating behaviors may improve with **opioid antagonists** such as naltrexone.

       (5) Atypical antipsychotics, such as risperidone, are occasionally indicated for acute stabilization of aggressive, self-injurious, or severely out-of-control behaviors.

    d. Adjunctive therapies, such as speech and language therapy, occupational therapy, and physical therapy, are often indicated.

8. **Prognosis.** Many autistic children develop grand mal seizures before adolescence. However, the prognosis for autistic disorder is better if the child has:
   a. A high intelligence quotient
   b. Reasonable language development
   c. Relatively mild symptomatology

B Childhood schizophrenia

1. **Clinical data.** Symptoms of childhood schizophrenia may include:
   a. Preoccupation with gory or grotesque fantasies
   b. Hallucinations (usually not prominent; visual hallucinations are more common in children than adults)
   c. Delusions (less common in children than adults)
   d. Propensity to digress, with poor attention span
   e. Responsiveness to individuals in the environment without consistent demonstration of sociability, reciprocity, or empathy
   f. Possible abnormal motor movements
   g. Unusual mannerisms

2. **Diagnostic criteria.** *DSM-IV* criteria are the same for children as for adults (see Table 2–1).

3. **Etiology**
   a. New studies continue to demonstrate a **genetic component** to the development of schizophrenia. Heredity alone, however, does not account for the etiology.
   b. A **grossly chaotic upbringing** with constant exposure to aggressive and sexual themes (e.g., chronic violence in the family) may contribute to schizophrenia-like symptoms.
   c. A **failure of repression** may also contribute to the development of symptoms. For example, a child who is repeatedly exposed to violence may be unable to repress sexual and aggressive fantasies. The ability to repress such fantasies normally occurs by age 6 years.
   d. Whether the prepubertal onset of schizophrenic-like symptoms in childhood represents an early onset within the same spectrum as the adult disorder or whether the prepubertal variant would be better described as **schizophreniform disorder** remains uncertain. Most likely, both alternatives occur clinically.

4. **Treatment**
   a. **Psychotherapy** may be helpful when environmental factors appear contributory. Family therapy may be indicated when disruption in the family is evident. When aggression and sexualized stimulation cannot be minimized in the home, out-of-home placement should be considered.
   b. **Psychiatric day treatment** may be indicated when the child's symptoms preclude his ability to function adequately in a public school environment.
   c. **Atypical antipsychotic medications** such as risperidone (0.25 to 1.0 mg/day) or olanzapine (2.5 to 5.0 mg/day) have been used beneficially.

5. **Prognosis.** The prognosis for individuals with childhood schizophrenia is generally more favorable than that for adult schizophrenia, provided adequate treatment and remediation of environmental deficits occur. This may be because the childhood disorder represents a diagnostic spectrum not fully continuous with the spectrum of the adult disorder. Nonetheless, studies indicate that at least 50% of individuals with childhood schizophrenia persist with significant symptoms and deficits into adulthood. A family history of schizophrenia worsens the prognosis.

C Symbiotic psychosis

1. **Clinical data.** Symbiotic psychosis is a disorder in which parents misperceive themselves as their child. The reciprocal is also usually true. Although this disorder usually occurs in mothers and their children, fathers are occasionally affected.

   a. A loss of ego boundaries (i.e., the inability to distinguish oneself from others) is apparent.

   b. Great anxiety at the threat of separation of the child from the parent is seen in both. Upon reuniting, the anxiety clears.

   c. The overlap between the parent and child can be manifested in almost any area (e.g., if parents diet, they assume that the child needs to diet).

   d. Although this disorder still is observed clinically, it is not specifically accounted for within the *DSM-IV*, in which it would be considered a psychotic disorder not otherwise specified.

2. **Etiology.** Parents who have **poor object relations** may see their child as an extension of themselves. **Borderline psychopathology** may predispose people to this disorder. Although the parent is the cause of the problem, the child usually manifests the symptoms (e.g., severe separation anxiety).

3. **Treatment.** Psychotherapy aimed at separating the child from the parent is needed. Parents sometimes require support to help them permit the separation and development of autonomy in the child. In certain refractory cases, an actual separation through out-of-home placement may be necessary.

4. **Prognosis.** Symbiotic psychosis carries the best prognosis of all the childhood psychoses, probably because its etiology is reactive and developmental rather than organically based.

V CHILDHOOD MOOD DISORDERS

Biologic markers, which are still being investigated, are even less valuable in identifying childhood depressive disorders than in identifying adult disorders.

A **Clinical data**   Depressive illness presents at all stages of development.

1. **Children between the ages of 7 and 30 months** may demonstrate **anaclitic depression.** The cause is a lengthy separation (>1 week) from caregivers with whom they have established an attachment relationship. Symptoms include listlessness, anorexia, psychomotor retardation, and sad facial expressions. The treatment is restitution of the relationship.

2. Depressed **preschool children** often demonstrate behavioral difficulties, such as hyperactivity and aggression, more than older children. These symptoms are often called **depressive equivalents.** Separation from caregivers or a poor sense of mastery over developmental tasks (e.g., toilet training) may be etiologic. Treatment should be aimed at changing the child's environment. Psychotherapy may help.

3. **Schoolchildren** may manifest the usual signs and symptoms of depression (e.g., vegetative signs, depressed mood). Biologic vulnerabilities and a sense of helplessness or incompetence may play an etiologic role at this age. Psychotherapy, especially cognitive-behavioral modalities aimed at helping the child feel a sense of competence in relation to her environment, may be helpful.

4. **Adolescents** may also demonstrate the usual signs of depression, especially a pervasive sense of boredom and lack of future orientation. The incidence of depressive disorders increases in adolescence, with girls affected more often than boys. In children and adolescents, the depressive mood is commonly expressed as **marked irritability.**

B **Diagnostic criteria**   *DSM-IV* criteria are the same for children as for adults (see Table 3–1).

C **Treatment**

1. **Psychotherapy.** Insight-oriented models aimed at grieving past losses and remediating early intrapsychic traumas have been used effectively in treating childhood mood disorders. Cognitive-behavioral models aimed at correcting cognitive distortions and reversing pervasive patterns of negativistic thinking have also been successful.

2. **Medication.** New research is beginning to document the efficacy of **antidepressants** as useful adjuncts in the treatment of depression in certain children and adolescents.

   a. Most often, medications should be used to augment ongoing individual or family psychotherapy.

   b. **Tricyclic antidepressants,** such as imipramine and nortriptyline, as well as the newer generation selective serotonin reuptake inhibitors (**SSRIs**) such as fluoxetine have been used effectively with children and adolescents. Because of their wider margins of safety and better side effect profile, the SSRIs generally are considered the first-line medications of choice.

    c. In 2004, the **U.S. Food and Drug Administration (FDA) issued a black box warning** that "antidepressants increased the risk of suicidal thinking and behavior (suicidality) in short-term studies of children and adolescents with major depressive disorder and other psychiatric disorders." Analyses of data showed that children and adolescents receiving antidepressants were two times more likely to show suicidal thinking and behavior during the first few months of treatment. No completed suicides occurred in any of the clinical trials. It is important to balance the FDA warning against the potential therapeutic benefit and risk of untreated psychiatric illness. Children and adolescents taking antidepressants should be closely monitored for clinical worsening, suicidality, and unusual changes in behavior.

    d. Parents must take the responsibility for administering the medication and for safeguarding the child and siblings from inadvertent overdosage.

D Associated mood disorders

1. **Manic-depressive (bipolar) illness** may present in early childhood. *DSM-IV* criteria are the same for children as for adults (see Table 3–2).

    a. Mood stabilizers, such as lithium, valproic acid, and carbamazepine, have been used effectively in children and adolescents.

    b. Hyperactivity (attention deficit hyperactivity disorder [ADHD]) may be **mistaken for mania;** however, major mood changes are not seen in hyperactive children.

2. **Suicide** may be a complication of a mood disorder in children and adolescents, as well as in later developmental stages.

    a. The **incidence** of suicide is increasing in preadolescents and adolescents (it has tripled among adolescents since 1970).

    b. Treatment. Depressed children should be carefully evaluated for suicidal ideation. When suicidal ideation is found, the child may require psychiatric hospitalization for acute clinical stabilization and his or her own safety.

VI TOURETTE DISORDER

A Clinical data Tourette disorder consists of recurrent, involuntary, purposeless motor movements accompanied by vocal tics (e.g., coprolalia, involuntary swearing, barking, and grunting). Motor tics may occur before or after the development of vocal tics. Psychological stress exacerbates the symptoms, but the cause, although unknown, is probably organic. Both ADHD and OCD occur with increased frequency among patients with Tourette disorder.

B Diagnostic criteria (Table 12–2)

C Epidemiology Tourette disorder is more common in boys. Onset is before the age of 21 years and often occurs in early childhood. Tourette disorder occurs in all socioeconomic classes and is considerably more prevalent than once believed. There is a spectrum of symptom severity, and previously undiagnosed individuals with more mild symptoms are now being appropriately diagnosed.

D Treatment

1. **Psychotherapy** is indicated when the tics cause psychological problems.

2. **Education** about the nature and course of the disorder for both the patient and the family is essential.

TABLE 12–2 Diagnostic Criteria for Tourette Disorder

Multiple tics, including both motor and vocal tics
Frequent tics, nearly daily, for a year or more, with no asymptomatic period of more than 3 months
Emotional distress or functional impairment as a result of the tics
Onset before age 18 years

3. **Medical treatment** includes the use of the following agents:
   a. **Haloperidol** suppresses the tics, and **pimozide** is an effective neuroleptic medication; however, it may cause cardiac arrhythmias. Atypical antipsychotics are now considered the treatment of choice.
   b. **Risperidone** has demonstrated effectiveness in suppressing tics.
   c. **Clonidine** has proved to be effective in some cases of Tourette disorder. Although highly sedating, clonidine does not have the dystonic and dyskinetic side effects of the neuroleptics. **Guanfacine** is a similar but less sedating alternative to clonidine.
   d. **SSRIs** such as fluoxetine may also be helpful.

VII SLEEP DISORDERS

A **Parasomnias** are sleep disorders that usually affect stages 3 and 4 of sleep, which predominate early in the sleep cycle. Thus, these disorders usually occur early in the night. Examples include the following:

1. **Somnambulism** (sleep walking) is exacerbated by psychological stress in some people but is normal much of the time. Alcoholism unmasks somnambulism in adults.

2. **Somniloquy** (sleep talking) has little clinical significance; however, if somniloquy is present, more significant parasomnias may also be present.

3. **Night terrors** are very common between the ages of 2.5 and 5 years, affecting 30% of children in this age bracket. Terrors are sometimes exacerbated by stress.
   a. **Night terrors should be distinguished from nightmares,** which occur during rapid eye movement (REM) sleep and whose content is remembered as a bad dream. Night terrors are characterized by:
      (1) Inconsolability of the child during the event
      (2) Absence of recall of the content of the dream
      (3) Absence of recall of the event the following morning
   b. **Treatment.** Although seldom necessary, night terrors may be treated by agents that suppress deep sleep, such as **chloral hydrate** or **benzodiazepines.**

4. **Nocturnal enuresis** (see VIII A 1) is generally caused by stress or to slow central nervous system (CNS) maturation. The disorder dissipates with increasing age and is, therefore, self-limited.

B **Narcolepsy** is characterized by REM-onset sleep.

1. Manifestations
   a. The entire sleep cycle is affected, resulting in **excessive daytime drowsiness and sleep attacks.**
   b. **Cataplexy,** a classic symptom of narcolepsy, is the loss of motor tone in response to an emotion (e.g., anger or excitement).
   c. On awakening, the patient may be transiently but completely paralyzed (**sleep paralysis**).
   d. **Hypnagogic hallucinations** are vivid auditory and visual hallucinations that occur at the onset of sleep. **Hypnopompic hallucinations** occur at the end of sleep.

2. **Treatment.** Agents that suppress REM sleep, such as psychostimulants and tricyclic antidepressants, provide some symptomatic relief for patients suffering from narcolepsy. **Modafinil** (Provigil) is an α_1-adrenergic receptor agonist that reduces the number of sleep attacks.

VIII ELIMINATION DISORDERS

A **Enuresis**

1. **Clinical data.** Children with enuresis continue to urinate at inappropriate times and places after the time when he should have been toilet trained (i.e., between the ages of 2 and 4 years). The disorder is much more common in boys.
   a. **Primary enuresis** is that which has never been interrupted by a period of good bladder control.
      (1) **Nocturnal enuresis** is a parasomnia that occurs during stages 3 and 4 of sleep.
      (2) **Diurnal enuresis** occurs during the waking hours.

   b. Secondary enuresis develops after at least 1 year of good bladder control. As in primary enuresis, the disorder may occur both during the sleeping and waking hours.

   c. The *DSM-IV* specifies that episodes occur at least twice weekly for 3 months or more. In addition, the condition is not diagnosed before the chronological age (or in developmentally impaired children, the developmental age) of 5 years.

2. Etiology

   a. Organic disorders may cause enuresis. These include:

     (1) Systemic illnesses, such as:

       (a) Juvenile-onset diabetes mellitus

       (b) Sickle cell anemia or sickle cell trait

       (c) Diabetes insipidus

     (2) CNS disorders, such as:

       (a) Frontal lobe tumor

       (b) Spinal cord lesion (e.g., spina bifida or spina bifida occulta)

       (c) Peripheral nerve damage

     (3) Anatomic disorders, such as:

       (a) Posterior urethral valvular dysfunction

       (b) Proximal genitourinary malformations

     (4) Urinary tract infections

     (5) Delayed CNS maturation After the age of 4½ years, as many as 10% of boys remain enuretic, often because of delayed maturation.

   b. Psychological factors account for most cases of secondary enuresis.

     (1) Acute stress can cause enuresis (e.g., the birth of a sibling, a family move, starting kindergarten).

     (2) Ambition. Enuresis sometimes occurs in very ambitious boys. Strength and quality of the urine stream may become equated with physical prowess. Micturition can then become conflicted, resulting in urination at inappropriate times.

     (3) Hostility can be expressed through the symptom of enuresis. Such an expression of hostility is nearly always unconscious: The child does not deliberately void at inappropriate times.

     (4) Family reaction to the enuresis sometimes causes more psychopathology than the psychological causes of the enuresis. The family may encourage enuresis unconsciously. The parents may take vicarious pleasure in the child's enuresis.

     (5) Preoccupation. Children who are too busy or preoccupied to remember to use the bathroom may suffer from enuresis.

3. Treatment may be necessary only sporadically. Because enuresis is a self-limited disorder, sometimes the best treatment is no treatment. Parents should be reassured that the disorder is a time-limited, normal developmental variant (especially the primary nocturnal pattern) that will ultimately be outgrown.

   a. Probing diagnostic procedures to search for an organic etiology, unless the preponderance of evidence points to such, **should be avoided.**

   b. The parents should be assured that the child is not purposefully wetting (enuresis is usually beyond the child's control). **Remedial measures** include:

     (1) Reduction of fluid intake after dinner

     (2) Awakening the child to urinate after 1 to 2 hours of sleep

     (3) Bladder exercises (having the child hold urine during the day for progressively longer periods of time)

     (4) Use of special feedback devices that set off an alarm upon urination in bed

   c. Medication is not considered first-line treatment.

     (1) Desmopressin, a synthetic antidiuretic hormone that may be administered either orally or as a nasal spray, may also offer symptomatic improvement.

     (2) Because of the time-limited nature of the disorder, drug holidays should instituted at least every 6 months to assess the need for continuing pharmacologic intervention.

   d. The child should be treated for any psychological stress. In refractory cases, long-term **psychotherapy** may be indicated.

B **Encopresis**

1. **Clinical data.** Encopresis is fecal incontinence beyond the period when bowel control should normally have developed. Most encopresis is unconscious and involuntary; only occasionally does it occur deliberately.
   a. **Primary encopresis** has occurred continuously throughout the child's life.
   b. **Secondary encopresis** develops after at least 1 year of good bowel control.
   c. The *DSM-IV* delineates two additional **subtypes:**
      (1) **With constipation and overflow incontinence**
      (2) **Without constipation and overflow incontinence**

2. **Etiology**
   a. **Organic disorders.** Hirschsprung disease rarely presents in older children as encopresis.
      (1) In Hirschsprung disease, the functional obstruction is proximal to the rectal vault so that no fecal obstruction is palpable on digital examination.
      (2) In the encopresis variant with constipation and overflow incontinence, however, the encopresis results from children avoiding evacuating their bowels and retaining feces.
         (a) This results in a fecal impaction that is readily identifiable within the rectal vault.
         (b) In these children, stool is passed around the impaction, often in small amounts.
   b. **Psychological factors**
      (1) **Unresolved anger at a parent** is sometimes expressed unconsciously through fecal incontinence. The child consciously and unconsciously perceives that his stool has a negative impact on the family.
      (2) **Regressive wishes** may be expressed by soiling in undernurtured and emotionally deprived children.
      (3) Fecal smearing may be a **psychotic symptom,** especially if the child is older than 4 or 5 years of age.
      (4) As is true with enuresis, parents can get vicarious pleasure from their child's symptoms.
      (5) When **autonomy and control battles** focus on toilet training at the age of 2 to 3 years and when parents are too punitive and unyielding in their approach to toilet training, conflicts over bowel evacuation develop in the child.

3. **Treatment**
   a. **Correction of fecal impaction** is necessary. A bowel regimen that consists of periodic cathartic administration to ensure that no impaction develops and to help regulate bowel control (e.g., administration of a bisacodyl suppository daily at the same time, immediately followed by placing the child on the toilet) may be beneficial.
   b. **Behavior modification** that reinforces continence is effective in some children (e.g., rewarding a child after a day of good bowel control or after evacuation in the toilet).
   c. **Psychotherapy** may be indicated. Occasionally, encopresis is a symptom of psychosis. The underlying disease should then be treated.
   d. **Family therapy** also is often indicated.

IX MASTURBATION

A **Definition**   Childhood masturbation involves genital manipulation and fondling. It is a universal behavior, not a disease. Nonetheless, many parents complain to the physician about this behavior in their children. An open attitude on the part of the physician is important in allowing the parents to express concern. Any notions that masturbation may cause growth retardation, mental retardation, or any adverse physical consequence should be dispelled.

B **Incidence**   Masturbation occurs in all children. It can develop before age 1 year. During the oedipal period (i.e., between the ages of 3 1/2 and 6 years), there is heightened focus on the genitalia.

C **Etiology**   Continuous masturbation may be a sign of severe understimulation, environmental deprivation, or excessive sexual stimulation or sexual abuse.

1. The parents should be queried about **other signs of self-stimulation** (e.g., rocking, head banging, hair pulling). The child should be enrolled in a stimulation program, and the situation should be followed up.

2. **Signs of child abuse** should also be sought. A detailed history of the child's exposure to sexual stimulation should be elicited. A careful physical examination may be indicated.

X THUMB SUCKING

A Incidence   Thumb sucking is more common in girls and is normal at transitional periods in the child's life (e.g., at bedtime, at times of separation from the parents). When it persists into the grade-school years, it more likely suggests underlying individual or family pathology.

B Treatment is usually not needed. If thumb sucking is chronic and occurs after the age of 31/2 years, however, it can cause changes in dentition.

1. Exploration of the nature of the child's relationship with the parents is usually indicated.
2. Thumb sucking in an older child can be a sign that the child is insecure or withdrawn. **Behavior modification** can be useful.
3. Coating the thumb with astringent agents has been of limited benefit.

XI SCHOOL PHOBIAS

A Definition   School phobias are defined as a fearful attitude toward and avoidance of school. In adolescence, they may herald the emergence of schizophrenia.

B Incidence   School phobias most commonly occur when a child is first introduced to school (at age 4 or 5 years) and in early adolescence, when children are required to shower at school after gym class. School phobias occur throughout childhood, however.

C Etiology   School phobia is best considered a symptom. It is caused by a variety of conditions, including:

1. Separation anxiety suffered by the child
2. Separation anxiety suffered by the parent
3. Malingering (e.g., the child has not completed a homework assignment)
4. A legitimate cause of fear at school (e.g., gangs, a cruel teacher)
5. Vulnerable child syndrome
6. Homosexual panic in an older child

D Treatment

1. Legitimate causes of fear should be evaluated for and eliminated when present. **The child should usually be sent back to school immediately** so that school avoidance is not reinforced by staying home.
2. **Psychotherapy** to treat the underlying disorder may be needed.
3. **Desensitization and other behavior therapy** modalities may be of benefit.
4. **Parental therapy** is necessary when the child is acting out the parent's anxiety about separating from the child.
5. Some cases are exceedingly refractory to treatment interventions and may even require **psychiatric hospitalization.**
6. **Anxiolytic medications,** such as the SSRIs, tricyclic antidepressants, buspirone, and occasionally, benzodiazepines, may offer acute symptom relief. They are usually unnecessary on an ongoing basis.

XII ATTENTION DEFICIT HYPERACTIVITY DISORDER (ADHD)

A Clinical data   Key symptoms of ADHD include a short attention span, difficulty concentrating, impulsivity, distractibility, excitability, and hyperactivity.

1. **Hyperactivity** is defined subjectively as an increase in motor activity to a level that interferes with the child's functioning at school, at home, or socially.

2. It is important to note, however, that symptoms of **attention deficit disorder may exist with or without hyperactivity.**

3. The *DSM-IV* distinguishes **three subtypes** of the disorder based on this differentiation:
   a. ADHD, predominantly inattentive type
   b. ADHD, predominantly hyperactive-impulsive type
   c. ADHD, combined type

B **Diagnostic criteria** (Table 12–3)

C **Etiology**

1. **Medication.** Sedative-hypnotics paradoxically cause hyperactivity in some children.

2. **Depression.** Sad feelings may be expressed by means of increased activity.

3. **Anxiety**

4. **Severe CNS disease.** A grossly abnormal CNS or a history of significant head trauma may cause hyperactivity.

5. **Constitutional hyperactivity.** Some children have a hyperactive temperament that is present from birth.

6. **An intolerant parent, teacher, or supervisor** may bring about factitious hyperactivity (i.e., the child is not truly suffering from increased motor activity).

7. **Specific learning disabilities** may be associated with hyperactivity.

8. Severe **language disorders**

9. There is an increased incidence of ADHD among children with **Tourette disorder.**

10. **Family history** is important; ADHD commonly runs in families.

D **Treatment**　Any underlying disorder should be treated (e.g., depression should be treated by means of psychotherapy, possibly in conjunction with antidepressant medication).

TABLE 12–3　Diagnostic Criteria for Attention Deficit Hyperactivity Disorder

Symptoms of inattention, such as:
- Lack of attention to details
- Difficulty sustaining attention for prolonged periods
- Not listening
- Difficulty following through or completing tasks
- Disorganization
- Avoidance of activities that require sustained attention
- Tendency to lose personal belongings
- Marked distractibility
- Forgetfulness

Symptoms of hyperactivity, such as:
- Fidgetiness or squirminess
- Difficulty remaining in seat, or sitting quietly
- Developmentally excessive activity level
- Difficulty engaging in nonaction activities
- Talking excessively

Symptoms of impulsivity, such as:
- Blurting out answers without raising hand or waiting for the end of the question
- Difficulty with "turn-taking" activities
- Frequent interruption or intrusion into others' conversations or activities

Presence of some symptoms before age 7 years

Significant functional impairment as a result of the symptoms

1. **Medications**
    a. **Stimulant medications** (e.g., **methylphenidate** administered orally in a divided dose of 5 to 60 mg/day) are effective. Alternate choices include **dextroamphetamine** and **dexmethylphenidate,** which have sustained-release preparations that provide more even blood levels and once-in-the-morning dosing. Growth curves should be followed on all children taking stimulant medications because appetite and growth suppression are the most common side effects.
    b. **Clonidine** and **guanfacine** have been shown to be effective alternatives to psychostimulants in many children. They may also be used effectively to augment psychostimulants in certain refractory cases. Aggression, hyperactivity, and impulsivity are more responsive than are the symptoms of inattention.
    c. **Antidepressants** such as **venlafaxine** and **bupropion** have been effective alternative agents in some children.
2. **Diet.** An alteration in the child's diet may be helpful, presumably because the emphasis on food alters a parent's relationship with a child in some meaningful way.
    a. Many parents of hyperactive children report that reducing the child's sugar intake reduces the hyperactivity.
       (1) These parents may pay more attention to their child, feel more in control of the problem, and spend more time with the child at mealtime as a result of changing the child's diet.
       (2) All of these secondary effects can be beneficial.
    b. No direct effects of diet on either the etiology or treatment of ADHD have been demonstrated, however.
3. **Behavior modification programs** are often beneficial. Despite the ADHD symptomatic deficits, children with this disorder must still be held accountable for their behavior and its consequences.
4. Although **psychotherapy** is not the mainstay of treatment in this disorder, it may be a useful adjunct to a comprehensive treatment plan in certain children.
5. **Environmental engineering** is of great benefit in ADHD. Because children with ADHD do not readily adapt to change or function well within highly stimulating environments, the environment around them should be constructed to minimize these distractions.
    a. Within the classroom, children with ADHD attend and concentrate better in the front row than in the rear.
    b. Study carrels are helpful because they block distracting stimuli.
    c. Children with ADHD function better with one-on-one instruction and in small groups rather than in larger groups.

XIII SPECIFIC DEVELOPMENTAL DISORDERS

A Clinical data   A wide range of disorders can interfere with a child's ability to perform certain intellectual functions. Children may suffer from specific reading, processing, writing, mathematical, and language disabilities (e.g., developmental dyslexia).

1. These disorders must be distinguished from both mental retardation and pervasive developmental disorders.
2. **Diagnosis** is established by documenting a mismatch between the child's performance on standardized measures of the skill in question and his or her intellectual capacity as measured by IQ testing.
3. The *DSM-IV* includes the following **categories and specific disorders:**
    a. **Learning disorders**
       (1) Reading disorder
       (2) Mathematics disorder
       (3) Disorder of written expression
    b. **Motor skills disorder** (developmental coordination disorder)
    c. **Communication disorders**
       (1) Expressive language disorder
       (2) Mixed receptive-expressive language disorder
       (3) Phonological disorder
       (4) Stuttering

B **Differential diagnosis** of specific developmental problems includes a variety of psychiatric conditions:

1. Depression
2. ADHD
3. School phobias
4. Other anxiety disorders
5. An interaction problem with the teacher
6. Childhood psychosis
7. Mental retardation
8. Pervasive developmental disorders

C **Treatment** is aimed at the underlying dysfunction. Learning disorders require academic remediation. The spectrum of services in this domain ranges from extra tutoring focused on the problematic academic skill (e.g., phonics tutoring for children with dyslexia) to placement in self-contained, special education classrooms for those with learning disorders.

1. **Motor skills disorder** may require occupational or physical therapy.
2. **Communication disorders** usually require intensive speech and language therapy.

XIV PROBLEMS OF ADOLESCENTS

A variety of disorders increase in incidence during adolescence (e.g., anorexia nervosa, adult schizophrenia, depression). Specific problems of adolescent development are discussed here.

A **Identity disturbances** Adolescents struggle to achieve a stable identity. Certain problems result when this aspect of development breaks down.

1. **Identity diffusion.** Adolescents have a poor sense of themselves and are easily swayed by the opinions of others.
2. **Peer-related disorders.** Some adolescents can be persuaded to do dangerous things (e.g., become sexually promiscuous, take drugs, drink alcohol, drive recklessly) to identify with their peer groups.
3. Problems with successfully resolving this developmental task may contribute to the development of an **identity problem, narcissistic personality disorder,** or **borderline personality disorder.**

B **Adult sexual development** In adolescence, adult sexual functioning is achieved, and sexual preferences are solidified.

1. **Homosexual behaviors** are commonly found in early adolescence. When they occur consistently throughout adolescence, however, they usually represent a true homosexual preference.
2. **Paraphilias.** The symptom expression found in exhibitionism, fetishism, frotteurism, pedophilia, sexual masochism, sexual sadism, transvestic fetishism, and voyeurism usually begins or heightens in adolescence.
3. **Pregnancy** may be the outcome of increased sexual promiscuity or may manifest from emancipation difficulties. For example, an adolescent who is struggling with separating from her family may become pregnant and turn the infant over to her parents for care. The infant thus replaces her and makes her emancipation easier.
4. **Sexually transmitted diseases,** including human immunodeficiency virus (HIV), are a risk of heightened sexual expression and activity during adolescence.

C **Separation** Adolescents negotiate emancipation from their family, and they redefine the parent–child and sibling roles and boundaries.

1. **Difficulty with emancipation** can be etiologic in several clinical disorders. For example:
   a. **Schizophrenia.** Psychosis becomes evident in many schizophrenics when they first leave home.
   b. **Anorexia.** The battle over food is actually a struggle for autonomy and independence in many individuals with anorexia.

    c. Depression. Separation and loss can trigger depressive feelings and even a major depressive episode in individuals so predisposed.

2. Difficult emancipation can lead to **mobilization of aggression** on the part of the adolescent, and intrafamily fighting ensues. Many adolescents believe that they will be able to emancipate successfully only through conflict.

3. **Incest** can develop to prevent a child from emancipating, and inappropriate sexual contact within a family sometimes signifies separation problems.

D **Treatment**   Special problems develop in the psychotherapy of adolescents.

1. **Labile allegiances.** Adolescents love the therapist one day and hate her the next day.

2. **Labile moods.** Because adolescents are in great hormonal and psychological turbulence, unstable moods frequently result.

3. **Communication difficulties.** Adolescents may not be comfortable with verbal communication but are too old for communication through play.

    a. Some adolescents **communicate by means of their behavior** (e.g., driving recklessly to signify anger or depression).

    b. Obstinacy may signify an emancipation problem because the individual refuses to take responsibility for himself.

4. **Overprotective parents** or parents with indistinct parent–child boundaries may meddle in an adolescent's treatment. In most cases, the adolescent should be seen at his or her own request in the service of developing autonomy even if it may, at times, be contrary to the wishes of the parents. When the parents are involved in the treatment of an adolescent, the confidentiality of the relationship between the physician and the adolescent is paramount. Parents should be notified, however, if the patient is:

    a. A danger to himself

    b. A danger to others

    c. Gravely disabled and unable to care for herself or to exercise appropriate judgment on her behalf

XV   CHILD ABUSE

Child abuse occurs when the individuals in a child's environment retard the child's development by hurting him or her.

A **Epidemiology**

1. Child abuse may be **physical, sexual,** or **emotional. Significant neglect** should be considered equivalent to abuse.

2. Approximately **15% of children who come to the emergency room with obvious trauma** have been abused.

3. **Parents who were abused** as children are at greater risk for abusing their own children.

4. Parents who are not overtly abusive may be **silently participating** in the abuse by failing to protect the child from the abusive parent (e.g., a mother who is physically present in the home yet is "unaware" of years of ongoing stepfather–daughter incest).

5. **Premature infants** are abused more often than full-term infants, probably at least partly, because of poor bonding.

6. **Reasons** for the abuse of infants often differ from those for the abuse of older children.

    a. Abuse of older children may be associated with psychosexual development (e.g., a 3-year-old soils her pants and is beaten).

    b. Abuse of infants occurs more frequently because their parents are emotionally needy and feel that the infant is taking attention away from them.

        (1) In this case, role reversal is also common. That is, the parent feels it is the duty of the child to meet the parent's emotional needs—to make the parent feel whole and good about him- or herself.

        (2) When the infant "demands" that her needs for basic care or nurture be met, conflict with the reciprocal "demand" by the parent results, and a potentially abusive situation ensues.

     (3) Likewise, when the parents' self-esteem is threatened by the perception that they are not good or effective parents (e.g., when the child cries), they are at increased risk for abusing the child.

     (4) Therefore, periods of normal infant fussiness (e.g., when hungry, sleepy, in need of diapering) or times when the infant is physically ill are potential crisis points for abusive parents and their infants.

  7. **Children with physical or developmental disorders** are at increased risk for abuse and neglect.

  8. The abused child often is the **scapegoat** for the individual pathology of other family members or for family pathology.

  9. It is **unusual for child abuse to begin after the age of 6 years,** with the exception of sexual abuse.

 10. Abuse occurs in **all socioeconomic** groups.

B **Effects on the child**

  1. Occasionally, **emotional development may be precocious.**

    a. The expectation that a child function as "a parent" (role reversal) causes some children to develop quickly.

    b. Fear of being abused for mistakes can also lead to precocious development and to **perfectionism** as a personality trait.

     (1) The precocity, however, tends to be superficial and defensive.

     (2) The underlying desire to be validated as a child for age-appropriate attributes is also usually apparent.

  2. Conversely, in some children, **development may be retarded** if the abuse is severe or enduring. In these cases, the destructive and deleterious impact of the abuse outweighs the child's ability to mount adaptive defenses against it.

  3. **Physical injuries** are a constant risk.

  4. **Emotional injuries** are an equally significant and consistent risk.

    a. These injuries may take the form of **low self-esteem and excessive guilt** that derive from the irrational acceptance of responsibility for the abuse (e.g., "I am bad or unlovable," rather than "My parent has a problem").

    b. **Chronic depression** and full-blown **posttraumatic stress disorder,** in which symptoms of the abuse are persistently reexperienced, may occur.

    c. Both **psychic numbing** and **chronic hyperarousal** are present.

  5. There is a **risk that the child may abuse his or her future offspring** when the abused child grows up and identifies with his or her parents.

  6. **Exposure to chronic violence** can increase aggression and antisocial behavior in abused children.

C **Treatment**

  1. **Suspected abuse must be reported** to the county protective services. If the child's health or life is in jeopardy, he or she should be removed from the abusive environment. If there is no improvement within 1 to 2 years after diagnosis, termination of parental rights should be considered.

  2. **Most abused children need psychotherapy.** Ultimately, the goal is to break what is often a multigenerational pattern of abuse in a family and to allow the child to grow into an adult who is capable of empathy, intimacy, and relational reciprocity in ways the previous generations were not. At times, the therapeutic relationship may be the first adult–child relationship that models a nonexploitative, noncontingent, emotionally available, and empathically attuned focus on the needs and well-being of the child.

  3. **Parents almost always need intensive, individual psychotherapy,** and often **marital therapy** as well. Parents may also benefit from **parent training classes** that educate them about normal development, appropriate limits and boundaries, and nonexploitative techniques for discipline and behavioral management. The knowledge base of parents is often erroneously assumed to exceed what is actually true.

BIBLIOGRAPHY

American Psychiatric Association: *Diagnostic and Statistical Manual of Mental Disorders,* 4th ed. Washington, DC, American Psychiatric Association, 1994.

Emde RN, Harmon RJ, Good WV: Depressive feelings in children: A transactional model for research. In *Depression in Children: Developmental Perspectives.* Edited by Rutter M, Izard D, Reed P. New York, Guilford Press, 1986, pp 135–160.

Garfinkle BD, Carlson GA, Weller, EB (eds): *Psychiatric Disorders in Children and Adolescents.* Philadelphia, WB Saunders, 1990.

Green M, Solnit AJ: Reactions to the threatened loss of a child: A vulnerable child syndrome. *Pediatrics* 34:58–65, 1964.

Klaus MH, Kendall JH: *Parent-Infant Bonding.* St. Louis, CV Mosby, 1982.

Lewis M (ed): *Child and Adolescent Psychiatry: A Comprehensive Textbook.* Baltimore, Williams & Wilkins, 1991.

Sadock BJ, Sadock VA: *Kaplan & Sadock's Synopsis of Psychiatry,* 9th ed. Baltimore, Williams & Wilkins, 2003

Spitz RA: Hospitalism: An inquiry into the genesis of psychiatric conditions in early childhood. *Psychoanal Study Child* 1:53–74, 1945.

Steele BF, Pollock CB: A psychiatric study of parents who abuse infants and small children. In *The Battered Child.* Edited by Helfer RE, Kempe CH. Chicago, University of Chicago Press, 1968, pp 103–145.

United States Food and Drug Administration, Public Health Advisory: *FDA Launches Multi-Pronged Strategy to Strengthen Safeguards for Children Treated with Antidepressant Medications,* Washington, DC, October 15, 2004.

Wiener JM (ed): *Textbook of Child and Adolescent Psychiatry.* Washington, DC, American Psychiatric Association, 1991.

Study Questions

Directions: *Each of the numbered items or incomplete statements in this section is followed by answers or by completions of the statement. Select the ONE numbered answer or completion that is BEST in each case.*

1. A 22-year-old woman has just delivered her first child, a healthy boy, by cesarean section under general anesthesia. When she awakens, she is frantic because she did not have the opportunity to "bond to her child." The physician's best course of action is to

- [A] reassure the patient that bonding is a lengthy process.
- [B] suggest that the mother breastfeed in order to offset the effects of poor postnatal bonding.
- [C] return in 1 day to see if the patient's concerns have dissipated.
- [D] recommend psychiatric counseling aimed at helping the patient bond to her child.
- [E] dismiss her concern as expectable, new-parent anxiety.

2. The etiology of childhood schizophrenia is most accurately described as

- [A] developmental.
- [B] environmental.
- [C] familial.
- [D] genetic.
- [E] multifactorial.

3. Anaclitic depression classically occurs

- [A] between birth and 6 months.
- [B] between 7 and 30 months.
- [C] between 31 and 48 months.
- [D] in elementary school ages (5 to 11 years).
- [E] in adolescence (12 to 18 years).

4. Which of the following statements about the etiology of encopresis is most accurate? The symptom often

- [A] is conscious and deliberate.
- [B] derives from delayed nervous system maturation.
- [C] indicates underlying gastrointestinal pathology.
- [D] derives from an underlying psychotic disorder.
- [E] derives from constipation and fecal impaction.

5. Which of the following statements regarding diagnostic criteria for learning disorders is most accurate?

- [A] They are usually associated with low-average intelligence.
- [B] It is an equivalent but less pejorative term than mental retardation.
- [C] Achievement testing and intelligence testing reflect differential profiles among individuals with these disorders.
- [D] They fall within the broader spectrum of pervasive developmental disorders.
- [E] Subtypes of the disorder include reading, writing, mathematics, history, and humanities.

QUESTIONS 6–8

A 7-year-old boy is brought to a child psychiatrist by his parents on a referral by the school where the child is in the second grade. The boy does not have a discipline problem, but he frequently answers questions without being called on and is often out of his seat without permission. His schoolwork is adequate, but the teacher believes he is capable of better. He has difficulty completing tasks and appears to spend much of the class time daydreaming.

6. Which additional piece of information would support the most likely etiology for his symptoms?

- [A] A history of head injuries
- [B] A history of neurologic symptoms

    C A history of tics

    D His medication history

    E Family psychiatric history

7. The most likely diagnosis is

    A Attention deficit hyperactivity disorder (ADHD)

    B Conduct disorder

    C Impulse control disorder

    D Learning disorder

    E Receptive language disorder

8. Regarding treatment, the best advice to the family would be that

    A he has a diagnosable disorder, so he should not be held accountable for his symptoms.

    B they should alter his diet immediately.

    C he needs intensive, probably long-term psychotherapy.

    D medications might be helpful.

    E they should probably not discuss his diagnosis with his teacher because it might be stigmatizing.

QUESTIONS 9–11

A 4-year-old girl is brought to the emergency department by her mother with a swollen and discolored forearm. Radiographs reveal an ulnar fracture. Her mother reports that the child had been jumping on the bed, lost her balance, and fell. The physician observes that the mother is apparently in her seventh or eighth month of pregnancy. He also observes that the child is quite thin and somewhat disheveled in appearance, and her hygiene is poor. When he asks if anyone else lives in their home, the mother acknowledges that her boyfriend does and then hastens to state, "But he wasn't even home when this happened."

9. After the radiographs, the physician's most appropriate next step is to

    A obtain a detailed developmental history from the mother.

    B insist that the mother's boyfriend come in to be interviewed.

    C interview the child separate from her mother.

    D examine the child's genitalia for signs of sexual abuse.

    E ask the hospital's child protection team to investigate.

10. Which statement best describes the physician's obligation to report the incident to the local child protective service agency?

    A If the physician suspects that the injuries might derive from abuse, then the incident must be reported.

    B If the physician finds additional evidence of deprivation and neglect, then he must report it.

    C If the physician finds additional evidence of physical abuse, then he must report it.

    D If the physician finds additional evidence of sexual abuse, then he must report it.

    E If in addition to the physician's findings, the child alleges abuse, then he must report it.

11. It is ultimately determined that the child's injury was inflicted by her mother's boyfriend. At this time, the most appropriate intervention with regard to the mother is to

    A remove the child from her care and place her in a foster home.

    B leave the child in her care as long as the perpetrator is not in the home.

    C insist on parenting classes as part of a court-ordered treatment plan.

    D evaluate her ability to effectively parent her yet unborn child.

    E be certain that her potential "silent" participation in the abuse is investigated.

12. The etiology of autistic disorder is best understood to be

    A infectious.

    B neurologic.

C psychogenic.
D psychologic.
E toxicologic.

13. Which of the following antidepressant medications would be the best second-line treatment for the symptoms of ADHD?

A Bupropion
B Fluoxetine
C Fluvoxamine
D Nefazodone
E Paroxetine

Directions: *Each set of matching questions in this section consists of a list of four to 26 lettered options (some of which may be in figures) followed by several numbered items. For each numbered item, select the ONE lettered option that is most closely associated with it. To avoid spending too much time on matching sets with large numbers of options, it is generally advisable to begin each set by reading the list of options. Then, for each item in the set, try to generate the correct answer and locate it in the option list, rather than evaluating each option individually. Each lettered option may be selected once, more than once, or not at all.*

QUESTIONS 14–17

Match the following medications with the correct clinical indication.

A Attention deficit hyperactivity disorder (ADHD)
B Bipolar disorder
C Encopresis
D Enuresis
E Tourette disorder

14. Risperidone

15. Methylphenidate

16. Valproic-acid

17. Desmopressin

QUESTIONS 18–21

Match the following childhood disorders with the most likely clinical etiology.

A Adult-spectrum disorder
B Maturational delays
C Neuropathology
D Parental pathology
E Parent loss

18. Narcolepsy

19. Feeding disorder of infancy or early childhood

20. Enuresis

21. Schizophrenia

Answers and Explanations

1. The answer is A [*II A, B*]. Bonding and attachment are processes that occur over a lengthy period. Although many parents worry that a cesarean section interferes with this process, simple reassurance is usually helpful. Breastfeeding would not necessarily offset any sort of aberration in bonding and attachment. At first, many new mothers feel that their infants do not belong to them. This feeling can last several days. Returning to see the patient is a good idea but should be done 3 to 4 days later; however, conditions can warrant returning sooner. When the mother is severely depressed, anxious, or psychotic, she should be evaluated for psychiatric treatment and follow-up. Sincere parental concerns should almost never be dismissed without discussion.

2. The answer is E [*IV B 3*]. Childhood schizophrenia is functionally understood as a regression to a psychotic state after previous attainment of better mental functioning. Suggested etiologies include a grossly chaotic upbringing with constant exposure to aggressive and sexual themes, with a subsequent failure of repression. Schizophrenia does occur in families; however, both genetic and environmental contributions may be involved. Growing research supports a genetic etiology continuous with the adult-spectrum disorder in many cases. Developmental factors may impact the expression of symptoms in childhood schizophrenia; however, they are not etiologic as in the pervasive developmental disorders. In short, childhood schizophrenia is best understood as deriving from the dynamic interaction of biologic, psychologic, and social factors.

3. The answer is B [*V A 1*]. Anaclitic depression is classically described as occurring between ages 7 and 30 months. During this phase of development, children are aware of who their primary caretaker is but do not yet have object constancy; that is, they lack the ability to maintain an image of their caretaker in the caretaker's absence. Therefore, they are vulnerable to lengthy separations (>1 week). Such separations from caretakers can result in a depressive syndrome that includes sad facial expressions, anorexia, apathy, and withdrawal from other individuals. The best treatment is to avoid prolonged separations. If that is not possible, a familiar individual or surrogate caretaker should be available to the child while the primary caretaker is away.

4. The answer is E [*VIII B*]. Soiling is only variably deliberate and is usually self-limited. Whereas enuresis often derives from delayed nervous system maturation, this is not true for encopresis, and it does not usually signify underlying gastrointestinal pathology. Although it may signify an underlying psychotic disorder within the child, this is not typically the case. The most common form of encopresis is in a child who retains feces, develops an impaction within the rectal vault, and experiences "overflow" soiling around the impaction.

5. The answer is C [*XIII A*]. The three subtypes of learning disorders are in reading, writing, and mathematics. Although mental retardation is often euphemistically referred to as a learning disorder, the term is used inaccurately in that context. The presence of a learning disorder does not suggest below-average intelligence. Although learning disorders fall broadly among the developmental disorders, they are not subsumed within the pervasive developmental disorders, which are characterized by pervasive developmental deficits in language, social relatedness, and behavior. Diagnosis of learning disorders is established by documenting a mismatch between cognitive potential (as demonstrated on intelligence tests) and academic performance (as demonstrated on standardized achievement tests).

6–8. The answers are 6-E, 7-A, and **8-D** [*XII C–D*]. Although both major (grossly abnormal central nervous system or history of significant head trauma) and minor (e.g., "soft" neurologic signs or nonspecific electrocardiographic changes) nervous system dysfunction may underlie the symptoms of attention deficit hyperactivity disorder (ADHD) in certain children, the most common etiology is a "constitutional" ADHD in the presence of a normal nervous system, often with a family history. A history of tics is important, both because Tourette disorder and ADHD can be comorbid conditions and because tics may be a side effect from stimulant medications that are commonly used to treat ADHD. Most children with ADHD do not have comorbid Tourette's disorder, however, nor do they develop tics as a side effect of treatment. Certain medications, particularly sedative-hypnotics, may result in paradoxic excitation, which causes hyperactivity in some children, but these medications are seldom used chronically in children.

ADHD is characterized by variable levels of hyperactivity along with impulsivity, distractibility, and attention and concentration deficits. Learning deficits secondary to inattention may be present; however, no primary learning deficits are derive from ADHD. Attentional difficulties are not characteristic of learning disorders. Conduct disorder may co-occur with ADHD, but it involves the repetitive and serious violation of multiple age-appropriate behavioral norms. Receptive language deficits do interfere with learning, but the learning difficulty derives from an inability to understand spoken language rather than from attentional deficits. Children with ADHD are behaviorally impulsive; this is to be distinguished, however, from impulse control disorders that are characterized by impulse disinhibition in discrete domains such as eating, substance use or abuse, gambling, stealing, fire setting, and violent outbursts.

Although the child has a diagnosable disorder, he still must be held accountable for his behavior and its consequences. Although many parents believe to the contrary, there is little empiric support for the notion that diet plays a role in this disorder, either etiologically or in terms of its treatment. Likewise, uncomplicated ADHD probably does not require psychotherapy, other than occasional behavioral interventions. Although stigmatization is always a risk of psychiatric diagnosis, the school would ideally be a partner in the therapeutic process, both to implement behavioral programs and to monitor overall therapeutic efficacy. Most children of ADHD are most effectively managed with medications, used at least adjunctively.

9–11. The answers are 9-C, 10-A, and 11-E [*XV C*]. Although the child's injury might have been sustained exactly as described by her mother, the physician must wonder whether nonaccidental trauma is involved. An interview with the child is essential. This should occur separate from the parent, and the child should be asked the source of her injuries. Questions should be otherwise nonleading and in language appropriate to her developmental level. Likewise, the responses of the child should be assessed in terms of their appropriateness to her developmental level. Developmental history may be important, insofar as there often is a history of problematic bonding between abused children and their parents. Likewise, children who physically or developmentally deviate from the norm are at increased risk for abuse. Nonetheless, obtaining a detailed developmental history is less urgent than hearing the child's own story. Although the physician must be sensitive to the potential for sexual abuse, a genital examination should be deferred until after the child is interviewed because it might not be indicated. A physician would not typically "investigate" a suspected perpetrator such as the mother's boyfriend. If that appeared necessary, it should be referred to the appropriate investigative agency (i.e., child protective services).

Reporting laws across the United States require that reasonable suspicions of abuse and neglect must be reported. Physicians are mandated to report under these circumstances and are civilly liable for failing to follow these reporting guidelines. Proof of abuse is not necessary, and neither is an inordinately high level of suspicion or direct allegations made by the child. Rather, any reasonable level of suspicion must be reported.

Abuse and neglect must always be viewed as reflecting adult pathology. The role of the perpetrator in the abuse is obvious. The role of other adults in the abused child's life is less obvious, however. At the very least, the "non-abusive" parent failed to protect the child from the perpetrator. In cases in which the abuse was known by the "non-abusive" parent or when the circumstances of the abuse were so obvious as to be impossible to miss, the "non-abusive" parent must be recognized as a silent and passive but equal participant in the abuse of the child. The child's immediate safety is the issue of first importance. Whether the child needs to be placed outside of her mother's care depends on her mother's "participation" in the abuse. Whether the mother needs a court-ordered treatment plan or needs to be evaluated in terms of her capacity to parent are issues to be addressed after the more immediate issues of current safety are addressed.

12. The answer is B [*IV A 4*]. Autistic disorder is a neuropathic disorder that commences in early childhood (before age 3 years) in which the child demonstrates disturbed relatedness to other human beings, inappropriate responses to the environment, and delays and oddities in language development. Findings that support the neurologic etiology of this condition include abnormal auditory evoked potentials, a high incidence of grand mal seizures during childhood, decreased nystagmus in response to vestibular stimulation, and a high incidence of comorbid mental retardation. Only occasionally are toxicologic agents (e.g., heavy metals) or infectious etiologies (congenital infections) suspected. Although once thought to be a psychogenic condition driven by parental psychologic factors ("icebox" parents who are cold, aloof, and detached), the organic etiology is now unequivocal.

13. The answer is A [*XII D 1*]. Bupropion, which is an antidepressant that may produce central nervous system stimulant effects, has also been demonstrated to be of some therapeutic benefit, particularly in individuals with ADHD and depressive symptoms. Fluoxetine, fluvoxamine, and paroxetine are all antidepressants of the SSRI family. Nefazodone is an antidepressant structurally unrelated to the SSRIs but with similar therapeutic effects. Although these medications are effective antidepressants and anxiolytics, they generally offer little benefit in the treatment of children with ADHD.

14–17. The answers are 14-E [*VI D 3 b*], **15-A** [*XII D 1 a*], **16-B** [*V D 1*], and **17-D** [*VIII A 3 c*]. Risperidone and clonidine have been used to treat the tics of Tourette disorder. Methylphenidate and dextroamphetamine have been used to treat the symptoms of attention deficit hyperactivity disorder (ADHD). Valproic acid, lithium, and carbamazepine are effective mood stabilizers useful in bipolar disorder. Desmopressin, an antidiuretic hormone, is useful in managing the symptoms of enuresis. There is no primary pharmacologic treatment for autistic disorder. Pharmacologic intervention in this disorder is aimed at specific target symptoms.

18–21. The answers are 18-C [*IV A*], **19-D** [*III C*], **20-B** [*VIII A*], and **21-A** [*IV B*]. Narcolepsy is a neurologic disorder, the symptoms of which derive from aberrations in the REM phase of the sleep cycle. Although feeding disorder of infancy or early childhood may derive from organic illness within the child, it is often secondary to parental pathology or pathologic parent–child interactions (e.g., nonorganic failure to thrive). Most often, enuresis, especially the primary nocturnal subtype, is a time-limited condition deriving from nervous system maturational delays, which the child will ultimately outgrow. Although childhood schizophrenia remains poorly defined, data indicate that at least 50% of individuals with childhood schizophrenia persist with significant deficits into adulthood. This suggests that there is some continuity with the adult-spectrum schizophrenia disorder; significant progress is being made in recognizing and defining the genetic contributions to this life-spectrum disorder.

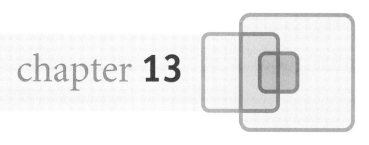

chapter 13

Legal Issues and Forensic Psychiatry

RICHARD L. FRIERSON

I INTRODUCTION

Legal issues pervade psychiatric practice to such an extent that forensic psychiatry has emerged as a subspecialty. Forensic psychiatrists engage in clinical practice and research in the many areas in which psychiatry is applied to legal issues. They routinely evaluate persons with mental illness and provide court testimony related to criminal and civil issues. They also provide consultation to general psychiatrists about the numerous legal issues that increasingly arise in general psychiatric practice. Therefore, psychiatrists must be familiar not only with advances in both pharmacologic and nonpharmacologic treatment but also with the legal issues that affect their patients and practice. These issues are divided into three areas: the legal regulation of psychiatry, criminal law, and civil law.

A Dual agency   Dual agency is serving both as a treator and an evaluator of a patient who is involved in a legal proceeding. Psychiatrists frequently encounter problems when their patients become involved in legal disputes, especially when patients or their attorneys seek to have a psychiatrist testify about the patient's condition and give an opinion related to the legal issue. For example, a psychiatrist treating a man who is involved in a divorce proceeding might be asked to testify about the patient's illness as it relates to child custody and give an opinion about the fitness of the man as a parent. These situations can be very damaging to the therapeutic alliance and the physician–patient relationship because an undesirable legal outcome for a patient can lead to feelings of distrust toward the treating psychiatrist. For this reason, dual agency situations should be avoided. In general, a psychiatrist should not be involved in both treatment of a patient and evaluation of that same patient for a court or attorney.

B Psychiatrists in court   When psychiatrists are subpoenaed, they should clarify their role before they appear in court to testify. They may assume the role of one of the two types of court witnesses: fact witnesses and expert witnesses.

1. **Fact witnesses** testify to events. For example, a psychiatrist called as a fact witness might testify to dates and type of treatment, diagnosis (or diagnoses) assigned, and medical record documentation. Fact witnesses are not allowed to give expert opinions about a patient's mental illness as it relates to a legal issue.

2. **Expert witnesses** testify to issues outside the knowledge of an average layperson. These witnesses must be qualified as experts after the court reviews their credentials. Expert witnesses may testify about the reasoning behind a diagnosis, a patient's prognosis, and how a patient's mental illness relates to the legal issue in dispute. For example, a psychiatrist called as an expert witness may be used to establish the standard of care in a malpractice suit or to determine a defendant's legal sanity in a criminal trial.

II LEGAL REGULATION OF PSYCHIATRIC PRACTICE

The practice of psychiatry, more than any other medical specialty, is regulated by both statutory and case law. Therefore, psychiatrists must be familiar with basic laws applicable to psychiatric practice in their jurisdiction. Although statutes vary from state to state, they are based in core legal principles.

A **Involuntary psychiatric hospitalization**   The first civil commitment law was passed in New York in 1788. Involuntary hospitalization statutes now exist in all 50 states. Because the U.S. Constitution provides individuals with "life, liberty, and the pursuit of happiness," denial of these freedoms requires due process and legal oversight. Commitment laws establish the criteria by which individuals may be involuntarily committed to a psychiatric hospital and the procedural safeguards to be used in this process. In most states, patients who are hospitalized involuntarily are afforded a formal hearing before or shortly after they are hospitalized. During this hearing, a judge (or jury) determines whether commitment criteria have been met based on the testimony of clinicians who have examined a particular patient. Almost all commitment statutes require that individuals be suffering from a *treatable* mental illness. The criteria used to determine whether involuntary psychiatric commitment is appropriate are based on one of the following legal doctrines:

1. **Police power.** This emergency commitment model, which is based in the government's authority to protect public safety, allows for hospitalization of patients if they are mentally ill *and* represent a danger to themselves or the public at large. A mentally ill person who is acutely suicidal or homicidal would fall under this model. This is the most common basis for psychiatric commitment laws in the United States. In most states, a physician, psychiatrist, or mental health professional determines if a patient meets commitment criteria, and the patient may be detained until a hearing is conducted in front of a judge or designated judicial reviewer. The reviewer ultimately decides if the patient is to remain hospitalized.

2. *Parens patriae.* Some jurisdictions also allow for commitment under a *parens patriae* model. Literally, *parens patriae* translates as "father of the country" and represents the government's role to act as a parent. This model allows the government to protect individuals who are mentally ill and who cannot take care of themselves or provide themselves with basic necessities, whether or not they are imminently dangerous to themselves or others. This model is designed to protect patients from their own impairments. For example, a psychotic individual who is too disorganized to find food or shelter could possibly meet commitment criteria under this model, even if this person is not acutely suicidal or dangerous to others. However, case law has established that hospitalization in such a case must represent the *least restrictive alternative* for treatment.

B **Voluntary psychiatric hospitalization**   Many states have statutes stating that individuals must be competent in order to voluntarily admit themselves to a psychiatric hospital. In these states, admitting psychiatrists should ascertain that patients understand, at the very least, the purpose of hospitalization and the criteria and procedures for release. Patients should also be competent to make basic treatment decisions (see II C 2).

C **Informed consent**   Many medical procedures require written informed consent, including psychiatric treatment with neuroleptic (i.e., typical antipsychotic) medications and electroconvulsive therapy (ECT). Informed consent has three basic elements: information disclosure, patient competence, and voluntariness.

1. **Information disclosure.** The amount of information to be disclosed to patients during the informed consent process depends on the risk associated with the treatment and the risk associated with the illness if it is left untreated. In general, the riskier the treatment, the more information patients should be given.
   a. Table 13–1 lists the types of information disclosed. Patients should always be afforded an opportunity to ask questions about the information presented to them.
   b. In more than half of the states, the standard for information disclosure is the **reasonable professional standard,** which means that the amount of information disclosed should be the amount that the majority of physicians practicing in that jurisdiction would normally disclose. The other states have adopted a **reasonable person standard,** meaning the amount of information disclosed should be the amount that any reasonable person would want to know before consenting to or declining treatment.

2. **Competency to consent.** Most adult patients are presumed to be competent to consent to treatment, and most minors are presumed incompetent, which means that they lack the ability to understand the information presented in the informed consent process. However, major mental illness can affect patients' ability to make informed decisions. This concern frequently arises

TABLE 13-1	Information Given to Patients When Obtaining Informed Consent

Description of the proposed procedure or treatment
Expected benefits of the procedure or treatment
Risks and side effects associated with the procedure or treatment
Advantages and risks associated with the absence of treatment
Available alternatives to the proposed treatment
Advantages and risks associated with alternative treatment options

in psychotic patients and elderly patients with dementia. Many clinicians question patients' competency when they refuse treatment. However, patients can just as incompetently consent to a medical procedure as they can refuse it.

    a. The elements of competency involved in informed consent are outlined in Table 13–2. Failure to consider patient competency may increase a clinician's liability, especially if a patient incompetently consents to a procedure that ends with a poor clinical outcome.

    b. If a patient is incompetent to consent to medical treatment, a substitute decision maker may be required. If the patient does not have a legally appointed guardian, most jurisdictions allow the closest relative to give informed consent. Other jurisdictions, especially when the treatment involves involuntary psychotropic medication, require a judge to order treatment.

3. **Voluntariness.** Informed consent must be given freely and voluntarily. Often the distinction between coercion and persuasion can be difficult. For example, if a clinician has withheld visitation or recreational privileges for an institutionalized patient because he refused to consent, the clinician would be coercive. The use of justified encouragement to a patient to accept treatment would not be considered coercive on the part of the clinician.

4. **Exceptions to informed consent**

    a. In **emergency situations** in which a delay in treatment could jeopardize the life of the patient or others, informed consent is not necessary. Although these situations are more common in other medical specialties, they do occur in psychiatry. For example, an acutely psychotic patient who is assaulting others or harming herself may be medicated acutely or restrained without obtaining consent.

    b. **Therapeutic privilege** allows for withholding informed consent if the clinician believes that the information disclosed would be harmful to the patient or significantly worsen the patient's condition. This exception has a high potential for abuse by clinicians and should be used cautiously. Note that withholding information because a clinician believes a patient would refuse treatment is *not* therapeutic privilege.

    c. A **waiver** of informed consent occurs if the patient indicates that he does not want to be told information related to the procedure or wants the clinician to make the decision for him. A patient waiver should be initially challenged by the clinician and clearly documented in the medical record.

[D] **Treatment refusal**   Psychiatric patients who refuse treatment present psychiatrists with a clinical dilemma. This situation most commonly occurs when psychotic patients refuse antipsychotic medication. In this case, the psychiatrist should carefully explore the reasons for refusal with the patient and work toward developing trust in the therapeutic alliance. If the patient's refusal is not a competently

TABLE 13-2	Elements of Competency in Informed Consent

The patient can communicate a choice.
The patient applies rational reasoning in making the choice.
The patient has the ability to understand the information presented by the clinician.
The patient understands the information, as evidenced by an ability to answer questions correctly about the information presented.

made decision, a substitute decision maker may be obtained (see II C 2 b). If the patient is competent to consent or refuse and continues to refuse, there are several options, including:

1. When clinically feasible, **discharge from the hospital** may be appropriate.

2. In a few jurisdictions, if the patient is civilly committed, involuntary treatment is permitted as long as the treatment is medically appropriate. Clinicians in these jurisdictions could seek **psychiatric commitment,** provided commitment criteria are met.

3. In some other states, committed patients are considered competent until judicially found incompetent. Clinicians in these states must abide by a **judicial ruling.** If a patient is deemed incompetent, a judge then decides whether to involuntarily medicate the patient using substituted judgment. In substituted judgment, several factors are taken into account, including the patient's previously expressed interest, the patient's religious convictions, the impact on the family, the drug's side effects, and the prognosis with and without treatment.

4. An **administrative review** may be necessary. In most states, involuntary medication may be allowed after administrative review, often by two or more psychiatrists, if it is found that a patient has a serious mental illness and is a danger to himself or others or is gravely disabled and can benefit from treatment.

E Confidentiality and privilege

1. **Confidentiality.** The physician–patient relationship is based on trust, and many patients routinely reveal intimate details of their lives to their treating clinicians. Confidentiality is the clinician's duty to prevent the communications received in the physician–patient relationship from being divulged to third parties. It is the clinician's obligation to maintain confidentiality, and courts have found clinicians liable for revealing patient information without the expressed written consent of the patient. This applies to information released to family members, other nontreating physicians, insurers and managed care companies, and medical researchers. Confidentiality also survives death.

    a. However, **exceptions to confidentiality** include:

    (1) **Emergencies.** In certain situations, release of confidential information to other health care providers may be necessary to guarantee a patient's immediate welfare. In these cases, which involve the most widely recognized exception to patient confidentiality, physicians are unlikely to be held liable if they genuinely believe they are acting in the patient's best interest.

    (2) **Voluntary or involuntary hospital admissions.** Psychiatrists may release information to a receiving hospital at the time of hospital admission.

    (3) **Certain infectious diseases, child abuse, and abuse of elderly and mentally or physically disabled individuals.** Most states have requirements mandating the reporting of certain diseases and child abuse. In addition, some states have passed legislation mandating the reporting of abuse of elderly or disabled individuals.

    (4) **Ancillary medical personnel.** Patient information can also be released to a physician's supervisor or other medical personnel involved in the direct care of a patient on a hospital ward. However, these ancillary staff members are bound by the same confidentiality expectations as the primary clinician.

    b. In some jurisdictions, **failure to abide by the reporting laws listed in II E 1 a (3) can lead to criminal charges against psychiatrists.** In general, previous crimes revealed by patients do not have to be reported.

2. **Privilege.** The patient's right to prevent a physician from testifying in a legal proceeding about material gained from the therapeutic relationship is known as privilege. If a psychiatrist receives a subpoena for records (i.e., a subpoena *duces tecum*), he or she should contact the patient and, with the patient's permission, the patient's attorney. If the patient does not want the records released, the psychiatrist should notify the attorney who sent the subpoena that the patient has invoked privilege, and the records cannot be released without a court order. It is ultimately up to the judge to decide whether the material subpoenaed is privileged and inadmissible. In the case of a deceased or gravely disabled patient, the psychiatrist may be obligated to claim privilege for the patient. Usually, if a patient places her mental status at issue in a legal proceeding (e.g., a patient sues her former psychiatrist), the patient cannot claim privilege.

F **Duty to third parties** Throughout the United States, courts are holding psychiatrists liable for damages to third parties as a result of acts on the part of their patients that led to injury to persons or property. Psychiatrists have been held liable for physical assaults by their patients, automobile accidents in which their patients were drivers, and more recently, "false memories" of childhood abuse uncovered in psychotherapy that led to subsequent disruption of family relationships.

1. A psychiatrist's liability to a third party was first found in the 1976 California Supreme Court case of *Tarasoff v. Regents of the University of California.* This case involved a college student who had told a university psychologist that he planned to kill his estranged girlfriend. After he killed Tatiana Tarasoff, her parents sued the University of California, alleging, in part, that the university was negligent in failing to warn a foreseeable victim. After several appeals, the California Supreme Court held that "when a therapist determines, or pursuant to the standards of his profession should determine, that his patient presents a serious danger of violence to another, he incurs an obligation to use reasonable care to protect the intended victim against such danger." **The court found that a psychiatrist has a duty not only to warn but to protect an intended victim as well.** In situations in which a patient threatens to harm an identified person, the psychiatrist should consider notifying the potential victim or the police or, if indicated, hospitalizing the patient.

2. Court decisions relating to the *Tarasoff* decision vary widely from state to state; some states have passed statutes that adopt a "*Tarasoff*" obligation to protect identified victims. In other states, appellate court decisions have also established this duty. Finally, many states have rejected this duty, and psychiatrists in those states can not be sued for failing to protect a known intended victim. Because of the variability regarding this duty across jurisdictions, psychiatrists should be familiar with the law in the state in which they practice.

III CRIMINAL ISSUES

The criminalization of mentally ill individuals has been an unintended side effect of deinstitutionalization, with more chronically mentally ill patients treated on an outpatient basis rather than in an inpatient setting; the Los Angeles County jail has been called the largest mental hospital in the United States. Mentally ill defendants present two main legal issues for trial courts: competency to stand trial and criminal responsibility.

A **Competency to stand trial (CST)** CST is a criminal defendant's ability to understand court proceedings and assist an attorney in the preparation of a defense. In the 1960 U.S. Supreme Court landmark case *Dusky v. United States,* the court held that in order for a defendant to be considered competent to stand trial, he or she must have "sufficient present ability to consult with his [or her] attorney with a reasonable degree of rational understanding" and "a rational as well as factual understanding of the proceedings against him [or her]." Table 13–3 lists the trial abilities that are routinely assessed in a CST evaluation. If a criminal defendant is found incompetent to stand trial because of symptoms that are treatable with psychotropic medication, the U.S. Supreme Court has held that involuntary medication may be administered if the proposed treatment is medically appropriate, if there is reasonable probability that it would restore competence, and if it would further legitimate governmental interests.

TABLE 13–3 Criteria Used to Evaluate Patient Competency to Stand Trial

The patient understands the pending criminal charge(s) and potential penalties that conviction could bring.
The patient appreciates the roles of court personnel (lawyer, judge, prosecutor, jury, and witnesses).
The patient knows the potential pleas available and understands the process of plea bargaining.
The patient is able to control his or her behavior in the courtroom.
The patient appreciates the significance of evidence and witness testimony.
The patient is able to be appropriately self-protective.
The patient is able to describe a desired legal outcome.
The patient is able to communicate effectively with his or her lawyer.

B **Criminal responsibility or legal insanity**   Unlike CST, there is no constitutional basis for the insanity defense. Consequently, although all states must have procedures to ensure defendants' competency, the recognition of a defense of insanity is not required. In response to John Hinkley's attempt to assassinate former U.S. President Ronald Reagan, several states have restricted the criteria for legal insanity or eliminated the insanity defense altogether. The insanity defense is rarely successful; fewer than 1% of felony prosecutions result in an insanity acquittal.

1. Determination of legal insanity requires that psychiatrists make a retrospective determination of a defendant's mental state at the time an alleged crime was committed. This can be difficult, especially if a long period has elapsed between the alleged crime and the time of the evaluation of criminal responsibility. It is most difficult when a defendant was acutely psychotic at the time of the crime but was subsequently treated and the psychotic symptoms have resolved before the evaluation. Consequently, in addition to a patient interview, evaluations concerning legal insanity require a review of police reports, defendant statements, witness and victim statements, the patient's psychiatric and medical records, and the defendant's functioning around the time of the alleged crime.

2. The statutory criteria for criminal responsibility (i.e., legal insanity) vary from state to state. Psychiatrists who perform these evaluations should be familiar with the legal definition of insanity in their particular state. Most states use one of the following three standards of legal insanity.
   a. The **McNaughten standard,** named for an 1843 English defendant, is the most widely used test of legal insanity in the United States. It requires that a person, as the result of mental disease or defect, failed to know the nature and quality of the criminal act he or she was committing or failed to know that the act he or she was committing was wrong.
   b. The **Model Penal Code,** also known as the **American Law Institute Rule,** states that a defendant should not be held responsible if a mental disease or defect impaired her capacity to appreciate the criminality of his or her conduct or to conform his or her conduct to the requirements of the law. It excludes illnesses that are manifested only by repeated criminal or antisocial conduct such as antisocial personality disorder or pedophilia.
   c. The **Durham rule,** the least restrictive of all insanity tests, merely requires that the crime is the product of a mental illness or defect.

IV   CIVIL ISSUES

Civil courts settle legal disputes that do not involve violation of a criminal statute. In general, civil litigation involves a tort, or civil wrong, done by one party to another. **Intentional torts** are wrongdoings done with prior knowledge that damages may result. For example, a psychiatrist or other specialist who becomes involved in a sexual relationship with a patient may be held responsible for an intentional tort and ordered to pay punitive damages to the patient. **Unintentional torts** involve **negligence,** the concept that the act led to an unreasonable risk of causing harm to another, although the act may not have been intended to cause such harm.

A **Guardianship and conservatorship**   Whereas commitment laws are designed to protect patients from immediate harm to themselves or others, conservatorship and guardianship laws protect patients from financial loss and other less immediate harm that may result if their mental illness or defect impairs their judgment and ability to make decisions.

1. **Guardianship.** A guardian is a person designated by the court to manage the property and rights of another individual and to make decisions related to the physical well-being of that individual. A guardian may make decisions related to financial matters, living arrangements, and physical needs, including, in some cases, medical treatment. In some states, a guardian is called the **committee of the person,** reflecting the global decision making involved in the guardianship role.
   a. Patients who are declared globally incompetent and in need of a guardian may lose many civil rights, including the right to vote, the right to own a firearm, or the right to have a driver's license. Consequently, patients undergoing guardianship proceedings are granted rights of due process, including the right to representation by an attorney. A petitioner must show the court, usually by clear and convincing evidence, that individuals lack substantial ability to

manage their property or provide for themselves or their dependents. Forensic psychiatrists may serve as experts to the court in these proceedings, describing specific patient impairments and the effect of impairments on patients' decision-making ability. The presence of psychosis, dementia, or other mental illness does not constitute incompetence per se, so a functional assessment must be performed.

   b. Traditionally, courts have appointed a guardian from the patient's family, usually with input from the patient. If a family member is not available, the court may appoint an attorney or other interested person to serve as guardian.

2. **Conservatorship.** A conservator, or limited guardian, is a person designated by the court to manage another person's financial affairs. Individuals in need of a conservator do not have to be declared globally incompetent. Therefore, they do not lose their basic civil rights. A conservator may pay bills, buy or sell property, and manage investments or other financial matters.

B **Testamentary capacity** The simplest of all competencies, testamentary capacity is an individual's capacity to make a will. The law presumes that a person is of sound mind when a will is signed. An evaluation of testamentary capacity at the time the will is signed can prevent challenges to the will by family members after the death of the testator (i.e., person executing a will).

1. To have testamentary capacity, individuals must understand the nature and purpose of a will, their assets (legally, the extent of their bounty), their natural heirs, and their relationship to their heirs. In addition, their decision-making abilities must be free of delusion.

2. Only a small percentage of contested wills are overturned. Most successful challenges involve proof of **undue influence,** the manipulation or deception of the testator by others to gain the affections of the testator.

C **Workers' compensation and psychiatric disability**

1. **Workers' compensation.** Workers' compensation laws are designed to reimburse an employee for medical expenses and loss of income resulting from a work-related injury. These laws are also designed to prevent litigation for work-related injuries. In most states, this compensation can last for up to 1 year after the injury. Most states bar compensation for self-inflicted injury or injuries occurring at work if the worker was under the influence of alcohol or drugs. This has led to increased drug screening by many companies. The three categories of claims for psychiatric injury can be described as follows:

   a. A **physical–mental claim** involves a physical injury that causes mental impairment. For example, an employee is physically injured in an industrial explosion and subsequently develops posttraumatic stress disorder (PTSD); he is unable to return to work after the physical injury heals.

   b. A **mental–physical claim** involves recurrent job stress that causes or aggravates a physical condition. For example, an automobile assembly technician who is required to work overtime subsequently develops a bleeding gastric ulcer requiring hospitalization. Mental–physical claims can be difficult to prove because of the issue of causality.

   c. A **mental–mental claim** occurs if job stress leads to the development of a mental condition. For example, a policeman who witnesses the murder of a partner in the line of duty is unable to return to work because of depression that develops after this traumatic event.

2. **Disability.** The Social Security Administration (SSA) administers two disability programs, Social Security Disability Income (SSDI or Title II) and Social Security Income (SSI or Title XVI). In 2005, more than 5.8 million people received some form of disability payment from the SSA, which has defined diagnostic categories of mental disorders for which disability payments may be awarded. In addition, functional disability must cause two or three of the following: restrictions in activities of daily living; difficulties with social functioning; deficiencies of concentration, persistence, or pace in the work environment; or repeated episodes of decompensation in the work setting, causing the worker to withdraw from work or experience a worsening of signs and symptoms of her mental impairment.

   a. SSDI provides cash benefits for disabled workers and their dependents if the worker has contributed substantially to the Federal Insurance Compensation Act (FICA).

   b. SSI provides minimal income for disabled individuals who have not contributed to FICA.

D **Psychiatric malpractice** Psychiatrists are less likely to be sued for malpractice than their physician counterparts. The most common psychiatric malpractice claims (in order of frequency of occurrence) involve, in order of decreasing frequency, incorrect treatment, suicide, improper diagnosis, and inadequate supervision of other mental health professionals.

1. **Negligence.** Most malpractice suits fall into the legal category of an unintentional tort. In malpractice actions, the plaintiff must prove the **"four Ds"** of negligence: **duty** on the part of the psychiatrist, if there existed a doctor–patient relationship; **dereliction** or breach of that duty, if the treatment provided failed to reach a standard of care; **damages** suffered by the patient; and **direct causation** that the breach of duty lead to the alleged damages.

   a. **Duty.** The concept of duty requires the existence of a physician–patient relationship. Thus, a physician must have agreed to treat a patient.

      (1) After duty has been established, it can only be ended by a medically indicated discharge or by transferring a patient to the care of another physician.

      (2) Duty may be excused in certain emergency situations in which a doctor–patient relationship was not previously established. To protect physicians (and others) from liability if they provide treatment to unconscious patients at accident scenes in emergent life-and-death situations, some states have enacted "good Samaritan" laws.

   b. **Dereliction.** If it is established that the treatment given by the physician fell below an acceptable standard of care, then dereliction has occurred.

      (1) Most successful malpractice suits use an expert witness (i.e., a physician in the same specialty) to testify that the defendant failed to provide care that meets a minimal standard of the profession.

      (2) In cases of outrageous physician conduct, an expert may not be needed. Such cases are known as *res ipsa loquitur,* which is translated as "the thing speaks for itself." Physical assault of a patient by a psychiatrist is an example of such a case. In this situation, the burden of proof shifts to the psychiatrist in proving that he or she was not negligent. Most malpractice insurers do not cover damages resulting from these actions.

   c. **Damages.** Physicians cannot be held liable for inadequate patient care, even if the care was grossly negligent, unless the patient has suffered damages. An expert witness is frequently used to establish the extent of damages a patient has suffered. In recent years, juries have had an increasing tendency to award large amounts of money for pain and suffering, leading to large increases in malpractice premiums.

   d. **Direct causation.** When damages have occurred, the plaintiff must prove direct causation; that is, if not for the actions of the physician, the damages the patient suffered would not have occurred. This is the most complicated element of a malpractice claim and often requires proof of proximate cause. The foreseeability of the harm done to the patient becomes a central issue in direct causation. For example, failure to hospitalize a suicidal patient with a history of serious suicide attempts and a current suicidal plan might not represent direct causation if the patient commits suicide 2 years after leaving the care of the psychiatrist; however, it might be direct causation if the patient committed suicide within days of seeing the psychiatrist.

2. **Malpractice prevention**

   a. In almost all malpractice suits, great attention is paid to the medical record. For this reason, good prevention against a successful malpractice action requires the maintenance of a thorough medical record that clearly documents the psychiatrist's reasoning behind treatment decisions.

      (1) Progress notes should be legibly written, dated, and signed.

      (2) A suicide assessment should accompany any change in an inpatient's status, including addition and removal of suicide precautions or changes in observation levels.

      (3) The purpose of medications and their target symptoms should be documented.

   b. Progress notes should never be used to criticize the treatment of other clinicians, and nursing notes should be reviewed regularly by physicians. Psychiatrists who supervise other mental health professionals may be liable for their negligence as well under a legal concept known as *respondeat superior.*

   c. The best prevention against malpractice claims is the maintenance of a healthy therapeutic alliance with patients. Patients may initiate a lawsuit based on a perceived attitude by a psychiatrist rather than a specific action. Careful attention should be given to patients who express dissatisfaction regarding their treatment. Patients' complaints should be discussed thoroughly with the patient in a noncondescending manner. A sincerely expressed apology after a clinical mistake may go a long way in averting a lawsuit.

BIBLIOGRAPHY

Dusky v. U.S., 362 U.S. 402 (1960).

Grisso T, Applebaum PS: *Assessing Competence to Consent to Treatment.* New York, Oxford University Press, Inc., 1998.

Gutheil TG, Applebaum PS: *Clinical Handbook of Psychiatry and the Law,* 3rd ed. Philadelphia, Lippincott Williams & Wilkins, 2000.

Gutheil TG: *The Psychiatrist in Court.* Washington, DC, American Psychiatric Press, 1998.

Rosner R (ed): *Principles and Practice of Forensic Psychiatry,* 2nd ed. London, Arnold, 2003.

Rosner R, Schwartz HI: *Geriatric Psychiatry and the Law.* New York, Plenum Press, 1987.

Sell V. U.S., 539 U.S. 166 (2003).

Simon RI, Gold LH: *Textbook of Forensic Psychiatry.* Washington, DC, American Psychiatric Publishing, 2004.

Tarasoff v. Regents, 17 Cal. 3d 425 (1976).

Zinermon v. Burch, 49 U.S. 113 (1990).

Study Questions

Directions: *Each of the numbered items or incomplete statements in this section is followed by answers or by completions of the statement. Select the ONE lettered answer or completion that is BEST in each case.*

1. A 42-year-old woman has been treated for major depression with psychotic symptoms with medication and weekly individual psychotherapy for 1 year after a serious suicide attempt. Because of low energy, poor ability to concentrate, and psychomotor retardation, she has been unable to return to work. Her application for disability under her company's disability policy was denied, so she has hired an attorney and has filed a suit against the company. Her attorney contacts the treating psychiatrist, requesting an opinion about the degree of her impairment and whether she is disabled under the policy guidelines. Which of the following actions should the treating psychiatrist take?

   A. Write a report to the attorney explaining the patient's impairments and degree of disability.
   B. Send the patient's medical records to the attorney.
   C. Call the patient and with her permission, the attorney, and suggest that they hire an independent psychiatrist to conduct a disability evaluation.
   D. Call the attorney and ask for a copy of the disability policy.
   E. Write a report to the attorney and company explaining only the patient's impairments.

2. Which of the following events is the most common cause of malpractice suits against psychiatrists?

   A. Breach of confidentiality
   B. Development of tardive dyskinesia
   C. Incorrect diagnosis
   D. Incorrect treatment
   E. Patient suicide

3. A male psychiatrist enters a sexual relationship with a married, depressed woman whom he is treating. After the treatment relationship and the sexual relationship end, she sues the psychiatrist, alleging that her depressive symptoms have worsened because of guilty feelings about the sexual contact and breakup of her marriage. She also alleges difficulty in trusting her current physician. The judge rules that expert testimony is not needed to prove that the sexual contact violated a professional standard of care under which of the following legal concepts?

   A. Direct causation
   B. *Res ipsa loquitur*
   C. *Respondeat superior*
   D. Unintentional tort
   E. Vicarious liability

4. Which of the following is an element in evaluation of competency to stand trial (CST)?

   A. The defendant has the ability to distinguish right from wrong.
   B. The defendant has the ability to behave according to the requirements of the law.
   C. The crime was a product of a mental illness.
   D. The defendant can communicate effectively with a lawyer.
   E. The defendant was delusional at the time of an alleged crime.

5. Which of the following psychiatric treatments requires that a psychiatrist obtain written informed consent from a patient?

   A. Behavioral therapy
   B. Group therapy
   C. Supportive psychotherapy
   D. Use of antidepressant medication
   E. Use of a typical antipsychotic medication

6. A 36-year-old homeless man with a history of schizoaffective disorder is brought to the hospital. He is hallucinating, and his thinking is grossly disorganized. His hygiene is poor, and he appears malnourished. He does not behave violently in the emergency department, he denies suicidal or homicidal thoughts, and he refuses admission. When asked about his family, he replies they have been replaced by look-alike "doubles"; he reports that "the CIA is involved." An examining psychiatrist finds that the patient is grossly psychotic but not imminently dangerous. Which of the following statements about the patient is correct?

- **A** His condition meets commitment criteria under a police powers model.
- **B** His condition meets commitment criteria under a *parens patriae* model.
- **C** His condition meets commitment criteria under the *Dusky* standard.
- **D** His condition does not meet commitment criteria for involuntary hospitalization under any model.
- **E** He can be involuntarily hospitalized only if he threatens suicide or homicide.

7. An acutely psychotic woman with schizophrenia is voluntarily admitted to the hospital. After a history and physical examination are completed, the psychiatrist orders antipsychotic medication, which the patient promptly refuses. Which of the following steps should the psychiatrist take next?

- **A** Contact a family member to consent to medication.
- **B** Give the medication over the patient's objections.
- **C** Consider the patient competent and convene an administrative panel to determine the need for involuntary medication.
- **D** Contact a judge to order involuntary medication.
- **E** Conduct an interview to determine if the patient is competent to consent or refuse medication.

8. A 50-year-old nurse witnesses her coworker and friend being shot and seriously wounded by an agitated patient in the emergency department. She subsequently develops posttraumatic stress disorder (PTSD) and is unable to return to work for 1 month. She is in need of financial assistance. What type of claim should she file?

- **A** Workers' compensation: mental–mental type
- **B** Workers' compensation: mental–physical type
- **C** Workers' compensation: physical–mental type
- **D** Social Security Disability Income (SSDI)
- **E** Social Security Income (SSI)

9. Which of the following series are the elements of an unintentional tort in a malpractice case?

- **A** Duty, dereliction of duty, documentation failure, and damages
- **B** Duty, dereliction of duty, damages, and direct causation
- **C** Dereliction of duty, damages, direct causation, and documentation failure
- **D** Duty, damages, direct causation, and documentation failure
- **E** Purposeful action to harm the patient, damages, and direct causation

10. Which of the following is a recognized exception to the clinician's confidentiality obligation and does not require patient consent to release information?

- **A** Providing information to a patient's employer
- **B** Providing information to a patient's attorney
- **C** Providing information to a deceased patient's spouse
- **D** Discovering that a patient may be abusing a child and reporting the abuse to a social service agency
- **E** Providing information to an insurance company

11. In *Tarasoff v. Regents of the University of California,* the California Supreme Court ruled that which of the following statements applies to psychiatrists?

- **A** They cannot be held liable for the malpractice actions of their employees.
- **B** They have a duty to warn intended victims.

C They have a duty to protect intended victims.

D They cannot be held liable for treatment rendered in an emergency.

E They have no duty to third parties.

12. An 82-year-old woman is referred for a testamentary capacity evaluation by her lawyer. She is able to quantify her assets of $500,000 and identify her two surviving children as natural heirs. She has decided to leave her assets to a local charity to begin an educational trust fund for abused and neglected children. She is leaving some family heirlooms to her two children and has divided these items equally. When asked about her decision, she states that each of her children inherited $1,000,000 at the death of another family member (this has been confirmed by her attorney), and she would like to leave her assets to someone who really needs them. Although her psychiatric examination reveals mild memory impairment, there is no evidence that this has caused problems in her daily functioning. Which of the following statements about this woman is correct?

A She has been unduly influenced.

B She lacks testamentary capacity because she is neglecting her children in the division of her assets.

C She lacks testamentary capacity because of memory impairment.

D She is in need of a guardian.

E She has testamentary capacity.

13. A legally appointed guardian is also known as which of the following?

A A committee of the person

B A conservator

C A curator

D A petitioner

E A testator

14. A conservator would be appointed to make which one of the following decisions?

A Whether to sell shares of a declining stock owned by the person in need of a conservator

B Whether to consent to a medical procedure

C Whether to allow another family member to live with the person in need of a conservator

D Whether to have the patient enter a nursing home

E The specifics of the will of the person in need of a conservator

15. A psychiatrist serving as a fact witness might not be allowed to testify about which one of the following things?

A The dates of psychiatric treatment of a patient

B The criminal responsibility of a patient charged with a crime

C The demeanor of a patient during a therapy session

D The observed behavior of family members toward a patient

E Comments the psychiatrist told another physician named in a malpractice suit

Answers and Explanations

1. The answer is C [*I A*]. It would be appropriate for the psychiatrist to send treatment records to the attorney or company but only after the patient has signed a release. The treating psychiatrist should avoid providing opinions about disability because a negative outcome for the patient (i.e., denial of disability in the litigation) could jeopardize the physician–patient relationship if the patient holds the psychiatrist responsible for the denial of disability. Such dual agency situations should be avoided.

2. The answer is D [*IV D*]. Improper treatment is the most common reason for lawsuits against psychiatrists, followed by suicide, misdiagnosis, and improper supervision of other mental health providers.

3. The answer is B [*IV D 1 b (2)*]. Expert testimony is not needed to establish dereliction of duty in a case of egregious misconduct by the psychiatrist, who, in this case, has a sexual relationship with a patient. The concept of *res ipsa loquitur* means that "the thing speaks for itself."

4. The answer is D [*III A, Table 13–3*]. The ability to communicate with legal counsel is one of the most important trial-related elements in an evaluation of competency to stand trial (CST). Distractors A, B, and C are standards used in determinations of criminal responsibility, depending in which state the crime occurred. The presence of delusions does not automatically impair CST unless it has a negative effect on a specific trial ability.

5. The answer is E [*II C*]. Patients should be provided information about all proposed treatments and should be afforded an opportunity to ask questions. Because neuroleptic medications carry the added risk of tardive dyskinesia, a potentially irreversible side effect, it is important to document the consent process in a written record. Traditional antidepressant indicators do not require written informed consent because they do not cause tardive dyskinesia.

6. The answer is B [*II A 2*]. The man could be involuntarily hospitalized in jurisdictions in which a *parens patriae* commitment model applies. This model allows involuntary hospitalization for patients whose mental illness is gravely disabling but who are not immediately dangerous to themselves or others, as long as hospitalization represents the least restrictive alternative. A police powers model would require that the patient is imminently dangerous to himself or others. The *Dusky* standard refers to competency to stand trial (CST), not involuntary hospitalization.

7. The answer is E [*II C 2*]. Before a substitute decision maker (family member or judge) is contacted, the patient should be assessed to determine if the patient is competent to give consent. A substitute decision maker should be used only if the patient is incompetent to make treatment decisions. Unless an emergent situation (assaultive or self-injurious patient) arises, medication cannot be given over the objections of a competent patient without administrative review (usually two or more psychiatrists). Disguising medication is unethical.

8. The answer is A [*IV C 1 c*]. This type of scenario would be a mental–mental claim under workers' compensation, in which a stressful work event led to psychiatric impairment. This patient would not be eligible for Social Security Disability Income (SSDI) or Social Security Income (SSI) until she has completed a workers' compensation claim and has been disabled for 1 year.

9. The answer is B [*IV D 1 a–d*]. The "four Ds" of a malpractice action are duty, dereliction of duty, damages, and direct causation. Although documentation is important in preventing malpractice claims, it is not a specific element of an unintentional tort.

10. The answer is D [*II E 1 a (3)*]. The exceptions to confidentiality are numerous. Most states have mandatory child abuse reporting laws. In addition, information can be released in emergent situations if physicians are acting in patients' best interest. Information can be released to physicians at a hospital that is accepting a transfer patient and to other professionals actively involved in the patient's treatment.

However, other releases require patient consent. Clinicians' obligation to maintain confidentiality continues even after patients are deceased.

11. The answer is C [*II F*]. *Tarasoff v. Regents of the University of California* states that psychiatrists have a duty to protect intended victims. This duty to protect might include warning potential victims, notifying the police, or hospitalizing a particular patient. Although some states have adopted the *Tarasoff* ruling, other states have specifically rejected it. Psychiatrists should be familiar with case law in their jurisdictions.

12. The answer is E [*IV B 1*]. This woman has testamentary capacity because she is aware of her natural heirs, the extent of her bounty (assets), and the nature and purpose of a will. There is neither evidence that this woman has been subject to undue influence nor evidence of a delusion. Memory impairment does not, by itself, preclude testamentary capacity. There is no requirement that patients leave their assets to their natural heirs; the patient is able to give a rational motive for her decision.

13. The answer is A [*IV A 1*]. In some jurisdictions, a guardian is called a "committee of the person," which is a reflection of a guardian's multiple decision-making capacities. A conservator does not make multiple decisions but merely controls a person's assets. A petitioner may file for the person to be declared incompetent and in need of a guardian, but the person may or may not be appointed by the court as the legal guardian.

14. The answer is A [*IV A 2*]. A conservator controls a person's financial affairs, including the management of investments. A conservator does not have the same global decision-making authority entrusted to a legal guardian. Decisions about living situations, including entering a nursing home and consenting to medical procedures, can be made by a guardian but not by a conservator.

15. The answer is B [*I B 1*]. In general, a fact witness may testify to person, place, dates, and events. A fact witness, even if the witness is a psychiatrist, may not render opinions regarding a legal issue unless specifically qualified by the court to do so. Testimony about criminal responsibility would require an expert witness, not a fact witness.

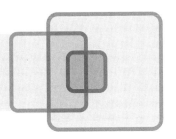

Drug Appendix

Antidepressants*	Starting Dose (mg)	Dose Range (mg)	Half-life (hours)
Tricyclic			
Amitriptyline (Elavil)	25 tid	50–300	15
Clomipramine (Anafranil)	25–100 qd	25–250	32
Desipramine (Norpramin, Pertofrane)	25 tid	100–300	17
Doxepin (Sinequan)	25 tid	75–300	7
Imipramine (Tofranil)	25 tid	75–300	7.6
Nortriptyline (Aventyl, Pamelor)	25 tid	75–150	26
Protriptyline (Vivactil)	5 tid	15–60	78
Trimipramine (Surmontil)	50 tid	150–600	24
Tetracyclics			
Amoxapine (Asendin)	50 bid	50–600	8
Maprotiline (Ludiomil)	25 tid	75–225	43
Selective serotonin reuptake inhibitors			
Citalopram (Celexa)	20	20–60	35
Escitalopram (Lexapro)	10	10–20	27–32
Fluoxetine (Prozac, Sarafem)	20	20–60	72
Fluvoxamine (Luvox)	50	50–300	15
Paroxetine (Paxil, Pexeva)	20	20–60	20
Sertraline (Zoloft)	50	50–200	26
Serotonin–norepinephrine reuptake inhibitors			
Duloxetine (Cymbalta)	20 bid	40–60	12
Venlafaxine (Effexor)	100	300 (rarely to 375)	5
Serotonin modulators			
Nefazodone (Serzone)	50	150–300	4
Trazodone (Desyrel)	50	75–300	7
Norepinephrine–serotonin modulator			
Mirtazapine (Remeron)	15	15–45	20
Dopamine norepinephrine reuptake inhibitors			
Bupropion (Wellbutrin)	150	300	3–4
Monoamine oxidase inhibitors			
Irreversible			
Isocarboxazid (Marplan)	10 bid	20–60	Unknown
Phenelzine (Nardil)	10	30–60	2
Tranylcypromine (Parnate)	15	15–90	2
Reversible			
Moclobemide (Aurorix, Manerix)	150	300–600	2

*Lower starting doses for elderly patients and individuals with anxiety disorders, especially panic disorders.
bid = twice a day; qd = every day; tid = three times a day.

Side Effects of Antidepressant Agents

Type of Agent	Sedation	Weight Gain	Sexual Dysfunction	Other
Tricyclic	Yes	Yes	Yes	Orthostasis, lethal overdose, anticholinergic
Tetracyclics	Yes	Yes	Yes	
Selective serotonin reuptake inhibitors	No	No	Yes	Nausea, insomnia, headache
Serotonin–norepinephrine reuptake inhibitors	No	Rare	Rare	Nausea, insomnia, headache
Serotonin modulators	Yes	Rare	Rare	Trazodone may cause priapism
Norepinephrine–serotonin modulator	Yes	Yes	Rare	Anticholinergic, increased serum lipids
Dopamine–norepinephrine reuptake inhibitors	No	No	No	Seizures; same as Zyban
Monoamine oxidase inhibitors	Rare	Yes	Yes	Hypertension, many potentially lethal drug interactions, dietary restrictions

Mood Stabilizers

	Usual Daily Dose (mg)	Serum Plasma Level	Notes
Carbamazepine (Tegretol)	400–1600	4–12 mg/ml	Liver function test and CBC
Divalproex (Depakote)	750–4200	50–100 mg/ml	Liver function test
Lamotrigine (Lamictal)	100–200	n/a	Liver function test and CBC
Lithium	600–1800	0.6–1.2 mEq/L	Renal and thyroid function tests and CBC

CBC = complete blood cell count; n/a = not applicable.

Antipsychotic Agents

	Usual Oral Dose (mg)	Approximate Equivalent Dose	Notes
Atypical			
Aripiprazole (Abilify)	10–30	5	Agitation, insomnia
Clozapine (Clozaril)	300–600	50	Agranulocytosis risk
Risperidone (Risperdal)	4–6	1	Cytochrome P450 effects; depot available
Olanzapine (Zyprexa)	10–30	2–3	Sleepiness, weight gain; IM available
Quetiapine (Seroquel)	200–800	100	Sleepiness, palpitations
Ziprasidone (Geodon)	80–240	80	Sleepiness, agitation; IM available
Conventional			
Phenothiazines			
Chlorpromazine (Thorazine)	300–600	100	High side effect profile
Piperidines			
Thioridazine (Mellaril)	300–600	100	Cardiac arrhythmia, retinopathy >800 mg
Mesoridazine (Serentil)	150–300	50	Prolonged Q-T interval
Pimozide (Orap)	2–6	1–2	Tourette disorder; do not use with stimulants
Piperzines			
Fluphenazine (Prolixin)	5–15	2	Depot available
Perphenazine (Trilafon)	32–64	10	
Trifluoperazine (Stelazine)	15–20	5	High side effect profile
Thioxanthenes			
Thiothixene (Navane)	20–30	5	Monitor for pigmentary retinopathy antemetic
Butyrophenones			
Haloperidol (Haldol)	5–15	2	Depot available
Dibenzoxapines			
Loxapine (Loxitane)	60–100	15	Similar to thiothixene: tardive dyskinesia
Molindone (Moban)	30–225	10	

IM = intramuscular.

Antianxiety Agents

	Starting Dose (mg)	Usual Dose (mg/day)	Approximate Dose Equivalent (mg)	Approximate Half-life
Benzodiazepines				
Alprazolam (Xanax)	0.25–1	1–4	0.5	12 h
Chlordiazepoxide (Librium)	5–25	15–100	10	1–4 d
Clonazepam (Klonopin)	0.5–2	1–4	0.25	1–2 d
Clorazepate (Tranxene)	3.75–22.5	15–60	7.5	2–4 d
Diazepam (Valium)	2–10	4–40	5	2–4 d
Lorazepam (Ativan)	0.5–2	1–6	1	12 h
Oxazepam (Serax)	10–30	30–120	15	12 h
Miscellaneous				
Buspirone (BuSpar)	10–30	30–60	n/a	2–3 h
Hydroxyzine (Atarax, Vistaril)	50–100	200–400	n/a	

Note: Selective serotonin reuptake inhibitors (SSRIs) and other antidepressant medications are indicated in the treatment of individuals with anxiety disorders:
  Obsessive-compulsive disorder: Clomipramine, SSRIs.
  Panic disorder: SSRIs, tricyclic antidepressants, alprazolam.
  Generalized anxiety: Buspirone, SSRIs, benzodiazepines.
  Stage fright: Beta-blockers.
  Social phobia: SSRIs, monoamine oxidase inhibitors, buspirone.
n/a = not applicable.

Index

Page numbers followed by the letter "t" designate tables; page numbers followed by the letter "Q" designate questions; page numbers followed by the letter "A" designate answers.